AF578324

# Laser Surgery in Gynecology and Obstetrics

Second Edition

# Laser Surgery in Gynecology and Obstetrics

Second Edition

**WILLIAM R. KEYE, JR., M.D.**
Associate Professor of Obstetrics and Gynecology
University of Utah Health Sciences Center
Salt Lake City, Utah

**YEAR BOOK MEDICAL PUBLISHERS, INC.**
CHICAGO • LONDON • BOCA RATON • LITTLETON, MASS.

1 2 3 4 5 6 7 8 9 0 YC 94 93 92 91 90



**Library of Congress Cataloging-in-Publication Data**

Laser surgery in gynecology and obstetrics / [edited by] William R.
Keye, Jr.—2nd ed.
p. cm.
Includes bibliographical references.
ISBN 0-8151-5033-4
1. Gynecology, Operative. 2. Obstetrics—Surgery. 3. Lasers in surgery. I. Keye, William R., 1943-
[DNLM: 1. Genitalia, Female—surgery. 2. Laser Surgery. 3. Pregnancy Complications—surgery. WP 660 L343]
RG104.L37 1990
618'.0459—dc20
DNLM/DLC
for Library of Congress

89-22408
CIP

Sponsoring Editor: Kevin M. Kelly
Assistant Director, Manuscript Services: Frances M. Perveiler
Production Project Coordinator: Carol A. Reynolds
Proofroom Supervisor: Barbara M. Kelly

*To my wife, Sue, and my children, Debbie and Jeff, for their support and encouragement.*

# CONTRIBUTORS

**Stephen L. Corson, M.D.**
*Clinical Professor*
*Department of Obstetrics and Gynecology*
*University of Pennsylvania School of Medicine*
*Attending Gynecologist*
*Pennsylvania Hospital*
*Philadelphia, Pennsylvania*

**James F. Daniell, M.D.**
*Clinical Associate Professor*
*Obstetrics and Gynecology*
*Vanderbilt University Medical Center*
*Nashville, Tennessee*

**Julian E. De Lia, M.D.**
*Associate Professor of Obstetrics and Gynecology*
*University of Utah School of Medicine*
*Salt Lake City, Utah*

**John Dixon, M.D.**
*Professor of Surgery and Medicine*
*University of Utah School of Medicine*
*Senior Consultant*
*University of Utah Laser Institute*
*Salt Lake City, Utah*

**Joseph Feste, M.D.**
*Associate Clinical Professor*
*Baylor College of Medicine*
*The University of Texas at Houston*
*Woman's Hospital of Texas*
*Houston, Texas*

**Milton H. Goldrath, M.D.**
*Assistant Professor of Obstetrics and Gynecology*
*Wayne State University*
*Detroit, Michigan*

**Edward V. Hannigan, M.D.**
*Frances Eastland Connally Professor*
*Department of Obstetrics and Gynecology*
*The University of Texas Medical Branch at Galveston*
*Galveston, Texas*

**Sue E. Huether, R.N., Ph.D.**
*Associate Professor*
*University of Utah College of Nursing*
*Salt Lake City, Utah*

**John Hunter, M.D.**
*Assistant Professor*
*University of Utah School of Medicine*
*Medical Director*
*University of Utah Laser Institute*
*Salt Lake City, Utah*

**Robert W. Kelly, M.D.**
*Omega International Institute*
*Metairie, Louisiana*

**William R. Keye, Jr., M.D.**
*Associate Professor of Obstetrics and Gynecology*
*University of Utah Health Sciences Center*
*Salt Lake City, Utah*

**Dan Lundergan, B.S.**
*Director of Professional Services*
*University of Utah Health Sciences Center*
*Salt Lake City, Utah*

**Dan C. Martin, M.D.**
*Clinical Assistant Professor*
*University of Tennessee at Memphis*
*Reproductive Surgeon*
*Department of Obstetrics and Gynecology*
*Baptist Memorial Hospital*
*Memphis, Tennessee*

**Gregory R. McArthur, Ph.M**
*Laser Consultant*
*Salt Lake City, Utah*

**Richard Reid, M.D.**
*Assistant Professor*
*Wayne State University School of Medicine*
*Director, Genital Dysplasia Clinic*
*Sinai Hospital of Detroit*
*Detroit, Michigan*

**Richard C. Straight, Ph.D.**
*Research Associate Professor of Medicine and Surgery*
*Director, Utah Laser Institute*
*University of Utah Health Sciences Center*
*Research Administrative Officer*
*Veterans Affairs Medical Center*
*Salt Lake City, Utah*

**Tung Van Dinh, M.D.**
*Professor, Department of Obstetrics and Gynecology*
*The University of Texas Medical Branch at Galveston*
*Galveston, Texas*

**V. Cecil Wright, M.D., F.R.C.S.(C)**
*Clinical Professor*
*Department of Obstetrics and Gynecology*
*The University of Western Ontario*
*London, Ontario, Canada*

**Roger B. Yandell, M.D.**
*Assistant Professor*
*Department of Obstetrics and Gynecology*
*The University of Texas Medical Branch at Galveston*
*Galveston, Texas*

# ACKNOWLEDGMENTS

I wish to thank my contributors for their scholarly, caring, and serious efforts; Carol Peck for her tireless typing and secretarial skills; Ruth Henson for her editorial advice and assistance; and Kevin Kelly at Year Book Medical Publishers.

*William R. Keye, Jr.*

# PREFACE

The revision of this text occurs in response to an increased interest in lasers by gynecologists and obstetricians and to the emergence of new experts in the field of laser surgery. It also reflects the greater acceptance of lasers in our specialty.

In the 4 years since the publication of the first edition of this text, laser surgical techniques have been refined, new delivery systems have been introduced, and the indications for lasers in obstetrics and gynecology have expanded. As a result, new chapters have been added describing the administrative aspects of establishing a laser unit, the application of lasers to the treatment of viral infections of the genital tract, the use of the frequency-doubled Nd:YAG laser, and the future of photodynamic therapy in gynecology.

While it is not yet imperative that every gynecologist be a laser surgeon, it is becoming more evident that the gynecolgist should be familiar with the physics, technology, and applications of lasers. Just as computers have become a routine part of our everyday lives, the laser will play an increasing role in patient care as we develop second- and third-generation lasers. The physician who becomes familiar with the lasers of the 1980s will be in a better position to respond to and take advantage of the developments in laser technology in the 1990s.

*William R. Keye, Jr , M.D.*

# CONTENTS

*Preface* *ix*

*Color Plates* *xvii*

**1 / Administration and Organization of a Laser Unit** *1*
*Dan Lundergan*

Program Development *1*
Data Collection *1*
Establishing and Evaluating Goals *2*
Evaluating Resources *2*
Program Design *3*
Organizational Structure and Distribution of Responsibilities *3*
Medical Laser Director *3*
Laser Coordinator *3*
Laser Safety Officer *4*
Engineer *4*
Educational Coordinator *4*
Quality Assurance Coordinator *5*
Committees *5*
Space and Design *5*
Certificate of Need *6*
Education and Training *6*
Credentialing of Physicians *6*
Support Staff *8*
Biotechnicians *8*
Administration *8*
Laser Safety Officer *9*
Finances *9*
Charging Structure *9*
Reimbursement *10*
Research *11*
Guidelines and Regulations *11*

ANSI Z136.3 *11*
Food and Drug Administration *11*
Occupational Safety and Health Administration *12*
Institutional Review Board *12*
Monitoring and Evaluation *12*
Conclusions *12*

## 2 / Laser Physics and Light-Tissue Interaction *14*
*Sue E. Huether*

History of Lasers *14*
Generating Laser Energy *14*
Laser System *18*
Types of Surgical Lasers *19*
Modes of the Laser *21*
Surgical Delivery Systems *22*
The Laser Beam Spot Size *23*
Power Density *25*
Understanding Superpulse *26*
Laser-Tissue Interaction *28*

## 3 / Laser Safety *35*
*Dan C. Martin*

Some Basic Safety Concerns *35*
Education and Credentialing *35*
ANSI Standards for the Operating Room *36*
Equipment Hazards *36*
Electrical Hazards *37*
Surgical Drapes *37*
Anesthetic and Cleaning Agents *37*
Protective Eyewear and Optical Filters *37*
Parfocus *38*
Pulmonary Hazards *39*
Carcinogenic Potential *39*
Protection of Surgeons' Hands *39*
Clinical Use in Gynecology *40*
External Genitalia *40*
Intra-abdominal Procedures *40*
Laparoscopy *40*
Photovaporization of the Endometrium *43*
Summary *43*

## 4 / Human Papillomavirus-Associated Diseases of the Lower Genital Tract: Implications for the Laser Surgeon *46*
*Richard Reid*

Basic Virology of the Papillomaviruses *47*
Taxonomy *47*
Virion Structure *47*

DNA Organization 48
Viral Genetic Function 48
Clinical Groups of Human Papillomaviruses 49
Cutaneous HPVs in the Immunocompetent Population 49
HPVs Affecting the Anogenital and Aerodigestive Mucosae 49
Cutaneous HPVs in Immunosuppressed Individuals 50
Stages of the Natural History of HPV Infection 50
Inoculation 50
Incubation Phase 51
Active Expression Phase 51
Host Containment Phase 52
Late Phase 54
Individual Differences in Disease Expression 54
Chronic, Latent Papillomavirus Infections 55
Minimally Expressed Papillomavirus Infections 56
Well-Developed Papillomavirus Infections 57
HPV and Genital Cancer: Causal or Casual? 60
Evidence Implicating HPV Infection 60
The Possible Operation of Other Co-carcinogens 60
The Prospects of Vaccination 61
Clinical Features of Preinvasive Vulvo-Vaginal Disease 61
Condylomata Acuminata 61
Maculo-Papular Lesions 63
Subclinical Papillomavirus Infections 63
Clinical Features of Preinvasive Cervical Disease 64
Exophytic Condylomas 64
Clinically Important, Minor-Grade Lesions 66
Clinically Inapparent, High-Grade Dysplasias 72
Laboratory Diagnosis of HPV Infection 73
Southern Blot Hybridization 75
Filter In Situ Hybridization 76
Dot Blot Hybridization 76
In Situ Hybridization 76
Polymerase Chain Reaction (PCR) 78
Therapeutic Principles 78
Preinvasive Cervical Disease (High Grade and Low Grade) 79
Benign Vulvo-Vaginal Condylomas 81
Vulvar Intraepithelial Neoplasia 82
Vaginal Intraepithelial Neoplasia 83
Idiopathic Vulvodynia 84
What Advantages Does The $CO_2$ Laser Offer? 88
Strategies to Limit Lateral Heat Conduction 88
Strategies to Aid Surgical Control 89
Other Surgical Strategies 90
Depth Control During Cervical and Vaginal Laser Surgery 90
Depth Control During Vulvar Laser Surgery 91

## 5 / Laser Therapy of the Vulva and Vagina *100*

*V. Cecil Wright*


Vulvar Intraepithelial Neoplasia *100*
- Lesion Locations *100*
- The Structure of Skin *104*
- Colposcopy of the Vulva *104*
- Principles of Laser Surgery for Vulvar Intraepithelial Neoplasia *107*
- Management of VIN Occupying the Hairy Areas *109*
- Combination of Laser Vaporization and Scalpel Excision *110*
- Healing and Postoperative Care *110*
- Results of Laser Surgery and Scalpel Excision for VIN III *113*

Vulvar Condylomata Acuminata *113*
- Principles of Laser Surgery for Vulvar Condylomata Acuminata *115*
- Laser Operative Technique for Vulvar Condylomata *116*
- Management of the Postoperative Patient *120*
- Anticipated Results *120*

Vaginal Intraepithelial Neoplasia *121*
- Clinical Histology and Anatomy of the Vagina *121*
- Vaginal Intraepithelial Neoplasia *122*
- Laser Surgery for VAIN *123*
- Laser Operative Procedure *124*
- Postoperative Care *124*
- Results of Carbon Dioxide Laser Surgery *134*

Vaginal Condylomata Acuminata *124*
- Technique of Laser Surgery for Vaginal Condylomata Acuminata *125*
- Condylomata of the Cervix *126*
- Postoperative Care *128*
- Results *128*


## 6 / Laser Therapy of the Cervix *130*

*Roger B. Yandell, Tung Van Dinh and Edward V. Hannigan*


Historical Perspective *130*

The Epidemiology of Cervical Intraepithelial Neoplasia *131*

The Biology and Natural History of Cervical Intraepithelial Neoplasia *132*

Non-Laser Therapy of CIN *133*
- Cryotherapy *133*
- Electrocoagulation Diathermy *134*
- "Cold" Coagulation *134*

Laser Treatment of CIN *134*
- $CO_2$ Laser Vaporization *134*
- $CO_2$ Laser Excisional "Cone" Biopsy *140*
- $CO_2$ Laser Excision Plus Laser Ablation (The Combination Procedure) for Endocervical and Ectocervical CIN *142*
- Follow-up After $CO_2$ Laser Surgery *144*
- Conization With Argon, KTP-532, and Nd:YAG Lasers *144*

Conclusion *148*

**7 / Intrauterine Laser Surgery** *151*
*Milton H. Goldrath*

The Treatment of Menorrhagia by Endometrial Photovaporization and Coagulation *151*
Preliminary Studies *153*
Clinical Studies *154*
Patient Selection *154*
Surgical Technique *155*
Results and Complications *156*
Histologic Follow-up *160*
Laser Metroplasty *161*
The Future of Intrauterine Laser Surgery *163*

**8 / Laser Surgery of the Fallopian Tube** *166*
*Robert W. Kelly*

Historical Review *166*
Laser Physics and Tubal Surgery *167*
Laser Instrumentation *168*
Accessories *171*
Animal Studies *173*
Clinical Uses *176*
Adhesiolysis *176*
Fimbrioplasty *178*
Destruction of Paratubal Cysts *178*
Neosalpingostomy *178*
Tubal Reanastomosis *179*
Linear Salpingostomy for Ectopic Pregnancy *180*
Tubal Reimplantation *181*
Clinical Results *181*
Advantages of Laser Surgery of the Fallopian Tubes *182*
Complications *183*
Training *183*
Summary and Conclusions *184*

**9 / Laser Laparoscopy: $CO_2$** *187*
*Joseph Feste*

Development of Prototypes for Carbon Dioxide Laser Laparoscopy *188*
Present Systems For Use of The Carbon Dioxide Laser Laparoscope *190*
Single-Puncture Laser Laparoscopy *190*
Double-Puncture Laser Laparoscopy *192*
Alternative Probes and Lenses *193*
$CO_2$ Laser Fibers and Wave Guides *194*
Clinical Applications *194*
Pelvic Endometriosis: Technique and Early Results *194*

Ablation of the Uterosacral Ligament for Dysmenorrhea (Laser Neurectomy) *199*
Laparoscopic Treatment of Polycystic Ovarian Disease *200*
Terminal Salpingostomy *201*
Adhesiolysis *203*
Salpingostomy for Ectopic Pregnancy *204*
Miscellaneous Uses *205*
Conclusions *206*

**10 / Laser Laparoscopy: Argon** *208*
*William R. Keye, Jr. and Gregory R. McArthur*

Instrumentation *209*
Results of Clinical Trials *213*
Surgical Techniques *214*
Destruction of Superficial Implants *214*
Destruction of Ovarian Endometriomas *215*
Adhesiolysis *217*
Neosalpingostomy *218*
Ectopic Pregnancy *218*
Advantages and Disadvantages *218*
Future Applications *220*
Conclusions *220*

**11 / Laser Laparoscopy: KTP** *222*
*James F. Daniell*

KTP Laser *222*
Initial Studies *224*
Clinical Trials *224*
Clinical Techniques for Laparoscopic Use *225*
Advantages of the KTP Laser for Laparoscopic Surgery *228*
Disadvantages of the KTP Laser System for Laparoscopy *229*
Safety Precautions and Training in Use of the KTP Laser *229*
Conclusions *230*

**12 / Laser Laparoscopy: Nd:YAG** *231*
*Stephen L. Corson*

Instrumentation *232*
Animal Studies *237*
Clinical Techniques *237*
Clinical Results *238*
Additional YAG Laser Laparoscopic Procedures *239*
Ovarian Wedge Resection *239*
Destruction of Non-endometriotic Ovarian Cysts *240*
Myomectomy *240*
Ectopic Pregnancy *240*

**13 / The Nd:YAG Laser in Fetal/Placental Surgery** *242*
*Julian E. De Lia*

Animal Studies *243*
The Sheep Experiments *243*
The Monkey Experiments *243*
Comment *246*
Conclusion *248*

**14 / The Future of Lasers in Gynecology: The Free-Electron Laser and Photodynamic Therapy** *250*
*Richard C. Straight, John Hunter and John Dixon*

Development of More Powerful Lasers *250*
Development of New Wavelengths *252*
Development of New Delivery Systems *253*
The Use of Lasers in Activating Photosensitive Reactions *254*
Mechanisms of Photodynamic Therapy *254*
Photochemical Mechanisms *254*
The Nature of Photodynamic Sensitizers *255*
The Pharmacology of Photosensitizers in Tumor Tissue *256*
Photobiological Reactions to Photodynamic Therapy *258*
Clinical Applications of Laser Tumor Photodynamic Therapy *259*
Factors Influencing Clinical Efficacy *259*
Gynecologic Applications of Photodynamic Diagnosis and Therapy *260*
Future Developments for Laser Photochemotherapy *261*
Non-thermal Effects of Lasers *263*
Summary *263*
Changing Role of Lasers in Gynecology *263*

*Index* *271*

# Color Plates

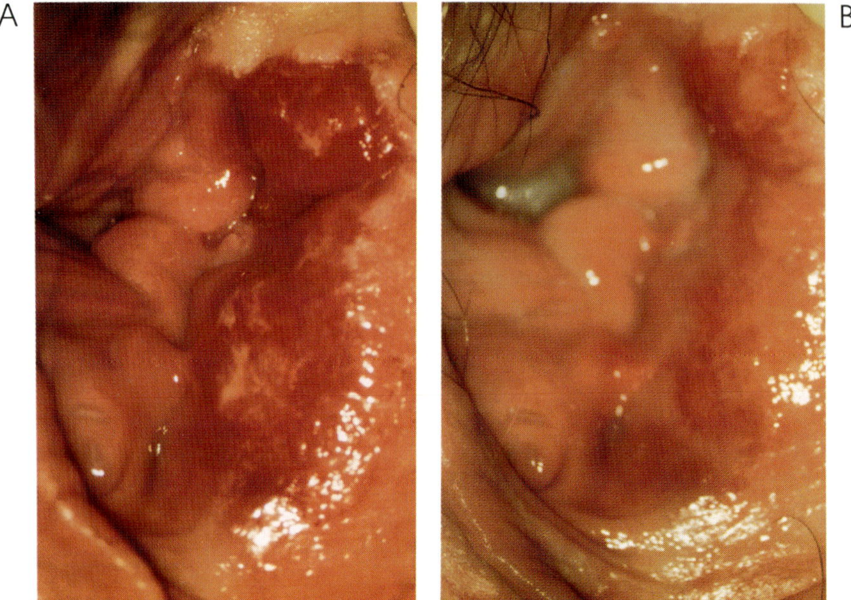


**PLATE 1.**—Intensely painful focus of vestibular erythema arising adjacent to the hymenal resection scar. **A,** after initial surgery. **B,** 2 months after argon-laser photocoagulation. (From Reid R, Greenberg M, Daoud Y, et al: *J Reprod Med* 1988; 33:523–532. Used by permission.)

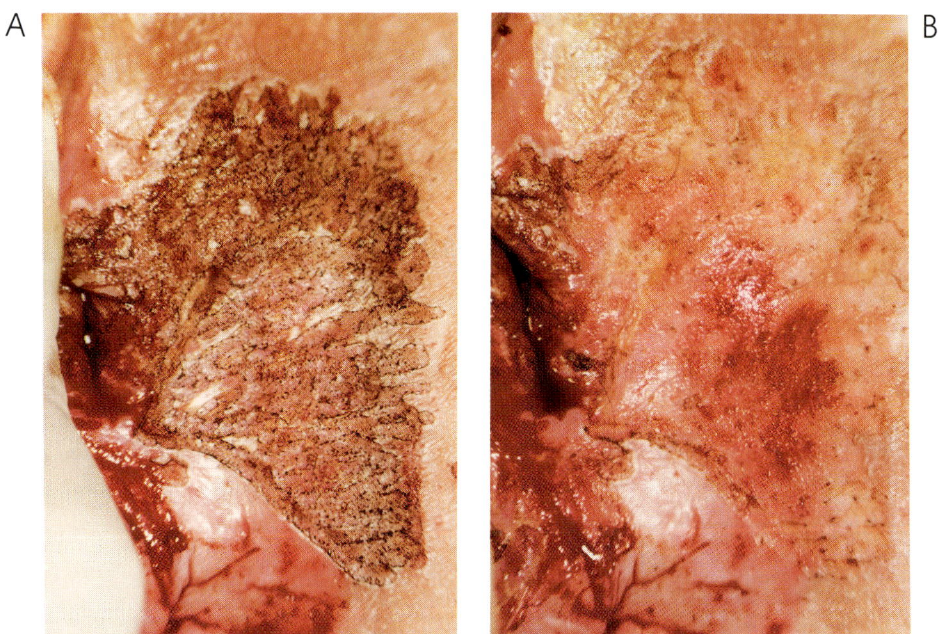


**PLATE 2.**—**A,** first surgical plane. A view through the operating microscope after initial "brushing" with the laser. Beneath the charred remnants of the surface sqaumes, the refractile remnants of plump keratinocytes in the proliferating zone of the epidermis can be seen. **B,** first surgical plane, after the epithelial debris has been wiped away with the moist gauze. This maneuver exposes the intact surface of the underlying corium. (From Reid R, Elfont E, Zirkin R, et al: *Am J Obstet Gynecol* 1984; 152:268. Used by permission.)

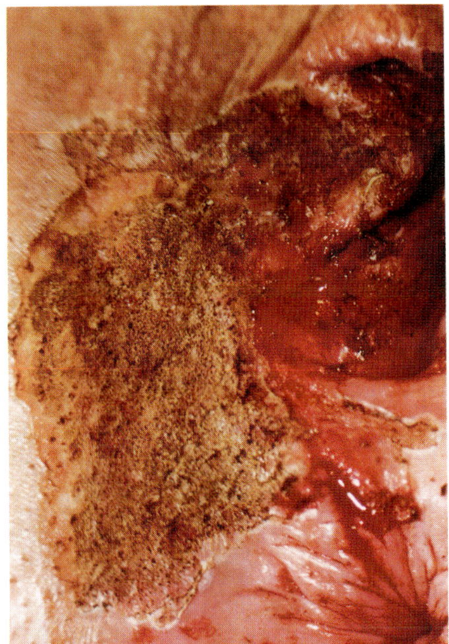

**PLATE 3.**—The second surgical plane. The exposed papillary dermis has been gently relased, sufficient to scorch (but not cut) the dermal surface. (From Reid R, Elfont E, Zirkin R, et al: *Am J Obstet Gynecol* 1984; 152:268. Used by permission.)

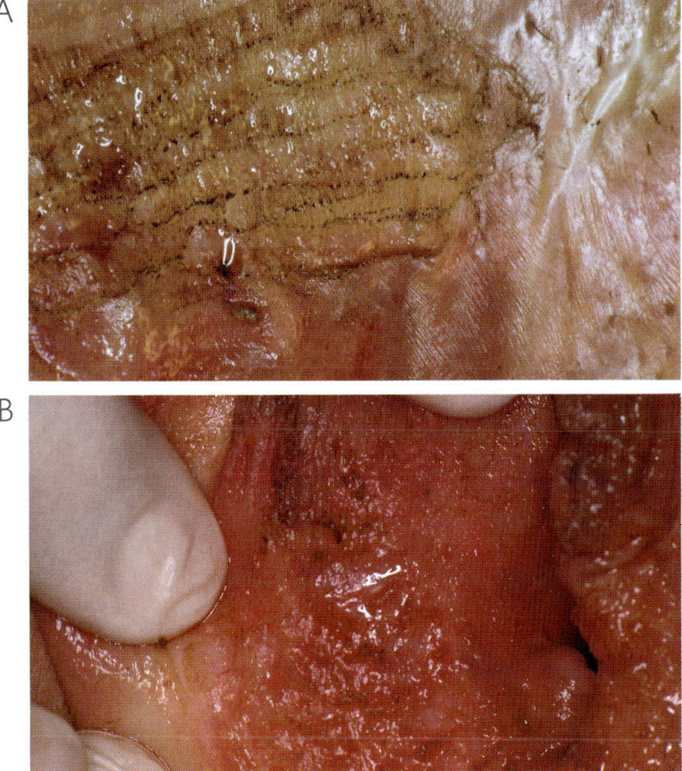


**PLATE 4.**—**A,** the third surgical plane. A slower, more deliberate movement of the laser beam has vaporized the upper half of the dermis, revealing a vertical pattern of fibers (the coarse collagen bundles of the reticular dermis). **B,** the deep collagen plates with attendant accurate blood vessels seen at the base of the third plane.

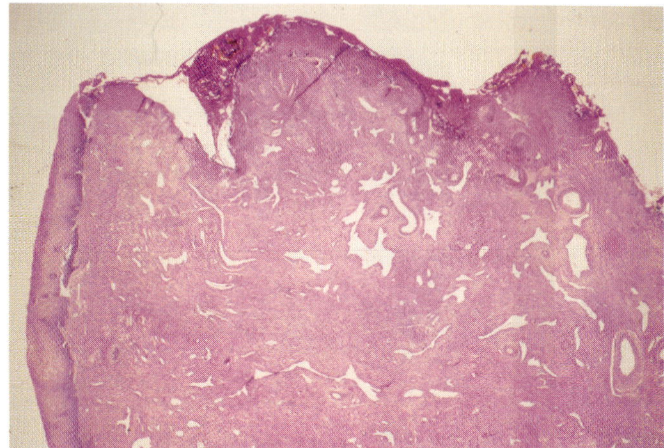

**PLATE 5.**—Carbon dioxide laser cone performed at the very low power density of 2,000 W/cm$^2$ in an effort to avoid excessive bleeding. Depth of coagulation necrosis is 400 microns (normal range is 50 to 100 microns).

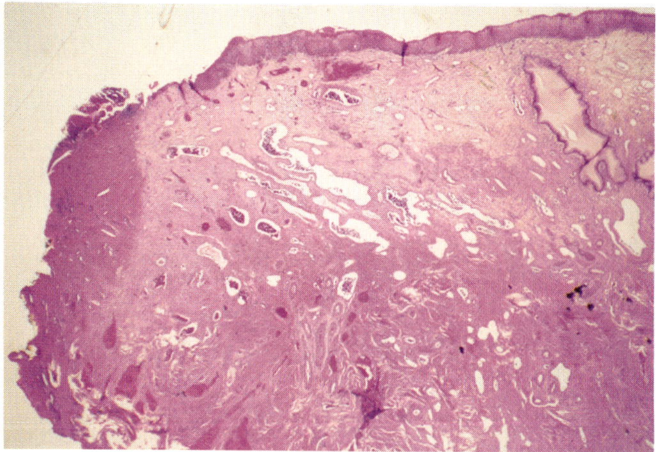

**PLATE 6.**—KTP-532 laser cone performed at less than optimal power of 8 watts. Depth of coagulation necrosis is 920 microns (range is 480 to 1,360 microns). Although this specimen is acceptable, new instrumentation allows power settings of 15 to 20 watts with a corresponding coagulation necrosis of 400 to 700 microns.

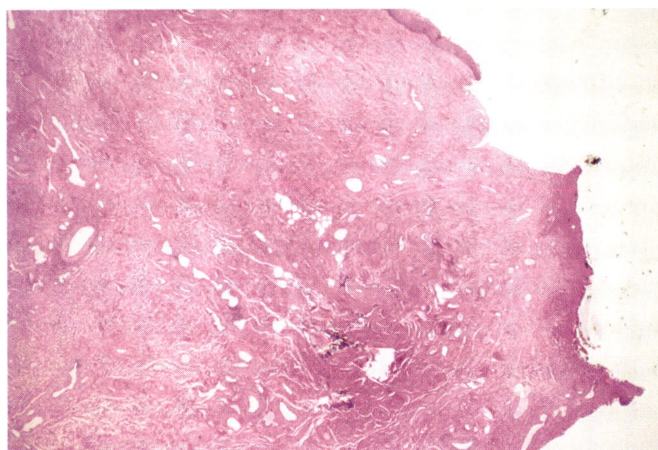

**PLATE 7.**—Nd:YAG laser cone. Depth of coagulation necrosis is 480 microns (range is 280 to 680 microns).

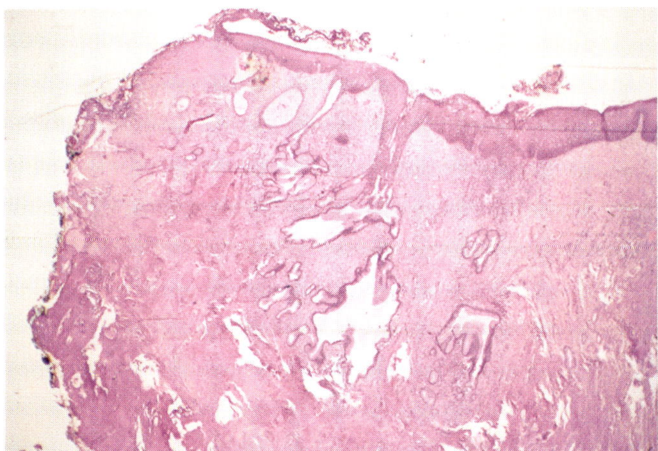

**PLATE 8.**—Argon laser cone. Depth of coagulation necrosis is 640 microns (range is 500 to 720 microns).

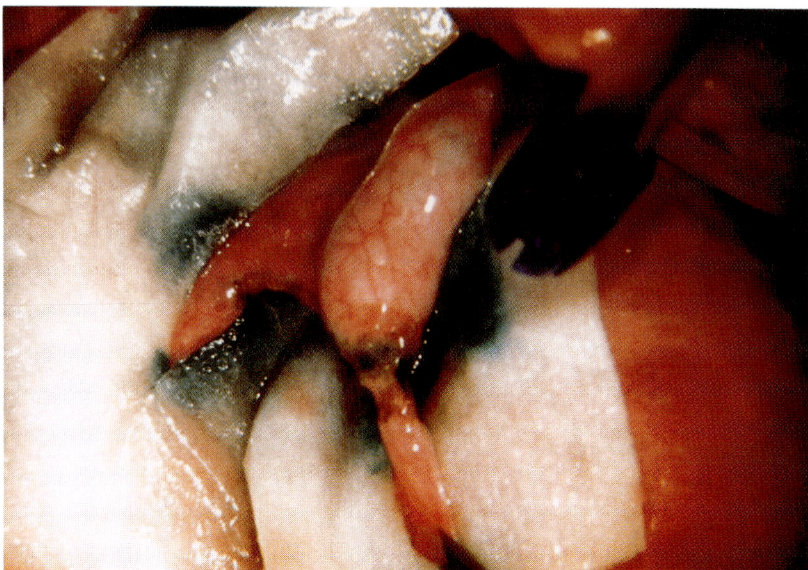

**PLATE 9.**—Preparation of the distal portion of the fallopian tube with the $CO_2$ laser prior to reanastomosis.

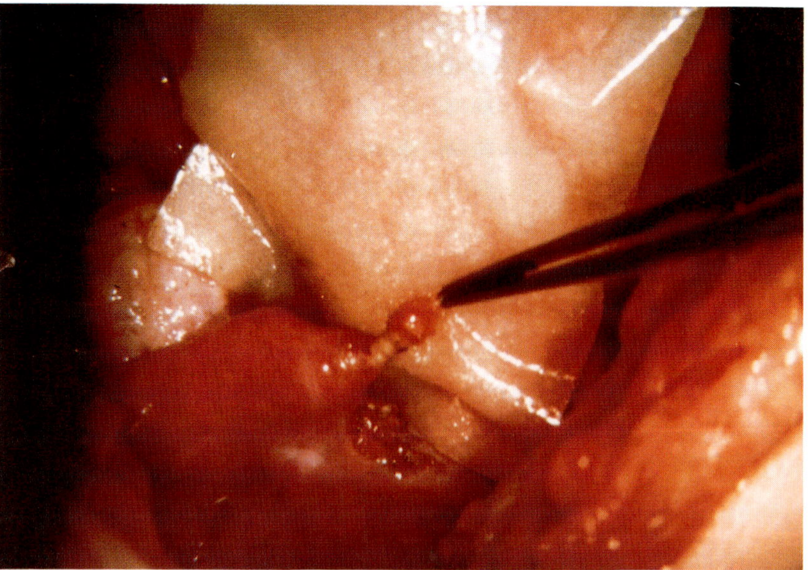

**PLATE 10.**—Preparation of the proximal portion of the fallopian tube with the $CO_2$ laser prior to reanastomosis.

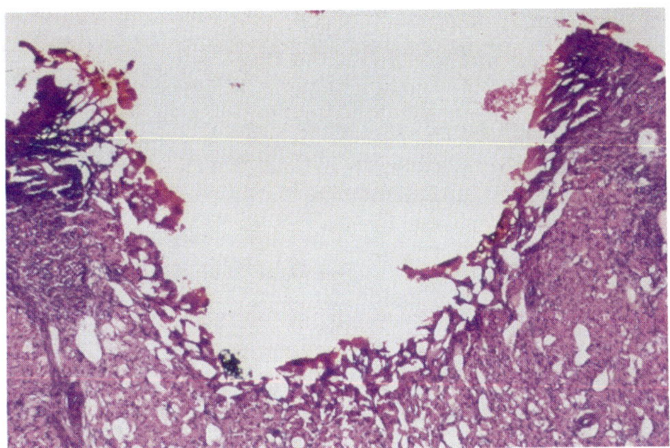

**PLATE 11.**—Immediate uterine lesion (rabbit) with 2 seconds at 20 watts with chisel probe (400×).

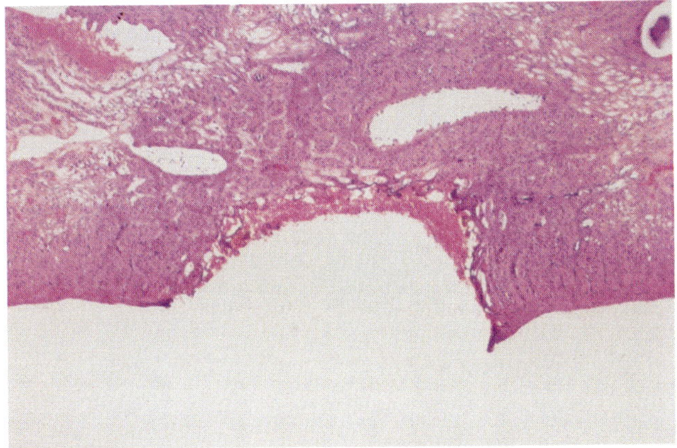

**PLATE 12.**—Acute ovarian lesion (rabbit) with 2 seconds at 20 watts with chisel probe (400×).

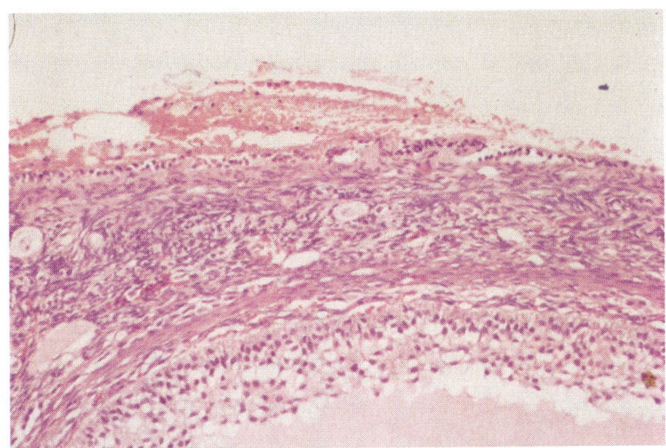

**PLATE 13.**—Rabbit ovary showing epithelial healing at 3 weeks (450×).

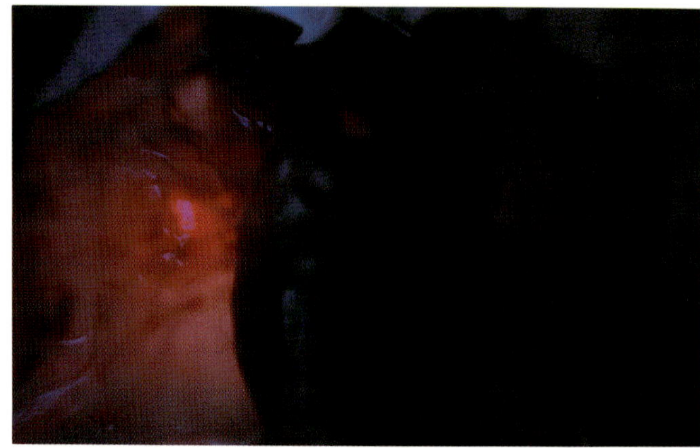

**PLATE 14.**—Red-light fluorescence of porphyrins localized in mouse S180 tumor and surrounding tissue involved in the host (Swiss-Webster) response to the growing tumor at 5 days after subcutaneous *(SC)* implant of $5 \times 10^6$ S180 cells. The host mouse was injected 24 hours earlier, intraperitoneally, with 20 mg/kg hematoporphyrin derivative (Photofrin I). The red fluorescence was produced by exciting the retained porphyrin with a broad-band black light (390 to 430 nm). The host response to tumor implant subcutaneously is similar to a wound repair response and includes neovascularization, deposition of fibrin and extracellular matrix components, and encapsulation of the growing tumor mass.

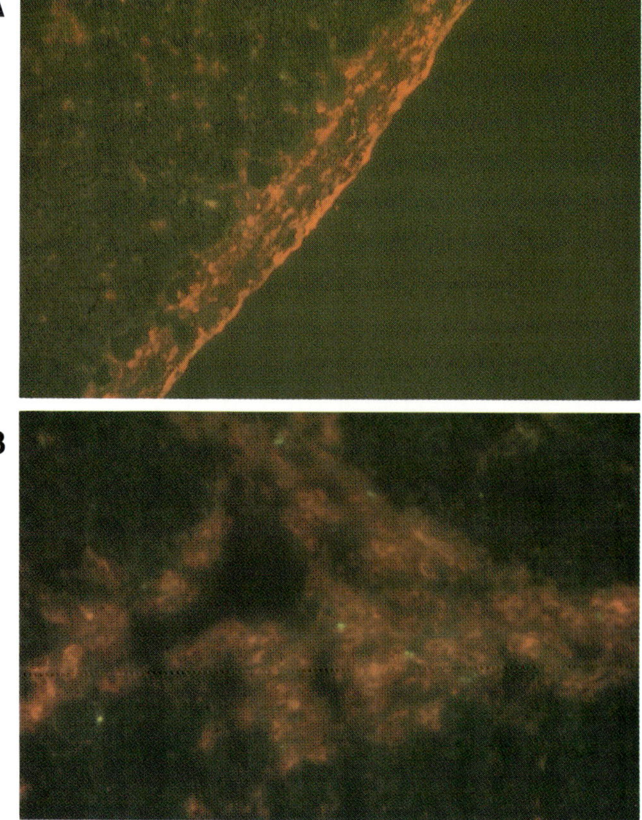

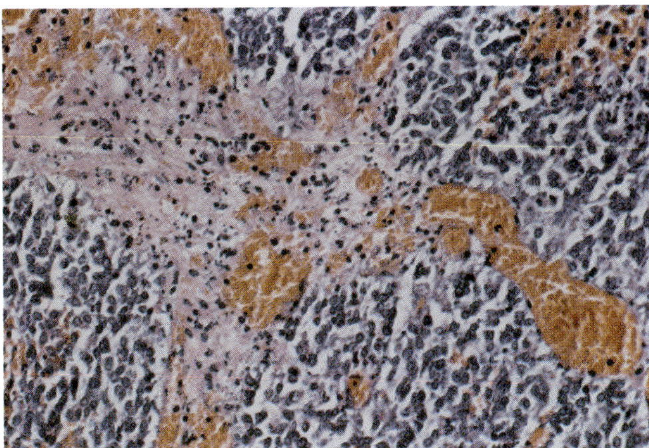

**PLATE 16.**—Hematoxylin-eosin-stained histological section of mouse S180 tumor 24 hours after photodynamic treatment showing extensive coagulation necrosis following microvascular disruption, hemorrhage, and intravascular coagulation. Microvascular effects are observed immediately during light exposure and are followed by interruption of blood flow and subsequent necrosis of the tumor mass.

←

**PLATE 15.**—Distribution of red fluorescent porphyrins in histological frozen sections of transplanted S180 tumor. The photomicrogram shows that the fluorescent porphyrin is not uniformly distributed throughout the tumor mass (green background) but is confined to the fibrovascular capsule surrounding the tumor (**A**) and the microvascular septae within the tumor (**B**).

Chapter 1

# Administration and Organization of a Laser Unit

Dan Lundergan, B.S.

Establishing a laser program is similar to establishing any hospital-based clinical program—goals, objectives, and actions must be clearly defined and implemented.[1] However, it also specifies some unique requirements. First, special safety needs must be considered, for both the medical staff and the patients. Second, a safe environment must be maintained in the face of a constantly changing technology. Third, because physicians and support personnel may not be trained in this new field, training programs are usually required. Fourth, a credentialing system is needed to ensure competence in laser surgery.

Although this chapter covers the basic format for the creation of a new laser program, the substantive content of the material should also prove helpful to those already involved in developing a laser program and even to those in fully established laser programs. This chapter addresses nine basic areas vital to the establishment of a new program: program development, program design, organizational structure and distribution of responsibilities, space and design, education and training, finances, research, guidelines and regulations, and monitoring and evaluation.

## PROGRAM DEVELOPMENT

### Data Collection

Collecting data is essential in determining the form and content of a future laser program. Valuable information can be obtained by researching the literature and by contacting laser companies, existing laser programs, and health-care professionals who are experienced in laser surgery. Contacting laser manufacturers is a good place to start, for in addition to technical information, they have user lists that identify current laser programs and laser users. From these sources it is possible not only to obtain information about the inner workings of laser programs but also to be directed to current laser publications, meetings, educational opportunities, training programs, and demonstrations. Next, one should contact individuals associated with several laser programs. Obviously, there are advantages in contacting programs that are comparable in volume, medical specialties, patient mix, and procedures.

## Establishing and Evaluating Goals

While in the planning stages, it is necessary to set realistic goals. To establish realistic goals, one must consider a number of economic and noneconomic factors. First, one must take a look at the economic impact of a laser program on the institution and determine whether lasers fit into the fiscal objectives of the organization. For example, it will be important to determine whether the institution can afford to fund the start-up costs of a laser program. It will also be important to determine at what point the initial costs will be returned and the program will become profitable. Next, the acceptance of a laser program by the community, the hospital, and individual physicians should be determined.[2] Finally, other non-economic items to consider are the public relations benefits of a laser program and the extent to which the laser program will increase the use of other institutional or hospital services. Demographic surveys, cost analyses, and reimbursement evaluation are procedures that can be used to obtain data to be used in evaluating these goals. Community demographics and existing surveys done by other hospitals and departments may also be helpful in justifying a new laser program.

## Evaluating Resources

Armed with this background information, internal and external resources should be evaluated.[3] A direct and useful means of obtaining information about human resources is a well-designed questionnaire directed to the following groups:

1. To physicians potentially involved in the program. This questionnaire is of value both in assessing and documenting a physician's degree of interest in and commitment to a laser program. Each physician can project the types and number of laser procedures and his preference for specific laser technology and may also be able to provide procedural logs, operating data forms and medical records to substantiate his projections. In addition, a letter of support may be important in justifying a laser program to the administration.
2. To the nursing and support staff. A questionnaire should assess the knowledge base of the staff and the extent of training needed.
3. To engineering staff. This questionnaire should verify the existing technical expertise of the engineering staff and affirm their cooperation to be trained in laser repair and maintenance.

The availability of space should also be assessed and compared to the projections for operating room space, as well as space for offices, storage, educational needs, and potential research. Attention should also be given to future expansion.

Often, the hospital, departments, or physicians may already own lasers. If not, it will be necessary to research the types of procedures to be performed and match them with the laser of choice for that purpose. Advice from other laser programs that have a similar mixture of laser specialists and procedures may be extremely valuable.

Among the external resources to be considered are consultants from the laser industry or other laser programs. Because consultants are expensive, it is economical to furnish a consultant with as much information as possible, especially about available resources, the limitations of the program, and prospective goals. Armed with this information, they can help design a laser program.

## PROGRAM DESIGN

Basically, there are three types of programs: (1) an integrated organization in which the laser program is one part of a bigger system, i.e., part of a hospital that assumes and shares responsibility for the personnel, budget, and equipment; (2) a dedicated organization that is located in a hospital but treated as a separate entity, i.e., the group or department is responsible for the laser unit and has an independent budget, equipment, and personnel; and (3) a free-standing laser organization that is independent of a hospital and is responsible for every aspect of its own operation. Currently, dedicated systems and disciplines are growing in popularity.

## ORGANIZATIONAL STRUCTURE AND DISTRIBUTION OF RESPONSIBILITIES

Paramount in the organizational structure is a clear and well-defined description of jobs and responsibilities and an environment that promotes clear and responsive communication. The following are possible job titles and assigned responsibilities in the organization of a laser unit.

### Medical Laser Director

The medical director is responsible for supporting the decisions made by the committees within the organization. He addresses key issues such as equipment purchases and program direction with other members in the organization. This individual is also responsible for the credentialing process and the approval of policies and procedures that affect the laser program. The laser director is usually a physician.

### Laser Coordinator

The laser coordinator should be someone who is knowledgeable about and committed to laser surgery. In light of the responsibilities involved with this position, the laser coordinator is usually a nurse. Responsibilities include:

1. Patient education.
2. Providing nursing input to physicians.
3. Implementing and enforcing laser policies.
4. Communicating problems to sales representatives or hospital engineers.
5. Interfacing with the laser safety officer.
6. Ensuring that an informed consent form is completed by a patient if the procedure is included in an FDA study.
7. Postoperative teaching.
8. Making follow-up phone calls.
9. Internal nursing staff education.
10. Personnel orientation programs for the laser.
11. Active involvement in the laser committee.
12. Keeping current on changes in the laser field in the nursing area.
13. Clearly understanding the Joint Commission on Accreditation of Hospitals'

(JCAH) criteria regarding laser surgery and the guidelines for use of lasers established by the American National Standards Institute (ANSI) in their document ANSI Z136.3.[4]

## Laser Safety Officer

The emergence of the laser safety officer (LSO) within the health care area will be solidified by the new ANSI Z136.3 document, which defines the LSO as "one who has authority to monitor and enforce the control of laser hazards and effect the knowledgeable evaluation and control of laser systems."[4] In the future it is anticipated that the LSO will become an essential part of every laser organization. More specific responsibilities are as follows:

1. To classify or to verify the classification of lasers and laser systems under the LSO's jurisdiction.
2. To evaluate the hazards of laser treatment areas, including the determination of nominal hazard zones.
3. To assure that the prescribed control measures are in effect and to recommend or approve substitute or alternate control measures when the primary ones are not feasible or practical and to periodically confirm the proper functioning of those control measures.
4. To approve standard operating procedures, alignment procedures, and other procedures that are requirements of the administrative and procedural control measures, i.e., preoperative, intraoperative, and postoperative checklists used by operating personnel.
5. To recommend or approve protective equipment (e.g., eyewear, clothing, barriers, screens) as required to assure personnel safety; to inspect protective equipment periodically to ensure proper working order.
6. To approve the wording on area signs and equipment labels.
7. To approve Health Care Laser Systems (HCLS) installation and equipment prior to use, to approve the modification of existing facilities or equipment, and to authorize laser technicians for performance of maintenance and service.
8. To assure that adequate safety education and training are provided to HCLS area personnel.
9. To determine the personnel categories for medical surveillance.

Additional recommended duties for the LSO are included in ANSI Z136.3.[4]

## Engineer

With the increase in cost of service contracts and the cost of "down" time for laser units, it is imperative that some in-house laser expertise be established for repairs and maintenance.

## Educational Coordinator

An effective educational program enhances the success of a laser center. This includes education for physicians, support staff, engineering, and even marketing personnel. The American Society for Lasers in Medicine and Surgery has established guidelines for education.[5]

### Quality Assurance Coordinator

The quality assurance coordinator provides documentation and checklists as necessary and ensures proper outcome.

### Committees

An advisory or steering committee can provide the visionary thinking needed to ensure a program's success (Table 1–1). Other possible committees for a laser program are the safety committee and the marketing committee.

## SPACE AND DESIGN

The space specified for a laser program depends on the type of laser chosen and its safety requirements. Lasers currently range from an 800-lb, refrigerator-size system to a portable, 40-lb, self-contained system. However, some types of lasers require only minimal room modification (i.e., the $CO_2$ laser requires only 110 volts at 60 Hz and no modi-

**TABLE 1–1.**
Hospital Laser Committee

- I. Suggested committee members:
  - A. Committee chairman
  - B. Representatives from subspecialties using lasers
  - C. Operating room head nurse
  - D. Endoscopic surgery head nurse (if applicable)
  - E. Bioengineering representative (if applicable)
  - F. Administrator
  - G. Laser safety officer (if other than any persons listed above)
- II. Committee responsibilities (tailored to meet individual institutional needs):
  - A. Definition of criteria for laser use privileges
  - B. Safety policies
    1. Personnel protection
    2. Prevention of electrical hazards
    3. Environmental safety
    4. Patient protection
  - C. Definition of start-up and shut-down procedures and assuring checklists have been properly reviewed and completed
  - D. Establish guidelines for maintenance
  - E. Develop patient consent forms that satisfy hospital, medical, legal, and FDA requirements
  - F. Develop laser documentation forms with checklists for equipment and nursing notes, and incident reports for accidents and equipment failure
  - G. Define responsibilities for staff with regard to laser use
  - H. Assist in laser budgeting and development of hospital charges for laser use
  - I. Design or renovate in order to accommodate laser systems
  - J. Evaluation and quality assurance
  - K. Outline in-house education and training of new employees and update information for existing employees
  - L. Oversee patient education activities (teaching pamphlets, etc.)

fication of power or plumbing). On the opposite end of the spectrum are the Nd:YAG and argon laser systems, which usually require window coverings and modifications of the power and plumbing systems. Prior to the construction or redesigning of an existing facility, the manufacturer should be contacted for a system's specific requirements. Additionally, the ANSI Z136.3 document[4] clearly reviews the minimal safety requirements for all systems and should be studied prior to construction or remodeling. This document mentions (1) window protection for wavelengths that transmit through glass, (2) a flashing light and safety signs located outside the control area (with appropriate signs in eye view), and (3) a hook for proper wavelength protection (goggles) to be hung outside of the room. Smoke evacuators are highly recommended. Some systems also specify external water systems. For your information, a layout plan of the Laser Lab Unit at the University of Utah Medical Center is presented in Figure 1–1.

### Certificate of Need

Some states require the Certificate of Need (CON) for the building of facilities and for the acquisition of major costly programs;[6] the purpose of the CON is to ensure consistency and to avoid needless duplication within a region. Local regulations should be checked before getting too far into the development process.

## EDUCATION AND TRAINING

Attention to quality education and training is vital to either a new or existing program. Above all, dedication to high standards of curriculum and faculty qualifications is imperative. The education program should be at least self-supporting. Revenues can be generated by grants from vendors as well as from tuition from physicians and nurses attending educational programs.

### Credentialing of Physicians

Credentialing for laser users is generally the responsibility of the governing board and administrative staff of the hospital or of the office-based group. They provide guidelines and document the credentialing process. Table 1–2 outlines the current recommended guidelines suggested by the American Society for Lasers in Medicine and Surgery.

Because it would be difficult to establish one standard to cover all disciplines, it is hoped that establishing minimal standards for credentialing may fall under each of the subspecialties within both the surgical and medical disciplines. According to Robert Ossoff, the credentialing process should be the responsibility of each subspecialty and its respective society.[7] However, as of 1988, few subspecialty societies have made such recommendations.

Prior to the participation of physicians, the guidelines for adequate training and training programs should be reviewed.[8] If physicians are sent to training programs at other institutions, obviously some committee or responsible individual must ensure that they receive adequate hands-on experience and training. Thereafter, a preceptorship program should be established so experienced laser surgeons observe physicians and supervise new physicians until they have demonstrated their expertise.

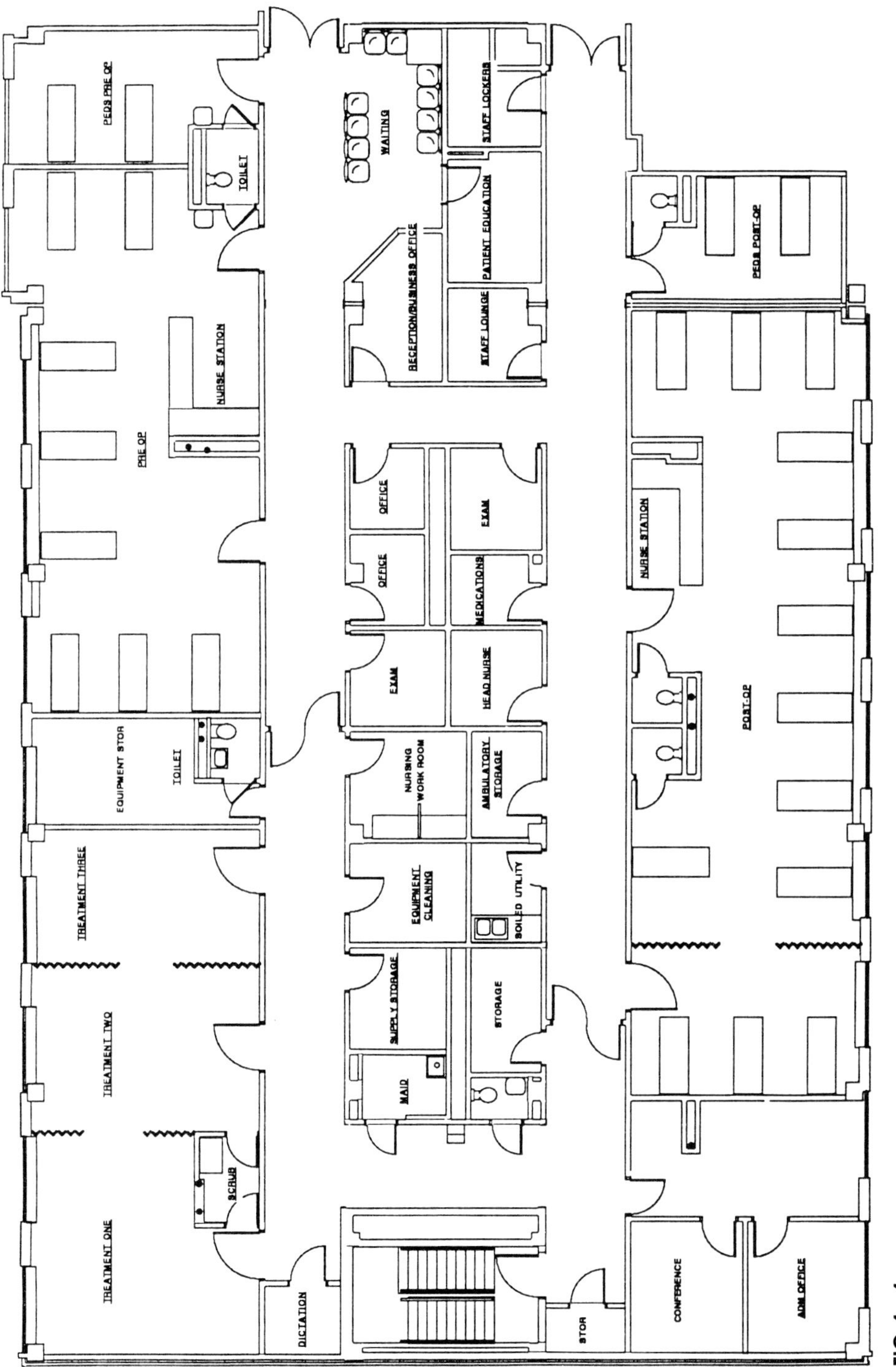


**FIG 1–1.**
Proposed ambulatory surgery/laser lab unit.

**TABLE 1–2.**

Standards of Practice for the Use of Lasers in Medicine and Surgery*

The following statement is proposed:

Hospital privileges are and must remain the responsibility of the hospital governing board. Those requesting privileges to use lasers shall meet all the standards of the hospital with regard to board certification, board eligibility, special training, ethical character, good standing, judgement, indications for application, etc.

In addition, the following laser training and experience is recommended:

1. This applicant shall review the pertinent literature and audiovisual aids and shall attend laser training course(s) devoted to teaching of laser principles and safety. These course(s) shall include basic laser physics, laser tissue interaction, discussions of the clinical specialty field, and hands-on experience with lasers. Such course(s) should be a minimum of 8 to 10 hours although courses ranging from 14 to 16 hours may be more appropriate for first-time attendees. Approximately 50% of the course time should involve hands-on training with the number of registrants assigned to each laser small enough (three to four) to ensure enough actual hands-on time.
2. The individual shall have spent time with an experienced operator in the specialty area involved when appropriate and practical. Such time may consist of several brief visits or a more prolonged stay, with a minimum of 6 to 8 hours of observation and hands-on involvement.
3. In lieu of the above, the applicant may present a letter from the program director of an accredited residency in which laser utilization is part of the experience obtained. Individuals in training are urged to obtain laser experience as part of their residency. As in 1 and 2 above, this must include a minimum of 6 to 8 hours of observation and hands-on involvement.

*Approved by the Board of Directors, American Society for Laser Medicine and Surgery, Inc, April 10, 1987.

## Support Staff

The credentialing of support staff is currently not well defined; it is the individual institution's responsibility to determine minimal standards for their support staff. At the University of Utah we require that laser nurses and laser support staff take a hands-on, 2-day course that involves all wavelengths, a post-course test, and a preceptorship. The ANSI Z136.3 document contains recently established specific guidelines for the credentialing of support staff.[4] Also, the Nursing Section of the American Society for Lasers in Medicine and Surgery, Inc., has specific guidelines for nursing personnel.[9]

## Biotechnicians

As outlined in the ANSI document,[4] technicians are now required to be credentialed if they maintain and repair laser systems. Training is available from manufacturers of specific wavelengths and models of lasers, and there are schools that provide 2-year training programs with specific technical training in the area of laser technology.

## Administration

Although no recommendations exist for the training of administrators within the area of medical laser surgery, this author recommends they have a working knowledge of this technology through participating, networking, reading publications, and attending meetings. However, their major responsibility is in the area of documentation. JCAH regulations suggest that hospital administrators establish adequate documentation, policy, procedures, and provision of laser safety meetings.

### Laser Safety Officer

The LSO is a relatively new position in the medical area with no defined training needs. However, the ANSI Z136.3 document outlines very specific roles for the LSO. Obviously, the LSO will need specific training to function effectively (see Tables 1–1 to 1–3).

## FINANCES

Budgeting for a laser program involves the same considerations as the budgeting process for any other piece of equipment or program. Consideration should be given to the cost of the equipment and to the period of time required for the equipment to pay for itself. Included in this payback period is the annual direct revenue to be generated by the equipment, the annual cost of the equipment and its maintenance, the cost of support staff, and the potential for attracting new patients and procedures.

Likewise, the space requirements for the laser program must be evaluated financially to see whether the laser program will maximize its returns on that space. If not, it may be necessary to extend the use of the laser space to other disciplines and procedures that do not involve the laser. An example of the costs associated with the establishment of a laser unit is shown in Table 1–3.

### Charging Structure

Below is an easy formula for figuring a charge for patient visits or procedures after accounting for laser depreciation.

$$\frac{\text{Total Purchase Cost}}{\text{Uses Per Year} \times \text{Years of Use}} + \frac{\text{Indirect Expenses}}{\text{Procedure}} + \frac{\text{Incidental Expenses + Profit}}{\text{Procedure}} = \text{Final Patient Charges per Procedure}$$

The *Total Laser Purchase Cost* includes all expenditures during the initial laser purchase and installation. It also may include the laser console, facility remodeling, accessory equipment (i.e., fibers, handpieces, etc.), a power meter (if desired), and training for the support staff.

**TABLE 1–3.**
Start-up Costs for a Laser Unit

| Item | Low Figure | High Figure |
|---|---|---|
| Equipment (one laser) | $ 20,000 | $ 100,000 |
| Supplies | 5,000 | 10,000 |
| Dedicated space | 0 | 10,000 |
| Training of personnel (nurses, physicians) | 2,000 | 10,000 |
| Power supply, water supply | 0 | 15,000 |
| Safety measures | 2,000 | 4,000 |
| Coordinator (1 FTE) | 20,000 | 25,000 |
| Service contract | 5,000 | 10,000 |
| Totals | $ 54,000 | $ 184,000 |

*Years of Use* is an evaluation of how long the laser will last and takes into account the normal wear and tear of the laser and the future obsolescence of the laser unit (usually 3 to 5 years). The University of Utah uses 5 years for the estimated laser life. Shorter life expectancies result in higher patient charges.

*Uses per Year,* derived from earlier questionnaire responses from physicians, should accurately estimate the annual number of laser procedures to be performed yearly with a specific laser.

*The Indirect Expenses* of a laser program include building depreciation, administrative and general services, support services (laundry, maintenance, plant operation, infection control). Our Laser Institute estimates approximately 24% indirect costs. Adjustments for bad debts may also be included in the indirect costs or may be a separate item in the accounting process. Depreciation of equipment is generally classified as an equipment charge, not an indirect cost. The indirect costs for equipment, such as education, service contracts, and goggle replacement, can be reported as equipment costs.

*Incidental Expenses + Profit* account for other incidental costs to the laser during its lifetime use, as well as a profit margin.

A hypothetical case is given to illustrate the use of the formula. The purchase price of a $CO_2$ laser is \$95,000, which includes \$85,000 for the laser and \$10,000 for additional handpieces (other than those included with the laser purchase), $CO_2$ wave guides, water inlet/outlet installation, and laser training for an operating room nurse and gynecology unit nurse. The estimated life expectancy is determined to be 5 years. A retrospective chart audit reveals that the laser could have been used 100 times per year on patients treated by a gynecologist. Based on these figures, the formula is:

$$\frac{\$95{,}000}{100 \text{ Patients per Year} \times 5 \text{ Years}} = \$190 \text{ Cost per Use}$$

A 30% increase was added to the \$190 patient charge to account for projected indirect laser expenses, incidential expenses, and profit. This brings the final patient charge to \$247.

In addition to the initial patient charge, it may be necessary to charge for the actual time of laser use. When the laser is used for longer procedures, the patient cost can be adjusted according to the actual time of laser use.

A standby charge for the laser may also be necessary. When the laser is reserved for possible use during an operative procedure but is not used, the patient may be charged for a "standby" fee. Although some argue that this is unfair, it is obvious that during this time the laser cannot be used by anyone else. This charge also discourages indiscriminate laser scheduling and reservation.

## Reimbursement

There are three basic types of payment for services rendered by health service provider organizations: cost-based, fixed, and charges. Cost-based payment reflects the actual cost of providing services and considers patient days, equipment charges, and tests.

A fixed payment (prospective payment) is when an organization receives a given annual premium regardless of the actual cost of providing service. Therefore, if the cost of services increases in a particular case mix, the organization loses money. This type of payment is currently used by health maintenance organizations (HMOs). In addition, Medicare patients are currently being shifted from a cost-based to a fixed payment system as a result of the passage of the Tax Equity and Financial Responsibility Act of 1982 (PL97-248) and the Social Security Amendments of 1983 (PL98-21).

Charges are made by some commercial payers and by self-payers. Invariably charges are higher than the actual cost of services to account for losses from individuals who do not pay.

The issue of reimbursement can either make or break a laser program. Therefore, particular attention must be given to the profit-loss margin and to the types of patient reimbursement for laser procedures.

## RESEARCH

Financial support for research within a laser center may be derived from grants and endowments and from the profits of educational programs. Additionally, financial backing may come from a manufacturer that furnishes equipment and supplies for a clinical research program with an intent to obtain FDA approval for a particular application or wavelength.

## GUIDELINES AND REGULATIONS

Current guidelines and regulations that affect a laser program are listed below.

## ANSI Z136.3

The American National Standard Institute Committee is composed of a group of volunteers with diverse backgrounds and a common goal of establishing guidelines for laser safety in the health-care environment. However, this document, the ANSI Z136.3, is a guideline, not a federal or state requirement, that attempts to provide a standard within the industry regarding hazard evaluation, classification, and control; laser safety; training programs; medical surveillance; and special considerations.[4] It also includes an appendix that reviews specific guidelines for each specialty. The purpose of this document is to provide technical and practical information with which to make informed decisions within the field of laser surgery and medicine.

In the future, the adoption of this document may occur within organizations such as OSHA and JCAH. From the vantage point of safety for patients and personnel and the standpoint of possible medical/legal difficulties, this document is strongly recommended as a viable guideline.

### Food and Drug Administration

The FDA controls laser systems at the level of the manufacturer. Their Performance and Specifications Document[10] outlines the regulated requirements for a laser system prior to market distribution within the United States. To meet these requirements, laser manufacturers must set up clinical trials and assure that an institutional review board or medical board is set up within each hospital or clinic involved in performing clinical trials prior to approval by the FDA; this board ensures that FDA guidelines are met during these premarketing clinical trials.

### Occupational Safety and Health Administration

Traditionally, OSHA stays an arm's length from the medical field, and very specifically away from lasers. They rely upon documents such as the ANSI Z136.3 and FDA requirements.[10] However, OSHA is becoming involved with medical issues such as the hazard of smoke plumes and other issues involving the health and safety of personnel. Certainly, attention to employee safety and protection and knowledge of the law are recommended.

### Institutional Review Board

The Institutional Review Board (IRB) is made up of medical and lay individuals within the community whose goal it is to provide direction for the use of investigational devices and drugs within institutions. They ensure that clinical and research safety protocols are followed and strive to protect patients through the use of informed consent forms and acceptable medical practice.

## MONITORING AND EVALUATION

After a laser program has been established, it is important to keep current on forthcoming changes within the laser industry and to react accordingly (e.g., an accessory piece of equipment may increase a program's ability to more adequately perform laser surgery or to expand its surgical role). Current publications should be checked continually for new and pertinent information on lasers. Also, networking with other laser programs and personnel may yield valuable information that will lead to changes.

The stability and success of a laser program requires that a periodic financial review be made. Patient charges should be evaluated to confirm that they are adequate and financial projections checked to determine whether they are accurate. While providing safety for all involved, the program should prove to be economically sound and practically feasible.

It is important to keep current on new safety information within the laser industry so as to assure the safety of one's own laser program. An LSO should recertify a successful safety program after adequately checking for compliance with new safety information and with the safety measures listed in the ANSI Z136.3 document.[4]

The yearly update of physician credentialing is necessary, as is the education and training for support personnel. Review should be undertaken of the case loads to assess any possible indication of an excessive complication rate. Patient complaints and dissatisfaction should always be examined.

Although a program evaluation is usually performed by internal personnel knowledgeable about current information and current standards and guidelines, outside consultants and safety experts also may be helpful here.

## CONCLUSIONS

It is challenging to add another dimension of patient treatment to the medical field and to explore the ever-increasing potential of laser surgery. Yet, focus must be maintained on the primary purpose of lasers in the medical environment—to meet patient needs. There is a challenge for laser programs to keep abreast of the new laser technology and equipment while running an economically feasible and safe program. The success of this challenge lies in insightful planning, trained and qualified personnel, adequate safety precautions, feasible economic planning, and clearly defined organizational positions and responsibilities.

## REFERENCES

1. Grey F, Mittelman H: Implementation and management of a laser program, in Apfelberg DB (ed): *Evaluation and Installation of Surgical Laser System*. New York, Springer-Verlag, 1986.
2. Thomas S: Marketing and public relations: Practical methods to ensure increased laser use, in Breedlove B, Schwartz D (eds): *Clinical Lasers—Expert Strategies for Practical and Profitable Management*. Atlanta, Georgia, American Health Consultant Books, 1985, pp 119–125.
3. Heinemann J: Foresight, planning only first steps in creating a laser clinic. *Clinical Laser Monthly* 1988; 5:65–68.
4. American National Standards Institute: *Safe Use of Lasers in the Health Care Environment, Z136.3*. New York, American National Standards Institute, 1988, p 1–61.
5. The American Society for Lasers in Medicine and Surgery, 813 Second Street, Suite 200, Wausau, Wisconsin 54401. Unpublished material, 1987.
6. Lundergan DK: Certificate of need may be required for laser departments. *Clinical Laser Monthly* 1984; 2:120–121.
7. Ossoff R: Anesthesia, special precautions and requirements, in Breedlove B, Schwartz D (eds): *Clinical Laser: Expert Strategies for Practical and Profitable Management*. Atlanta, Georgia, American Health Consultant Books, 1985, pp 207–221.
8. The American Society for Lasers in Medicine: *Suggested Outline for Specific Laser Courses*. Unpublished material, 1987.
9. The American Society for Lasers in Medicine: *Nursing By-Laws, Nursing Section*. Unpublished material, 1987.
10. Code of Federal Regulations, CFR: 21 CFR 1040.10, 1987.

Chapter 2

# Laser Physics and Light-Tissue Interaction

Sue E. Huether, R.N., Ph.D.

This chapter provides an introduction to the properties and generation of laser light and light-tissue interactions. This information is basic to understanding safety principles and energy delivery through the various surgical delivery systems. "Laser" is an acronym for Light Amplification by Stimulated Emission of Radiation and represents an intense beam of light with a particular wavelength. The unique properties of laser light allow selective tissue effects with a precision not achieved using traditional surgical instruments. Medical lasers in common use today are non-ionizing and are used for both diagnostic and therapeutic applications.

## HISTORY OF LASERS

In 1917 Einstein proposed the concept of stimulated emission, a concept that formed the basis for lasers.[1] In addition, Planck's Quantum Theory and Bohr's Theory of Spontaneous Absorption and Emission of Radiation contributed to the development of lasers. In 1954, Townes developed the first maser (microwave amplification by stimulated emission of radiation)[2] and, in 1958, together with Schawlow, proposed the principles for developing stimulated emission of light.[2] In 1960, Maiman developed the first laser, using a ruby crystal as an active medium.[3] The helium:neon laser was the first gas laser and was developed by Javan, Bennett, and Herriott in 1961.[4] By 1964, Patel had developed the first $CO_2$ laser,[5] and the neodymium:yttrium-aluminum-garnet (Nd:YAG) laser was developed by Geusic and colleagues.[6] The argon-ion laser was invented by Bridges and colleagues in 1965.[7] Organic dye lasers, invented by Sorokin and Lankard in 1966,[8] are now tunable to a variety of wavelengths from near ultraviolet to near infrared. Frequency-doubling of the Nd:YAG laser to the green was possible by the late 1960s and has been recently produced using potassium-titanyl-phosphate (the KTP laser).[9]

## GENERATING LASER ENERGY

The laser works according to the properties of light and electromagnetic radiation. Light is composed of photons (particles or quanta of energy) and is propagated with wave-like motion. The electromagnetic spectrum represents the frequency and wavelength distribution of atomic energy. The most commonly used medical lasers, the $CO_2$ and Nd:YAG lasers, are infrared lasers while others such as the argon and KTP are in the visible portion of the electromagnetic spectrum (Fig 2–1). Ordinary white light is in the visible part of the electromagnetic spectrum and represents a random or incoherent combination of multiple frequencies or colors. In contrast, laser light is monochromatic, that is, it contains a single frequency (or a very narrow spectral band), and is coherent with all the photons in phase with one another, both in space and time (Fig 2–2). Finally, laser light is collimated, that is, all rays are virtually parallel to one another. As a result of collimation, there is very little divergence over long distances. This allows the beam to be easily controlled or focused. Laser light is also very bright or intense because the energy is condensed into a very narrow frequency distribution (Fig 2–3). Laser brightness and intensity are the results of collimation and small beam diameter.

Atomic activity is used to produce the laser light of the medical lasers used today. Atoms are capable of absorbing energy when they are in a ground or resting state (Fig 2–4, A). The energy absorbed may be electrical, chemical, thermal, or light energy and is

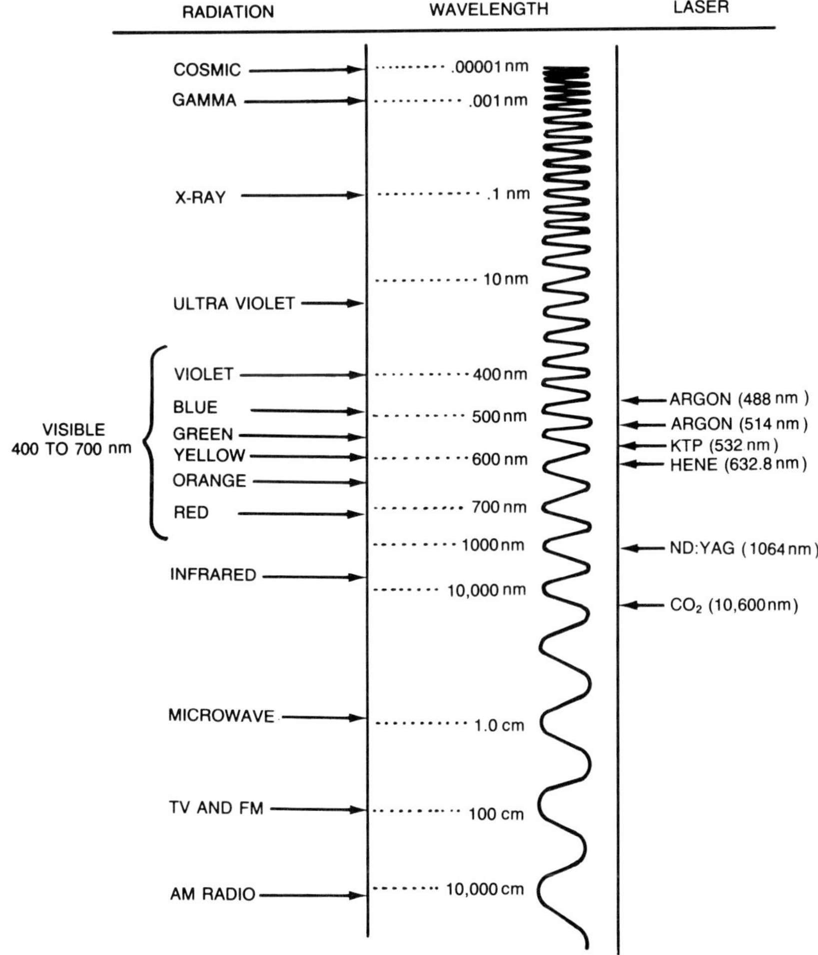


**FIG 2–1.**
The electromagnetic spectrum showing varying types of lasers, including laser output, and their associated wavelengths.

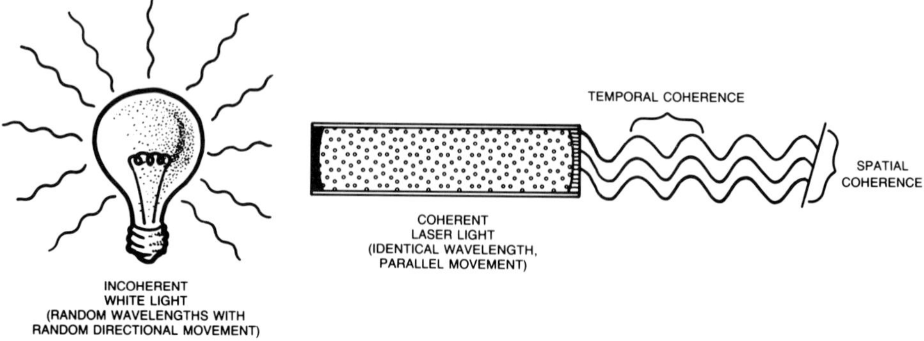


**FIG 2–2.**
A comparison of coherent versus incoherent light.

known as the source energy. When source energy is directed into an atom it is spontaneously absorbed, and the atom makes the transition from a resting state to an excited state (Fig 2–4,B). Electrons orbiting the nucleus move to outer orbits or change their pattern of vibration or rotation. The energy level of the atom is related to the orbital location of its electrons. Atoms remain in an excited state for only a millionth to a billionth of a second and then return to the ground or resting state (Fig 2–4,C). During this orbital transition, spontaneous emission of photons occurs.

Stimulated emission of radiation requires atoms to be in a metastable state (a pause from a second to a millionth of a second at a particular orbital position) in the transition from an excited state to a resting state. If an atom in a metastable state encounters a photon of a particular wavelength, the atom is stimulated to give up its energy. Instead of being absorbed, the stimulating photon continues to be propagated. The end result is two photons of identical wavelength moving in phase through space and time (Fig 2–4,D).

If a high population of atoms in an excited state is stimulated further by the right photons, a chain reaction of stimulated emission occurs. Sustained stimulated emission of

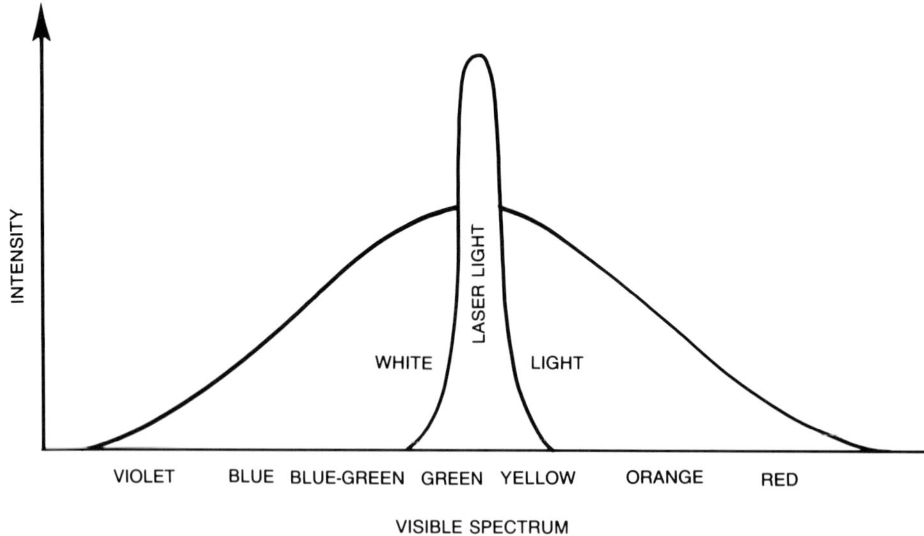


**FIG 2–3.**
A comparison of spectral purity of a hypothetical green/yellow laser beam with normal white light.

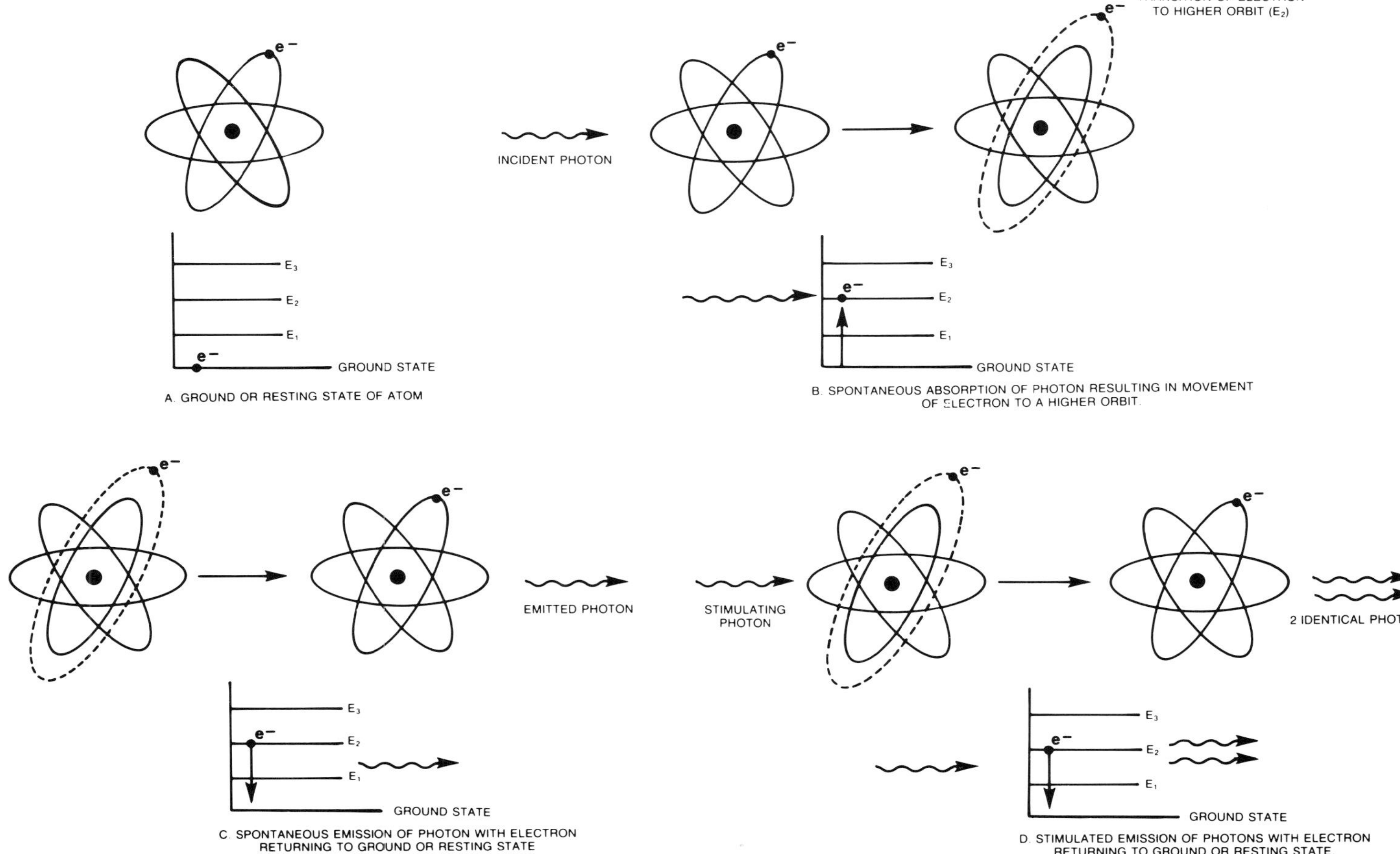


**FIG 2–4.**
Absorption, and spontaneous and stimulated emission of radiation.

radiation requires that there continually be more atoms in an excited state than in a resting state; this is known as a population inversion. A population inversion is achieved by exposing atoms to a source energy and pumping them to higher energy states. When the population inversion is established, atoms begin the cascade to the resting state with a spontaneous emission of photons. The spontaneously emitted photons may then collide with atoms in a metastable state, stimulating them to emit an identical photon. These photons then collide with other atoms, and a chain reaction of stimulated emission is initiated.

Although each photon pair created by stimulated emission is moving in the same direction, other stimulated photon pairs may be moving in a different direction. To achieve collimation, the random directional movement of photons must be changed to a parallel beam. This requires a resonator, which organizes the photons into a coherent and collimated beam by reflecting them off curved mirrors at either end of the resonating chamber by repeated passes through the cavity, each time creating a path more toward the optical axis. This causes the amplification process and aligns the photons before allowing them to emerge through one mirror, which is partially reflecting and partially transmitting.

## THE LASER SYSTEM

The components of a laser system include an energy or pumping source, a lasing or active medium, and an optical or resonating chamber (Fig 2–5). The pumping source can be electrical, chemical, thermal, or optical energy. The active medium can be a solid, liquid, or gas (e.g., the Nd:YAG crystal, a liquid dye, or argon or $CO_2$ gas), and the gas can be permanently sealed or flowing. The composition of the lasing medium determines the wavelength output and name of a particular laser. The medium is located within the resonating chamber (the laser tube), which has a cylindrical structure with a fully reflecting mirror (99%) on the posterior end and a partially reflecting mirror for light emission on the anterior end. The population inversion necessary for the chain reaction of stimulated emission occurs within the resonating chamber. Some photons are lost from the side of the

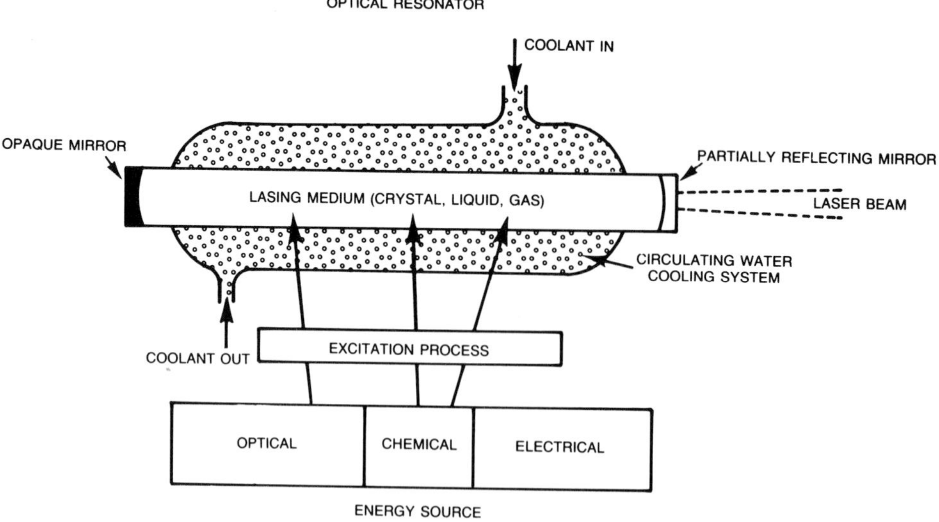


**FIG 2–5.**
Laser system components.

cylinder as heat, but photons moving horizontally are reflected back into the medium. A resonating beam of light develops and, as more atoms are stimulated to release photons and the photons are reflected back and forth through the cavity, the beam is organized and amplified (Fig 2–6).

The maximum energy output of a laser is a function of the length of the resonating chamber and the amount of lasing medium. Because a large amount of heat can be lost from the laser tube, some lasers require a continuous flow of cooling water (e.g., some argon, Nd:YAG, and KTP laser designs), whereas others may have a closed recirculating cooling system or are aircooled (e.g., most $CO_2$ lasers). The efficiency of a laser is the ratio of the beam power to the pump power; most medical lasers have a low efficiency (i.e., a small power output in relation to the pumping power). Efficiency is usually reported as a percentage of the input power.

## Types of Surgical Lasers

There are many types of lasing media. These require different pumping sources and the combinations produce different wavelengths. Lasers are usually named for their active media (Table 2–1). Those most commonly used in medicine and surgery are the carbon dioxide ($CO_2$), argon (Ar), Neodymium:yttrium-aluminum-garnet (Nd:YAG), potassium-titanyl-phosphate (KTP), and the "tunable dye," which produces laser energy from an organic fluorescent material dissolved in a common solvent such as rhodamines in alcohol and fluorescein in water.[10] The helium:neon (HeNe) laser is often used to produce a finder beam for invisible beam lasers.

The $CO_2$ laser contains a medium of $CO_2$, nitrogen, and helium gases. Pumping is accomplished by an electrical discharge (dc or rf) in the gas mixture, which can be sealed or flowing. The output wavelength is in the far infrared (10,600 nm). $CO_2$ lasers require alternating current of 110 volts, operate at an efficiency of 10% to 15%, and are cooled by internal fans and recirculating coolant fluids.

Because this infrared wavelength is invisible, a visible helium:neon aiming beam is included in the laser device; this aiming beam is coaxial with the surgical laser beam. The aiming beam indicates the surgical beam path.

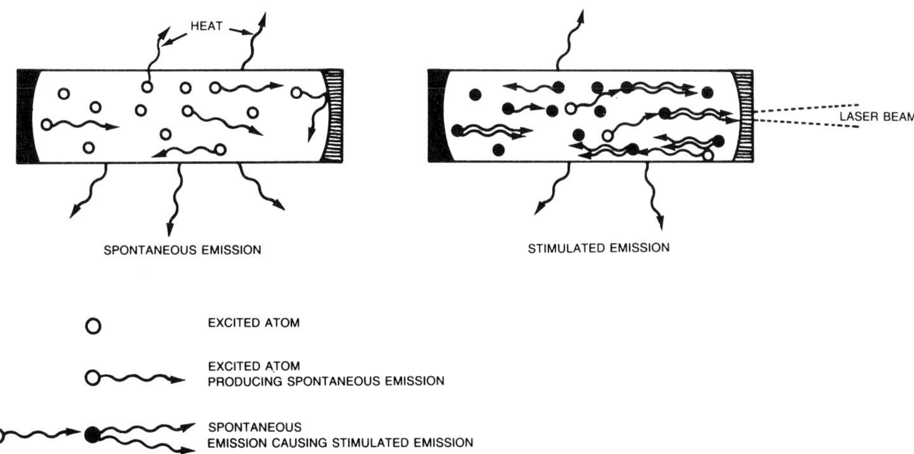


**FIG 2–6.**
Stimulated emission and amplification occurring within the resonant cavity to produce the laser beam.

**TABLE 2–1.**
Types and Characteristics of Lasers

| Laser | Active Medium | Wavelength | Pumping Source | Power Output | Preferential Absorbance | 99% of Energy Absorbed in Tissue Depth |
|---|---|---|---|---|---|---|
| Argon | Argon ion gas | 418 nm and 514.5 nm | AC discharge | <1.0 – 25 watts (20 watts to pump dye laser) | Hemoglobin | 1–2 mm |
| $CO_2$ | $CO_2$, nitrogen helium gases | 10,600 nm | DC discharge or RF discharge | <1.0 – >100 watts | Water | 0.1–0.3 mm |
| Nd:YAG | Neodymium yttrium aluminum garnet crystal | 1,064 | Optical-pumping with flash | <1 – >100 watts | Dark or black color | 7 mm |
| KTP | YAG beam frequency-doubled by a KTP crystal | 532 nm | As with Nd:YAG | <1.0 – 16 watts | Hemoglobin, melanin | 1–3 mm |
| Dye | Dissolved organic material | 400–800 nm | Argon or krypton laser | <1 – 4 watts | (Visible) photo-sensitized cells, pigmented lesions | |
| HeNe | Helium | 632.8 | | 0.001 – 0.025 | About the same as Nd:YAG | |

The argon-ion laser's active medium (ionized argon gas, permanently sealed) is pumped by the discharge of high-density electrical current (dc or rf) at low voltages. The output wavelengths are in the blue range of the spectrum at 488 nm and the green at 514.5 nm. The argon laser uses alternating current electricity and those producing more than a few watts of power are water cooled, requiring access to running water and a drain. This laser operates with an efficiency of less than 1% and because of this has a limited maximum power output of around 25 watts. But the argon laser achieves desirable photocoagulation effects at an output power of as little as two watts. Typical continuous wave surgical argon lasers, which can photocoagulate and vaporize, produce 15 to 25 watts.

The Nd:YAG, a solid-state laser composed of a neodymium-doped YAG crystal, is optically pumped by a krypton arc flash lamp. It operates at about 2% efficiency or less. This laser produces an invisible beam with a wavelength of 1,064 nm in the near infrared range; this beam can be continuous or pulsed. It requires an aiming beam, uses 208 volt electricity, and flowing or recirculating water, depending on the design. Typical surgical units generate up to 80 to 100 watts of power.

The KTP laser is a frequency-doubled Nd:YAG laser, producing a 532-nm visible green beam by passing the Nd:YAG laser's output through a potassium-titanyl-phosphatic crystal. This laser requires 208 volts of AC electricity, is cooled by inflowing water, and operates at less than 1% efficiency.

In the tunable dye lasers, the active dye is an organic fluorescent material which is excited by a flash lamp or another laser beam. Typically, these devices produce lower power output beams of specific wavelengths for cutaneous absorption by pigmented skin or activate photosensitive dyes in photodynamic therapy of malignant tissues.

## Modes of the Laser

The longitudinal (or axial) mode of a laser is a function of the distance between the resonating mirrors and determines photon wavelength. The optical cavity is structured to optimize the amplification of only one frequency in order to maintain monochromatic output.

Light output from a laser is often generated in short pulses lasting about a millisecond, or the output can be a continuous wave (CW). The temporal output is known as the temporal mode of the laser. The carbon dioxide, argon, KTP, and Nd:YAG lasers are continuous wave lasers. Some lasers, such as the Nd:YAG, can also operate in a Q-switched mode. In the Q-switched mode, energy is stored in the resonating cavity during pumping by inserting a shutter between the lasing medium and the partially reflecting mirror, and is then released in a single high-energy pulse or burst (i.e., within a picosecond in megawatt range). Pulsed delivery of the light can be achieved from settings on the instrument panel as pulses per second (PPS) or as a pulse duration or pulse width in tenths of a second to milliseconds.

Mode locking is used in some types of lasers to synchronize the phase relationships of the axial or resonating modes in the laser chamber. The synchronization is achieved by the use of a shutter or bleachable dyes. Locking the modes together results in a "beat" or a train of pulses with a high peak power (megawatts) from a picosecond to a nanosecond duration. Q-switching and mode locking attain power outputs that exceed those of CW or pulsed lasers. The tissue impact of high-energy short-duration pulses can create plasma formation if the power density exceeds $1 \times 10^{10}$ W/cm$^2$ and can cause acoustical shock waves with selective mechanical disruption of cell and tissue membranes.

The transverse electromagnetic mode (TEM) defines the spatial energy distribution pattern across the face of the beam. Various TEM configurations are illustrated in Figure 2–7. Most contemporary surgical lasers have a fundamental mode configuration ($TEM_{00}$) with a Gaussian or normal distribution of energy across the beam, which has no cool spots and is round. The smallest effective beam diameter and hence the highest power intensity occurs with a $TEM_{00}$ beam, i.e., no cool spots either vertically or horizontally.

Early lasers produced intensity profiles with maximum intensity some distance from the true center and less intensity at the center, yielding a footprint in the target looking like a doughnut. This was called the doughnut mode TEM and was designated $TEM_{01}$. Other spatial profiles can occur as well.

A Gaussian beam is symmetrical, and the spatial profile is sustained when the light is projected through lenses. The energy pattern of the beam will have a mirror image effect in tissue (Fig 2–8). Distributed mirror alignment in the laser tube or articulating arm of the $CO_2$ laser or damage to the optical fiber of the argon or Nd:YAG laser can alter the beam profile and thus change the laser effects in tissue.

## Surgical Delivery Systems

Delivery of the beam from the output port of the laser's resonating chamber onto the surgical site is accomplished by one or a combination of four basic schemes: transmission through a flexible optical fiber of varying diameter (from 60 to 600 μm), reflection from a series of mirrors in an articulated arm, direct irradiation from the resonator via lenses and mirrors, or through hollow-core wave guides. Most visible and near-infrared beams are transmitted by fibers of optical glass or quartz. Mid- and far-infrared (e.g., $CO_2$) beams utilize direct opto-mechanical coupling, articulated arms, or hollow-core wave guides. The latter are only recently available and can be flexible, though not as narrow or flexible as fibers, allowing 90 degrees of arc without significant loss of power.[11]

Somewhere in the delivery scheme the collimated laser energy coming out of the laser

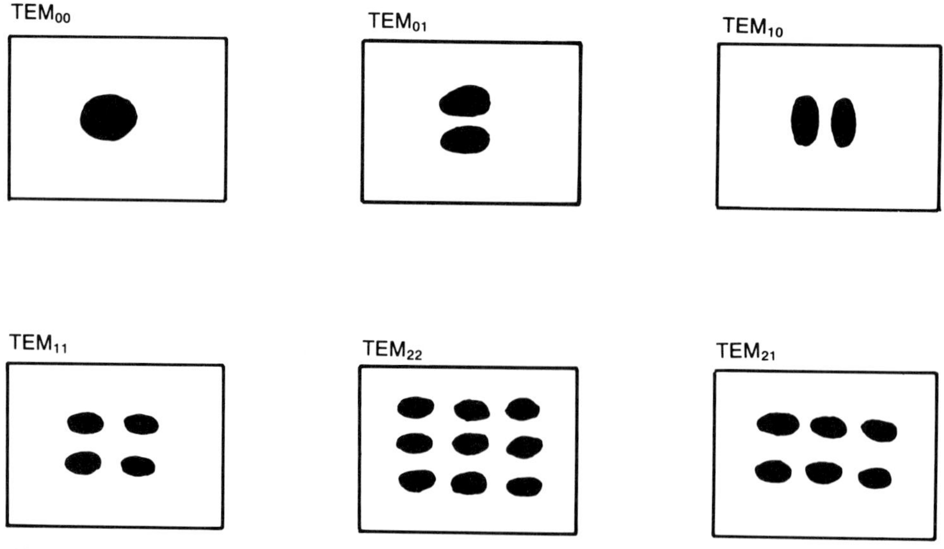


**FIG 2–7.**
Transverse electromagnetic mode (TEM) patterns. $TEM_{00}$ represents a Gaussian distribution with the energy concentrated in the center of the beam. The subscripts indicate vertical and horizontal cool spots (e.g., $TEM_{01}$ has no vertical and one horizontal separation).

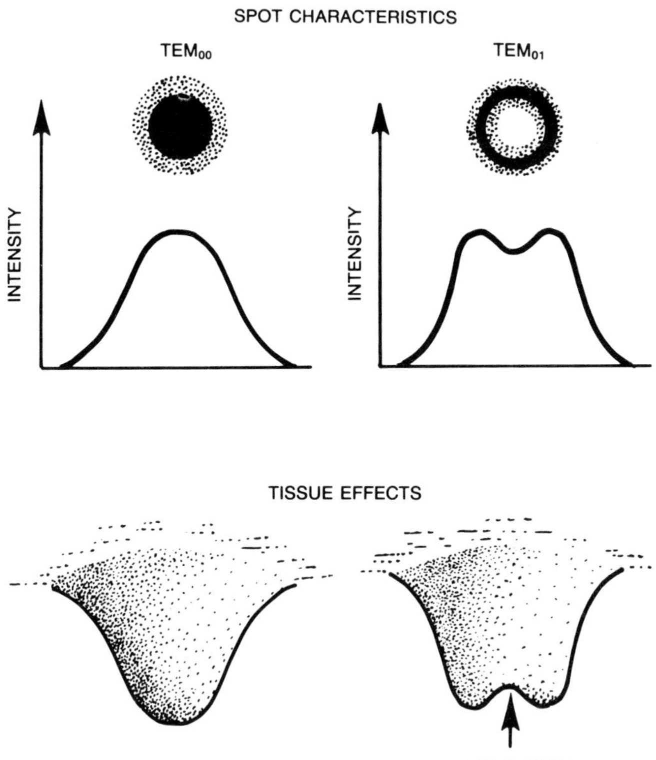


**FIG 2–8.**
The effect of the TEM on crater shape in tissue.

tube is focused at least once by a laser lens and concentrated in a small surface area. In the $CO_2$ laser surgical system with direct irradiation, the beam is focused as it exits the resonator, then it is reflected off a gimbaled mirror onto the target, which should be at the focal length of the lens. With an articulating arm, the unfocused beam is transmitted to either a focusing handpiece or to a micromanipulator attached to an operating microscope, which contains the focusing lens and a reflective mirror attached to a joystick or to an endoscope with a focusing lens. Either way, the surgical beam and its visible finder or aiming beam are moved over the surgical target by the surgeon who simply manipulates the joystick or moves the endoscope. With hollow-core wave guides, the $CO_2$ laser beam is focused by a handpiece or endoscope coupler containing the lens (Fig 2–9).

Laser beams transmitted by fibers are focused as they enter the fiber to decrease diameter and increase intensity. At the output end of the fiber, the beam diverges. This diverging beam may be refocused by a handpiece if necessary. Most laser beams are used surgically in non-contact mode. Recently, however, artificial sapphire "focusing" tips have been developed to concentrate Nd:YAG beams; these enable contact laser surgery with special handpieces or contact endoscopic laser surgery with tips fitted to the fiber's end.[12]

## The Laser Beam Spot Size

Collimated laser energy coming out of the laser tube is focused by a laser focusing lens and concentrated in a small surface area (Fig 2–10). Some beam divergence occurs

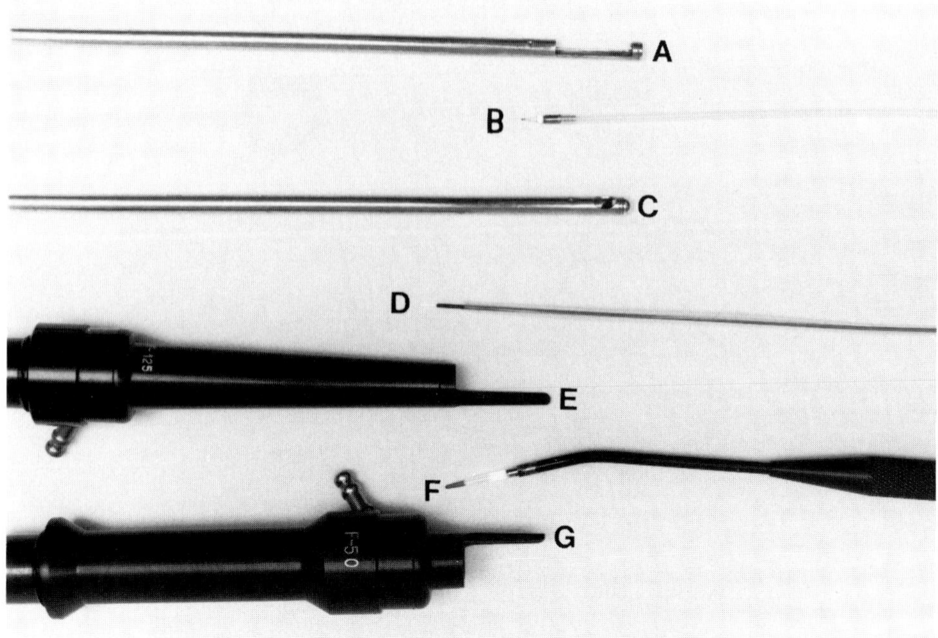


**FIG 2–9.**
Various end beam delivery instruments for $CO_2$ and Nd:YAG lasers.

as the beam enters the focusing lens. The minimum effective laser beam diameter (d) produced by a particular laser and optical system is a function of the focal length (F) of the laser focusing lens and the beam divergence ($\theta$); that is $d = F\theta$. The divergence is a function of the wavelength and the unfocused beam diameter; that is, $\theta = 4\lambda/\pi D$ where $\lambda$ is the wavelength and D is the beam diameter entering the lens. The minimum beam diameter and the highest power concentration occur at the focal plane of the laser lens. For a $TEM_{00}$ laser beam, the effective diameter of the smallest spot is given by $d = 4F\lambda/\pi D$,

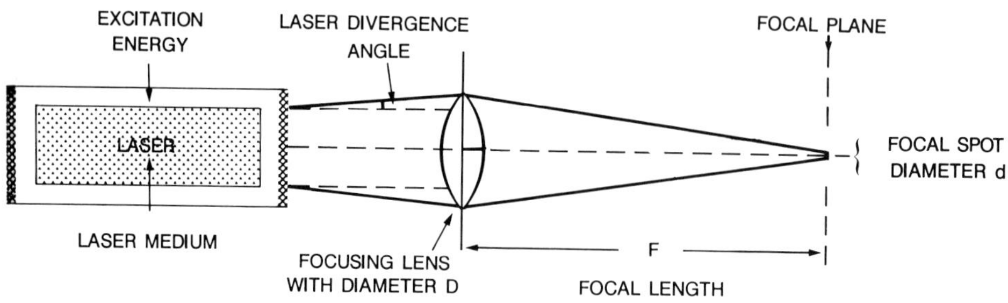


**FIG 2–10.**
Configuration for focusing the laser beam with a lens of sufficient diameter to capture all the beam energy as it exits the optical cavity. The focused beam has a focal spot of diameter *(d)* at its focal length *(F)*. (From Wright VC, Riopelle MA: *Gynecologic Laser Surgery: A Practical Handbook*. Houston, Biomedical Communications, 1982. Used by permission.)

where $\lambda$ = the wavelength produced by the laser, D = the unfocused laser beam diameter as it enters the focusing lens, and F = the focal length of the lens.

Since the beam divergence is fixed for any particular laser system, for clinical applications the laser surgeon will need to manipulate the spot size of the effective laser beam diameter by changing the focal length of the laser focusing lens: the longer the focal length, the greater the beam diameter. A laser with a 300-mm focusing lens attached to an operating microscope with an objective lens of 300 mm gives an approximate effective laser beam diameter of 0.5 mm. The laser surgeon can increase the beam diameter by employing the variable-spot-size mechanism. This mechanism alters the diameter of the laser beam where it enters the focusing lens. A small focused laser beam (0.2 to 0.5 mm) is used for cutting, a larger beam (2 to 2.5 mm) for in situ destruction by vaporization, and a larger (3 to 5 mm) beam for coagulation. Handpieces for freehand delivery (F = 125 mm) produce a miniscule beam diameter of approximately 0.2 mm. With handpieces or endoscopes of fixed focal length lenses, the beam diameter is enlarged by defocusing the lens, i.e., moving the unit away from the target. With a contact tip the spot size is changed by interchanging fiber tips.

Surgical laser beams are usually described by their diameters, but it should be noted that the more important aspect is focal spot area. This is because the beam intensity varies with the area (or the square of the diameter) when power in the beam is constant (see Fig 2–10).

## Power Density

The thermal effects of the light-tissue interaction are a function of several variables operating simultaneously: (1) energy output in watts, (2) beam diameter, (3) duration of exposure, (4) absorption and scattering ratios of the different laser wavelengths at the different tissue interfaces, and (5) thermal conduction in tissue (i.e., the effects of blood flow and tissue temperature). For a given laser-tissue combination, the quantitative aspect of the laser effect depends on power density.[13] The power of a laser beam (P) is measured in watts and the power density defines the power of the beam per unit area. Power density varies across the beam because of the TEM, and therefore a more useful way to describe the intensity of a beam is by average power density ($P_a$). Because the Gaussian (or $TEM_{00}$) laser beam's intensity diminishes at its periphery to negligible levels, not all of the actual beam creates a defect. Within the effective spot diameter, $d_e$ (a convention established by physicists that describes the distance between opposite points of a concentric circle where intensity drops to 1/e2 times the maximum power in the center), 86% of total beam power is transmitted; 14% is on the periphery, outside the circle of diameter $d_e$ (Fig 2–11). Because only 86% of the power is within the effective beam area, effective power ($P_e$) is 0.86P, where P is total watts in the beam. Effective beam area ($A_e$) is $r^2$, where r is effective beam radius, $d_e/2$, measured in millimeters by a microruler after a 10-watt one-tenth second test-firing. Therefore, average power density ($P_a$) is effective power ($P_e$) divided by effective area in square millimeters:

$$P_a = P_e/A_e = 0.86\ P/\pi\ r^2 = 0.86\ P/\pi\ (d_e2/4) = 4 \times 0.86\ P/\pi d_e^{\ 2} = 1.10\ P/d_e^{\ 2} = \text{watts/mm}$$

To convert watts per square millimeters (above) to the more conventional watts per square centimeter, the numerator must be multipled by 100, yielding:

$$P_a = 110\ P/d^2 \text{ in watts/cm}^2$$

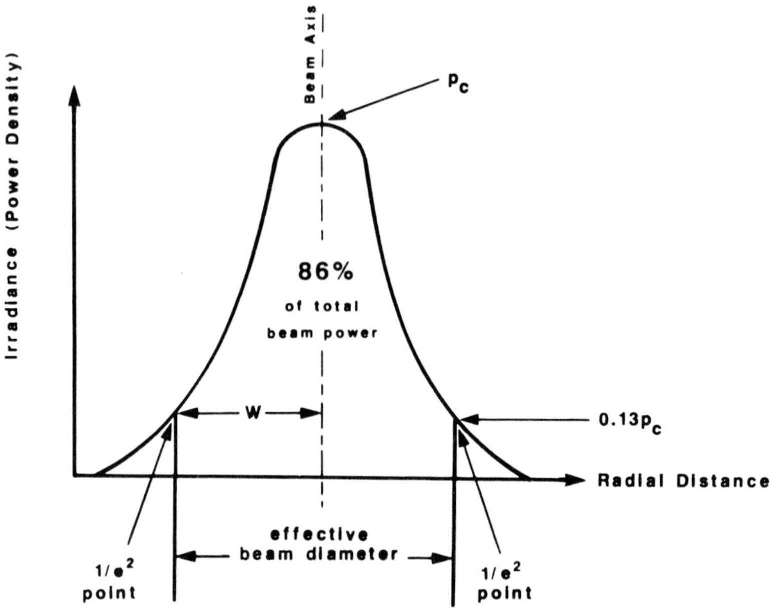


**EFFECTIVE DIAMETER OF A GAUSSIAN BEAM**

**FIG 2–11.**
The effective diameter of a Gaussian laser beam between points where maximum intensity at the center ($P_c$) drops to a level of $P_c/e^2$. (From Wright VC, Riopelle MA: *Gynecologic Laser Surgery: A Practical Handbook.* Houston, Biomedical Communications, 1982. Used by permission.)

To simplify matters, one can ignore the extra 10% and use the following formula:[13]

$$P_a = 110\ P/d^2 \text{in W/cm}^2$$

To calculate the average power density for a beam, measure the beam diameter in millimeters, square that figure and divide that amount into the product of 100 and the watts read off the power meter.

It is important to remember that power density varies inversely with the square of the effective laser beam diameter. This means that doubling the beam diameter will increase the area four times and, more important, will decrease the power density to one-fourth its original level. The smaller the effective beam diameter (spot size), the greater the power density will be when other factors are held constant. A larger spot diffuses the power, creating a more superficial effect (Fig 2–12). Table 2 summarizes the power density at different watts and spot sizes. When exposure time or pulse duration is considered, time is included in the calculation as seconds and measured in joules (watt seconds). Radiation time or duration of exposure is important for controlling the desired tissue effects and for preventing excess tissue damage. With the $CO_2$ lasers, the use of higher peak powers at high repetition rates (as discussed under the superpulse section) has a more precise cutting effect with less peripheral thermal conduction, although there is some variation with different tissue elements.[14]

## Understanding Superpulse

Most $CO_2$ lasers operate in the continuous-wave temporal mode (CW). Employing this mode, the laser surgeon controls the application time by depressing a foot pedal to activate

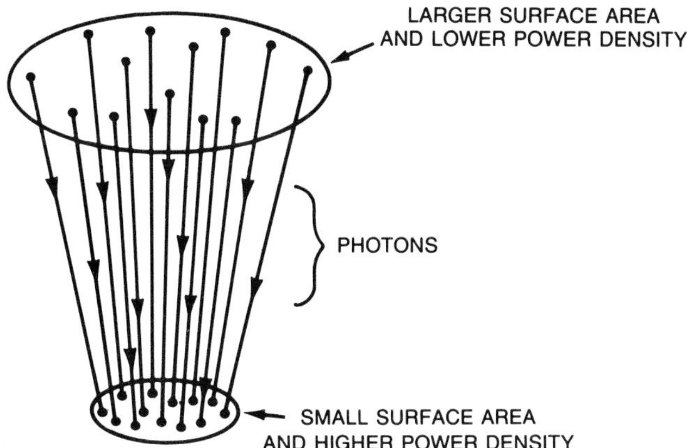


**FIG 2–12.**
The effect of reduced focal spot size or beam intensity for constant input power as a function of focal spot area.

the laser or open the output shutter. Actual tissue exposure time (the time a beam remains in contact with a particular target cell population) is controlled by moving the beam with the joystick or handpiece. The power and power density remain uniform throughout the application unless the power is changed on the control panel by the operator or the spot size is varied. In superpulse temporal mode, the output beam is produced in the form of a train of pulses with a controlled rapid repetition rate (frequency in hertz) and short pulse duration or width (seconds). Between the successive pulses, there is a pause that allows the tissue to cool. The amount of heat conducted into the surrounding tissue is less than that in the continuous mode setting because thermal damage is a function of exposure time and the use of superpulse minimizes exposure time. Superpulse efficacy begins to decline when the duration of a pulse exceeds about one-tenth (or 10%) of the time before the pulse is repeated.[11]

There is also a limit to the usefulness of pulse width or duration of exposure. If the superpulse width becomes too long, the peak power per pulse declines very rapidly. Optimum pulse durations usually range between 200 and 400 microseconds (0.2 to 0.4 milliseconds, 0.0002 to 0.0004 seconds). The duty factor (or duty cycle) is obtained by multiplying the frequency (in hertz) by the pulse width (in seconds). For example, a surgical laser system with a combination of a 200-microsecond (0.0002 second) pulse width and a repetition rate of 400 hertz yields a duty factor of 0.08, or 8%. Above a duty factor of 10%, the usefulness of superpulsing begins to diminish because cooling time is lessened and the effect becomes more and more like the continuous-wave mode. The peak power of

**TABLE 2–2.**
Power Density Values Calculated From Effective Spot Diameter and Power*

| | Effective Spot Diameter (mm) | | | |
|---|---|---|---|---|
| Power (Watts) | 0.5 | 1.0 | 1.5 | 2.0 |
| 10 | 4,000 | 1,000 | 444 | 250 |
| 20 | 8,000 | 2,000 | 888 | 500 |
| 30 | 12,000 | 3,000 | 1,333 | 750 |
| 40 | 16,000 | 4,000 | 1,778 | 1,000 |
| 50 | 20,000 | 5,000 | 2,222 | 1,250 |

*From: Wright VC, Riopelle MA: *Gynecologic Laser Surgery: A Practical Handbook.* Houston, Biomedical Communications, 1982. Used by permission.

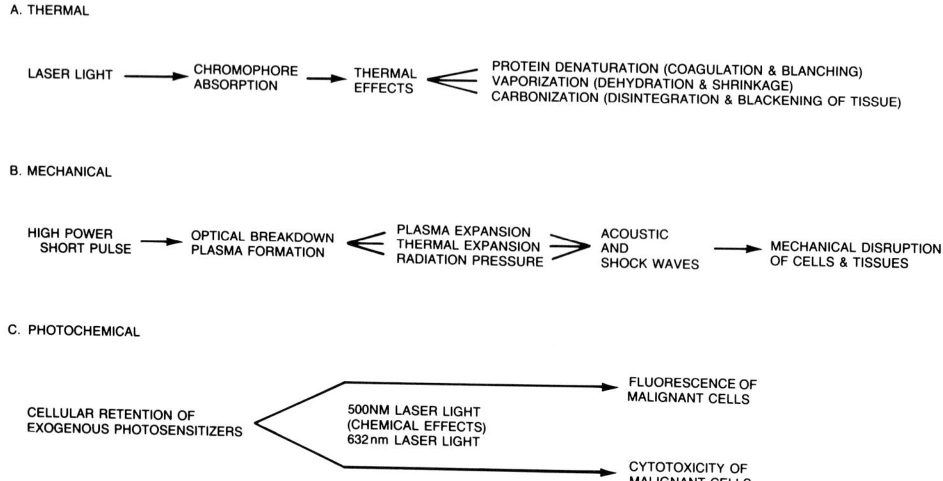


**FIG 2–13.**
Summary of basic qualitative laser effects in tissue.

the superpulse is calculated by dividing the average power by the duty factor. In turn, the average power is calculated by multiplying the peak power by the duty factor.

Energy per pulse is a useful measurement to employ when comparing one laser machine or superpulse setting with another. The higher the energy per pulse, the more tissue volume that is incised or destroyed for a given repetition frequency with a stationary laser beam. The energy per pulse (expressed in joules) can be computed by dividing the average power by the repetition rate.

## LASER-TISSUE INTERACTION

Medical or surgical laser radiation causes three types of effects on living tissue: thermal, mechanical, and chemical (Fig 2–13). As a particular laser wavelength strikes a particular type of tissue, some of the beam will be reflected off the surface and some amount of incident power will be converted to other forms of radiation, such as heat or fluorescence. Some energy will be transmitted through the tissue or be scattered within it by the rays being bounced off particles, molecules, or cells. Each scattered ray will subsequently be rescattered in another direction, and eventually absorption of the remaining energy will take place. Most absorbed energy, either at the tissue surface or within it, is converted to heat, some of which can flow from the impact site by conduction or convection (e.g., in vasculature), and some power can be converted into mechanical energy, causing disruption of tissue. The proportion of laser light that is absorbed, scattered, transmitted, or reflected by tissue is wavelength-dependent and is also dependent upon the absorptive properties of the different tissues (Fig 2–14).

The amount and type of absorption of laser radiation is also wavelength-dependent. In the visible and near infrared range virtually no absorption occurs in biologic molecules unless chromophores are present. Therefore, tissues without artificially introduced chromophores (such as dyes or photosensitizers) do not absorb argon, HeNe, dye, or Nd:YAG laser wavelengths except for the erythrocytes and melanocytes, which contain hemoglobin

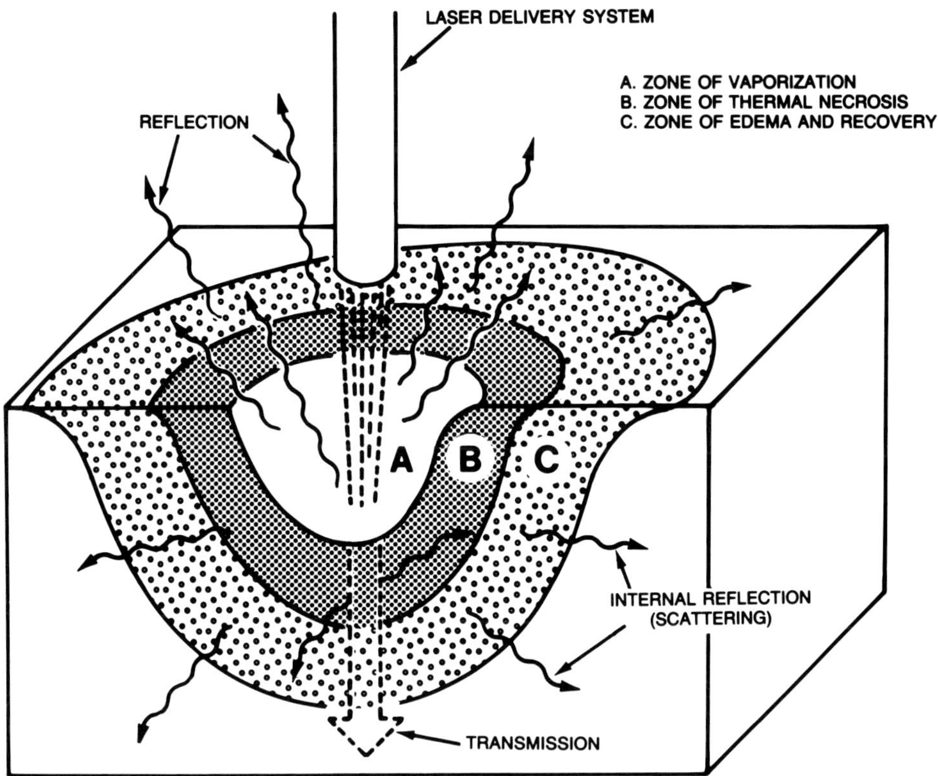


**FIG 2–14.**
Reflection, scattering, absorption, and transmission of laser energy within tissue and zones of injury reduced. Not all tissue effects occur with every wavelength-tissue type combination.

and melanin. In the far infrared range, all biological material is absorptive to a lesser or greater extent, depending upon its water content.

The absorption coefficients of hemoglobin, melanin, and water as functions of wavelengths are illustrated in Fig 2–15. The blue-green argon and KTP laser beams are maximally absorbed by hemoglobin and to a lesser extent by melanin but are transmitted

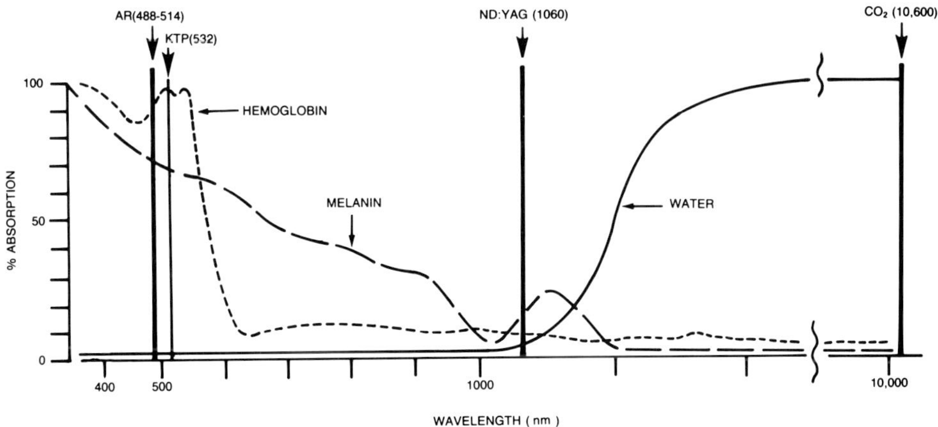


**FIG 2–15.**
Absorption as a function of wavelength for hemoglobin, melanin, and water for the visible and infrared regions of the spectrum with laser wavelengths indicated.

through water. Because these wavelengths are maximally absorbed by blood in the capillary beds, this laser is most effective for coagulation or vaporization of superficial vascular lesions, vaporization of strongly pigmented tissue, or coagulation of small vessels. Because the Ar wavelength is transmitted benignly through clear fluid, it can be used on the retina through the vitreous humor. The argon and KTP lasers have seen limited application to date in gynecology.[15, 16] Photochemolysis and photochemosynthesis, used for tumor localization and selective tumor cell destruction, occur at extremely lower power densities and employ photosensitizers plus pure light of a particular wavelength (visible through near infrared) to match the absorption spectrum of the sensitizer. Hematoporphyrin-derivative (HPD) and 630-nm dye laser light are used in combination to effect photochemotherapy for unresectable malignancies in which the sensitizer is selectively absorbed by tumor cells; those cells are then destroyed by producing singlet oxygen when exposed to the laser light.[17-19] Application of photoradiation therapy in gynecology is just beginning.[20]

For wavelengths of 400 nm or longer and at power densities within surgical ranges, almost all laser light is converted to heat and absorbed in some fashion. This range of wavelength includes argon, KTP, HeNe, Nd:YAG, and $CO_2$ laser output.

The Nd:YAG laser beam is strongly reflected by soft tissue; up to half of the incident power of a non-contact beam can be lost. This wavelength is also generously scattered within tissue, making it difficult to predict the exact depths of thermal injury being created. Also, the maximum tissue effect can actually be located under the surface of the tissue being irradiated. Continuous exposure can create a pocket in tissue with sufficient pressure caused by steam formation to actually explode. These potential difficulties com-

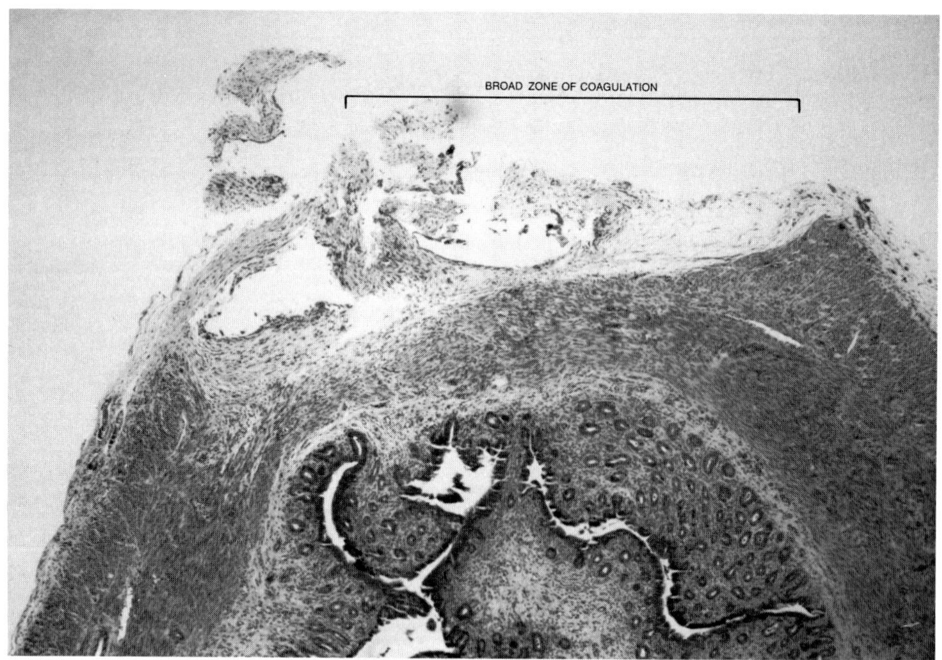


Nd: YAG 25 WATTS
(Non contact)

**FIG 2–16.**
Tissue effects of Nd:YAG laser at 25 W (non-contact) in rabbit uterus. Note the broad zone of coagulation compared to the much narrower zone illustrated in Figure 2–17. (Courtesy of WR Keye, Jr, MD, University of Utah Department of Obstetrics and Gynecology.)

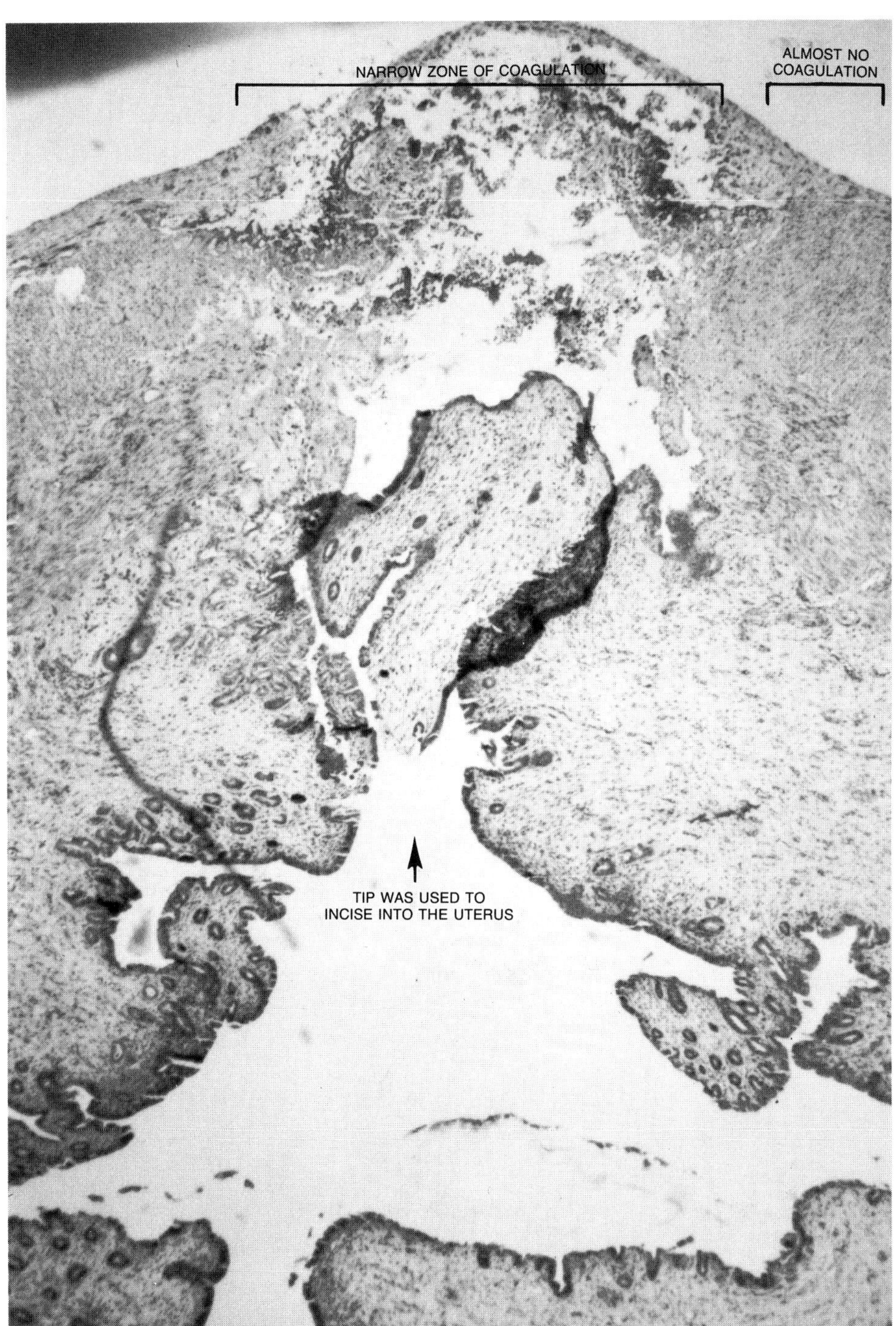


Nd:YAG 25 WATTS
(Conical Tip)

**FIG 2–17.**
Endometrial ablation with Nd:YAG laser using a contact tip. Nd:YAG laser at 25 watts with conical tip in rabbit uterus. Note the narrow zone of tissue coagulation. The effect is more like that of a $CO_2$ laser (precise cut) than the Nd:YAG laser without contact tip. (Courtesy of WR Keye, Jr, MD, University of Utah Department of Obstetrics and Gynecology.)

plicate Nd:YAG laser surgery and require that special precautions be taken by surgeons. Nd:YAG energy is more strongly absorbed by dark or black substances. In the non-contact mode, this beam, delivered to near the target surface by fiber, is used for volumetric coagulation of tissue, thereby taking advantage of the scattering (Fig 2–16).

Utilizing contact mode, the variously shaped tips can be used to effectively concentrate the divergent beam coming out of the optical fiber. Some pointed tips can be used like a scalpel with a tissue effect approaching that of the $CO_2$ beam. Vaporization occurs at the center but with a larger zone of thermal injury at the periphery because of scattering. The tips significantly reduce the incident beam reflection and lower the output power required to accomplish the same task with a non-contact mode. They also allow incision (Fig 2–17) and provide surgeons with the familiar tissue contact. The Nd:YAG laser is used predominantly in gynecology for hysteroscopic ablation of the endometrium.[21]

As is apparent from the absorption curve, the $CO_2$ laser is maximally absorbed by water. Since 80% to 85% of most biological tissue volume is water, the $CO_2$ energy has a very superficial penetration almost everywhere. Ninety percent of the incident power is absorbed in 0.03 mm of soft tissue; 99.9% in 0.1 mm. Virtually all the energy is converted to heat that evaporates superficial cells, producing a vapor plume of smoke and carbonized particles, a sterilized crater, and an extremely minute zone of thermal necrosis surrounding the vaporized crater. A finely focused $CO_2$ beam can remove tissue volumes as small as 25 to 50 cubic micrometers or in large amounts with larger beam diameters. Because of this, the $CO_2$ laser provides excellent cutting and vaporization characteristics for all colors of tissue. As tissue is vaporized, smaller blood vessels and lymphatics up to a diameter of 0.5 mm are sealed, often resulting in hemostatic surgical procedures.

Because of the $CO_2$ beam's ability to incise, excise, and destroy in place virtually all types of soft tissues, this laser is truly the workhorse laser in gynecology. Attached to the operating microscope or colposcope, it is valuable for lower genital viral dysplastic and neoplastic lesions (Fig 2–18);[22] with the microscope or laparoscope it is used within the pelvis for a variety of disorders.[23]

In summary, individual lasers are selected for specific surgical purposes because of the wavelengths produced and the wavelength-tissue combination. Sometimes a compro-

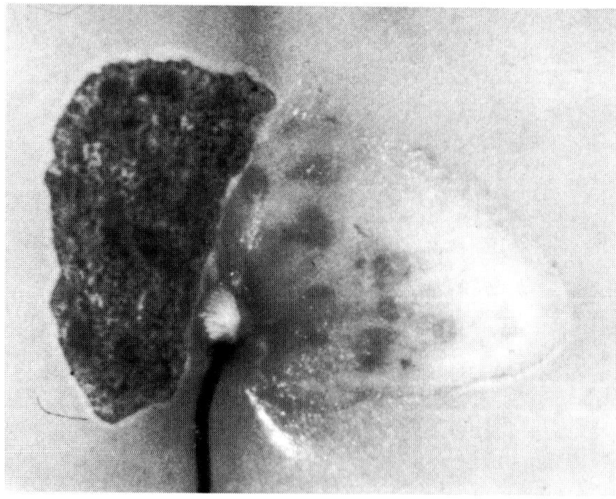

**FIG 2–18.**
Immediate post-treatment of anal condyloma acuminatum with a $CO_2$ laser at 12 to 15 watts, beam diameter 1.5 mm. The right side has been debrided. (Courtesy of James Gosewehr, MD, University of Wisconsin Department of Obstetrics and Gynecology.)

mise of wavelength is necessitated by the availability of a delivery system. The argon, KTP, Nd:YAG, and $CO_2$ lasers have all been used for gynecological surgery, much of which is described in the following chapters. The quality of the surgical defect can be minimized by limiting exposure time, either by rapid beam movement, by use of superpulse settings, or by interrupted exposures. The more time a beam is in constant contact with an area of tissue, the more conduction of heat will occur and increase the zone of thermal necrosis, negating the precision and minimal damage to surrounding cells. The surgeon must be familiar with the various kinds of laser-tissue interaction, the degree to which tissue color affects absorption of different wavelengths, the effect of power density and the use of contact modes, and the particular hazards associated with each wavelength, delivery system, and target.

## REFERENCES


1. Einstein A: Zur quantentheorie der strahlung. *Physio Z* 1917; 18:121–128.
2. Schawlow AL, Townes CH: Infrared and optical masers. *Physiol Rev* 1958; 112:1940.
3. Maiman TH: Stimulated optical radiation in ruby masers. *Nature* 1960; 187:493–494.
4. Javan A, Bennett WB Jr, Herriott DR: Population inversion and continuous optical maser oscillation in a gas discharge containing a HeNe mixture. *Phys Rev Lett* 1961; 6:106.
5. Patel CKN, McFarlane RA, Faust WL: Selective excitation through vibration energy transfer and optical maser action in $N_2$-$CO_2$. *Physiol Rev* 1964; 8:470-473.
6. Geusic JE, Marcos HM, Van Uitert LG: Laser oscillations in Nd-doped yttrium aluminum yttrium gallium and gaddinium garnets. *Appl Phys Lett* 1964; 4:182.
7. Bridges WB, Chest AN: Visible and UV laser oscillation at 119 wavelength in ionized Ne, Ar, Kr, Xe, 0 and other gases. *Appl Opt* 1965; 4:573.
8. Sorokin PD, Lankard JR: Stimulated emission from an organic dye, chloro-aluminum-phthalocyanine. *IBM J Res Dev* 1966; 10:162.
9. Liu YS, Denz D, Belt R: High-average-power intracavity second harmonic using $KT:OPO_4$ in an acouto optically Q-switched Nd:YAG laser oscillator at 5kHz. *Opt Lett* 1984: 9:76.
10. Fuller TA: Operating characteristics of surgical lasers and delivery systems, in Shapshay SM (ed): *Endoscopic Laser Surgery Handbook.* New York, Marcel Dekker, 1987, p 131.
11. MacDougall TW, Saunders PE, Maklad MS: Flexible $CO_2$ laser transmitting waveguide (Abstract 211). *Lasers Surg Med* 1988; 8(2):190.
12. Daikuzono N, Joffe SN: Artificial sapphire probe for contact photocoagulation and tissue vaporization with the Nd:YAG laser. *Med Instrum* 1985; 19:173–178.
13. Fisher JC: The power density of a surgical laser beam: Its meaning and measurement. *Lasers in Medicine and Surgery* 1988; 2:301–315.
14. Walsh JT, Follett S, Anderson RR, et al: Pulsed $CO_2$ laser tissue ablation: Effect of tissue type and pulse duration on thermal damage. *Lasers in Surgery and Medicine* 1988; 8(2):108–117.
15. Daniell JF, Miller W, Tosh R: Initial evaluation of the use of the potassium-titanyl-phosphate (KTP/532) laser in gynecologic laparoscopy. *Fertil Steril* 1986; 46(3):373–377.
16. Keye WR, Matson GA, Dixon J: The use of the argon laser in the treatment of experimental endometriosis. *Fertil Steril* 1983; 39:26.
17. Dougherty TJ, Kaufman JE, Goldfarb A, et al: Photoradiation therapy for the treatment of malignant tumors. *Cancer Research* 1978; 38:2628–2635.
18. Berns MW, Wilson M, Rentzepis P, et al: Cell biology of hematoporphyrin derivative (HPD). *Lasers Surg Med* 1983; 2:261.
19. Wilson BC, Patterson MS: The physics of photodynamic therapy. *Phys Med Biol* 1986; 31(4):327–360.
20. Ward BG, Forbes IJ, Cowled PA, et al: The treatment of vaginal recurrences of gynecologic

malignancy with phototherapy following hematoporphyrin derivative treatment. *Am J Obstet Gynecol* 1982; 142(3):356–357.

21. Goldrath MH, Fuller TA, Segal S: Laser photo-vaporization of the endometrium for the treatment of menorrhagia. *Am J Obstet Gynecol* 1981; 140:14–19.
22. Wright VC, Riopelle MA: *Gynecologic Laser Surgery: A Practical Handbook*. Houston, Biomedical Communications, 1982.
23. Baggish MS (ed): *Basic and Advanced Laser Surgery in Gynecology*. Norwalk, Conn, Appleton-Century-Crofts, 1985.

Chapter 3

# Laser Safety

Dan C. Martin, M.D.

Like any surgical instrument, a laser must be used with skill, discretion, and common sense. Although improved techniques and equipment can help decrease complications, these may also result in a rapid expansion in the types of techniques and the numbers of physicians using them. It is essential this expansion be associated with an emphasis on safety. Moreover, growing confidence and expertise with the new equipment should not lead to a relaxation of safeguards.

Lasers have been used with excellent clinical results but have also been associated with skin rashes, skin burns, retinal swelling, pneumothorax, ocular hemorrhage, emergent laparotomies, colostomies, pulmonary explosions, blindness, and death.[1–4] This chapter is for the practicing gynecologic surgeon who wishes to avoid these complications. For more comprehensive information, particularly for those physicians responsible for safety, texts on safety are available and are listed among the references of this chapter.

## SOME BASIC SAFETY CONCERNS

### Education and Credentialing

An adequate education is the single greatest factor in the development of surgical judgement and technique.[5] Education is needed for any type of surgery. Education and understanding are even more important with highly technical equipment. The use of lasers may be learned from a combination of gynecologic laser courses and laser preceptorships. Practice on surgical or other specimens in the operating room or laboratory is essential. One advantage of practice in the hospital operating room is that the surgeon can use the equipment in a familiar setting.

Education and credentialing in surgery are a responsibility for hospitals, surgical centers, and other controlling groups. In general, privileges are granted in specific areas (e.g., external genital, intra-abdominal, laparoscopic, or hysteroscopic) for a specific laser. This occurs after a specified combination of education prerequisites which often include a two-day, hands-on course and operating room exposure to three to ten cases as an observer or precepted surgeon. Guidelines for credentialing and course content are found in Appendices C and D of "American National Standard for the Safe Use of Lasers in Health Care Facilities" (ANSI Z136.3-1988).[6] This publication is useful to all involved in credentialing, education, and safety.

Currently, no minimum standards for laser education have been drawn up, but months of work are needed to achieve competence. While learning progresses, surgeons should anticipate that they will be better surgeons with the older techniques than with the newer laser techniques. During this learning time, physicians should be prepared to return to the older techniques when these appear to be better for the patients.

## ANSI Standards for the Operating Room

The American National Standards Institute (ANSI) uses industry volunteers to establish consensus standards in various fields. What standards there are for the use of lasers have been used by the Occupational Safety and Health Administration (OSHA) as the basis for issuing laser safety violations.[7] The following ANSI Z136.1 standards for the use of class IV lasers are adapted from "American National Standard for the Safe Use of Lasers" (ANSI Z136.1-1986).[8]

I. Direct supervision is required by an individual knowledgeable in laser technology and safety.
II. Location is such that access to the area by spectators requires approval.
III. Appropriate warning signs are posted:
   a. The word "DANGER" should be on all signs and labels associated with the laser system.
   b. In addition, a sign such as "Laser Radiation: Avoid eye or skin exposure to direct or scattered radiation" should be prominently displayed.
   c. When using infrared wavelengths that cannot be seen, the word "Invisible" should be included in the warning sign.
IV. Any potentially hazardous beam should be terminated in a beam stop of an appropriate material that is highly absorbent, nonreflecting, and fire resistant.
V. Use only diffusely reflective materials, such as dull-surfaced instruments, in or near the beam path when feasible.
VI. Use safety latches or interlocks to prevent unexpected entry of personnel into laser-controlled areas.
VII. Cover or restrict all windows in areas with levels above the ocular maximum permissible exposure.

## Equipment Hazards

The mechanical shutters of lasers are kept closed until the laser is ready for use. When the laser is in use, the shutter of the aiming beam is kept open at all times. With the $CO_2$ laser, closure of the aiming beam shutter does not mean that the laser operating beam shutter is closed. Even though the helium:neon beam is not visible, the $CO_2$ beam can still be activated and will function.

Room lights should be positioned so that they will not interfere with the motion of a rigid laser arm. Interference has the potential for damaging either the laser arm mirrors or the room light. This damage could interfere with the proper function of the unit or contaminate the operative field.

The counterbalanced articulated arm of the laser is potentially a source of trauma for the surgeon. These arms are frequently at head height and have been responsible for superficial head lacerations. Fiber-equipped lasers avoid this problem.

The knuckles of the laser-articulated arm must be kept tight. When these knuckles are loose, the laser may become erratic in its motion across the target surface and loss of control may result. A stockinette drape can be applied to the laser attachment arm when draping is needed for sterility. This can be held in place with rubber bands attached to the various points on the laparoscope and the knuckles can be tightened through the drape, if necessary.

Pedals for the laser and for any auxiliary equipment (such as microscopes or cautery) should be on different sides of the surgical table to prevent unintended activation of the laser. The surgeon should avoid the use of any other pedals unless absolutely necessary.

## Electrical Hazards

There is a potential danger from the high power densities inside the main power box of the laser. Voltages in this box may exceed 15,000 V and can cause pain, burns, ventricular fibrillation, and death.[2] Because these high voltages are stored and present even after the equipment is unplugged,[9,10] panels protecting this area should be removed only by a skilled technician.

## Surgical Drapes

Surgical drapes should be fire retardant and, when feasible, should be wet. Ignition of these drapes can result in burns to the patient, surgeon, or other personnel. These drapes can be ignited by the laser, by cautery, or by high-intensity photographic lights.[9, 11, 12]

## Anesthetic and Cleaning Agents

Alcohol, ether, and combustible anesthetic gases should not be used in association with the laser. These materials may be ignited and can cause burns. A fire extinguisher should be kept in the room or nearby, with the location known to operating room personnel.

Care must also be taken in the choice of the cleaning solutions used on both the patient and the laser, and these solutions must be thoroughly rinsed off after use. Vaporization of the solutions creates a plume containing the chemical remnants from the solution. The plume from chlorhexidine (Hibiclens) has caused dermal rash in both a surgeon and a nursing assistant when vaporized with the laser.[1, 10]

## Protective Eyewear and Optical Filters

Because the eye is the most delicate organ commonly exposed to laser injury, all personnel should wear protective eyewear with side panels that are appropriate for the laser in use. For non-laser light sources, the blink reflex and the eye's normal aversion response to high brightness (0.25 seconds) protect the eyes. However, laser energy is so intense that protective eyewear is needed.[13] The level of protection needed is related to the applicable maximum permissible exposure (MPE) and the boundaries of the nominal hazard zone (NHZ). For laser use with lenses in place, the NHZ is 2.37 m for the $CO_2$ laser, 6.37 m for a continuous wave Nd:YAG laser, and 33.6 m for helium neon, argon, KTP or other visible lasers.[6]

The glasses and other filter devices for a specific laser are usually available from the manufacturer of the laser. Information regarding the wavelength, optical density, and safety applications should accompany the glasses.[6] Unfortunately, these glasses or goggles may reduce the quality and quantity of the field of vision, alter color vision, or make the laser beam invisible; however, do not interchange these glasses. An adequate optical density to protect the operating room personnel and patient from accidental exposure should be balanced against the need for adequate visualization for effective surgery.

Energy from the $CO_2$ laser is absorbed in the cornea and can cause denaturation and coagulation of the proteins in the epithelial layers of the cornea, resulting in corneal opacification; fiber-transmitted lasers generally focus on the retina (Fig 3–1). In addition, when using the clear glass for a $CO_2$ laser, the helium:neon laser can be transmitted to and focused on the retina. It is possible that 10 seconds of focused helium:neon laser exposure will damage the retina.[11] The MPE for visible lasers is less than 0.003 watts/cm$^2$ for a 0.25 second (aversion response time) exposure.[6] Although the lenses of the microscope or endoscope are sufficient to protect the eyes from a $CO_2$ laser, the Nd:YAG, KTP:532, and argon lasers can be scattered and transmitted back through lens systems or fiberoptics.[6, 14–16] Specific filters are needed to protect the surgeon's eyes from this hazard.[17] These filters take the form of glasses, lens caps, and interlocking shutters. The effect of scatter can also be decreased by using sapphire tips with the Nd:YAG laser.[18]

## Parfocus

The microscope should be parfocused prior to attachment of the laser to the microscope. Parfocus is performed by focusing the microscope head distance at the highest

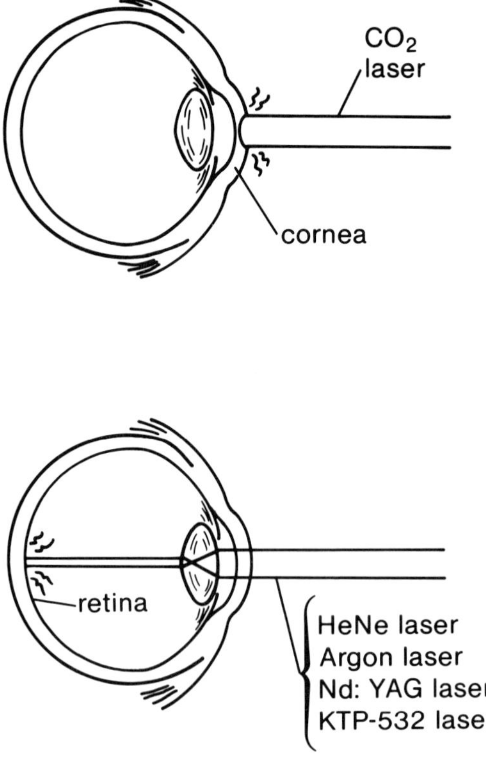


**FIG 3–1.**
Eye damage can occur with any type of laser. In general, the $CO_2$ laser will damage the cornea while the other lasers will damage the retina. (From Martin DC (ed): *Intra-abdominal Laser Surgery*, ed 2, in preparation. Used by permission.)

power and the eyepieces at the lowest power. This series may need to be repeated. When parfocusing is completed, it should be possible to move through the powers of the microscope without changing the distance of the microscope head to the target. If it is necessary to change the focus of the laser when the powers are changed, the microscope is not parfocused. This may result in inadvertent changes of the power density and spot size. Changing the power density and spot size will alter the tissue effect and could potentially compromise the intent of the surgery.

## Pulmonary Hazards

Adequate suction must be available to collect all the carbon plume from the operating field to prevent the plume from being inhaled by operating room personnel. Most of this carbon plume, particularly those particles less than 1.1 micron in diameter, would be deposited in the alveoli after it enters the lungs. Early studies demonstrated that 3% of particles were greater than or equal to 9 microns while 77% were less than or equal to 1.1 microns.[19] More recent studies at greater than or equal to 6,000 watts/cm$^2$ have a particulate distribution of 0.1 microns to 0.8 microns.[20] Although less mutagenic than smoke from an electrical coagulator,[21] this material has been shown to be mutagenic in *Salmonella typhimurium* (Ames Test)[19] and is similar to cigarette or other particulate smoke.[22]

Intact viral DNA of papillomavirus has been confirmed in the vapor of laser-treated verrucae.[23] Although the viral particles of this study were not shown to be viable, the potential infective nature remains. Furthermore, plume from a pulsed laser contains viable cells.[24] This contrasts with other studies showing that the smoke plume from malignant tissue vaporized by a continuous $CO_2$ laser does not contain viable cells.[25, 26] In addition, there appears to be additional protection from the human immunodeficiency virus (HIV) and hepatitis virus due to their fragile nature. HIV is inactivated at 57°C and may be destroyed due to exposure to the 100°C heat of vaporization of water.[27]

The suction line has a filter within it to prevent the carbon from entering and damaging the hospital vacuum system. The filter must be changed after each operation and may have to be changed more often if it becomes obstructed during long procedures. In addition, standard filters may not be adequate for 0.1-micrometer particles[28] and standard masks are inadequate[20] and may be limited to particles greater than or equal to 0.3 microns. Positioning the suction is important. Suctioning at less than or equal to 1 cm removes 98.6% of all particles while suctioning at 2 cm removes only 50.7% of particulate matter.[19]

## Carcinogenic Potential

There has been no increase in carcinogenic potential or atypical changes demonstrated in tissue remaining after use of the $CO_2$ laser.[3, 29, 30] Furthermore, there have been no reports of carcinogenicity of similar carbonized material left after cautery.

## Protection of Surgeons' Hands

The microscope gives the greatest control over the beam and has the least potential for inadvertent misdirection. It has, however, been responsible for the most damage to surgeons' hands. This has most commonly occurred in workshops by trained microsurgeons who roll their hands through the operating field while doing microsurgery. Because of the long depth of field, the invisible beam can easily cut when hands are allowed to wander through this field. The concept of no-touch surgery must be mastered to use the microscope effectively.[31]

## CLINICAL USE IN GYNECOLOGY

### External Genitalia

General anesthesia should be considered for most laser surgery of the external genitalia, for unexpected motion by the patient has caused laser lacerations.[1] Vulvar surgery should be performed with protection of the vagina and rectum by moist sponges soaked in saline and packed into these areas. These moist sponges will prevent penetration of the laser. When possible, all other healthy tissue should be covered with soaked sponges. With respect to the concern about igniting methane gas, preoperative laxatives may help evacuate the lower bowel and decrease the amount of gas.[11]

### Intra-abdominal Procedures

Gynecologists accustomed to a large margin of safety in the use of lasers for external use will need to reorient themselves to the decreased margin in the abdomen. This is particularly true of the use of hand-held attachments with their increased mobility. The freehand attachment should be kept on a wet towel when it is not actively in use.

Backstops are frequently used to prevent the penetration of the $CO_2$ laser beam (Fig 3–2). These are generally metal rods, soaked sponges, or water solutions. Pyrex, quartz, and glass rods have fractured under the rapid heating produced by the laser and are currently avoided. Etched metal rods will cause some reflection of the beam and should not be used in the immediate vicinity of such delicate tissue as the small bowel, where reflection may cause damage. The depth of penetration can also be limited by using pulse and superpulse settings of the laser. Fiber-directed lasers have an intrinsic limitation on their effective zone of vaporization and coagulation (Fig 3–3). This limitation provides protection to organs outside the coagulation zone. On the other hand, if the fiber is moved away from the tissue during vaporization, then unintended coagulation can occur.

When mirrors are used for redirecting the beam inside the abdomen, they should be used with great care. The mirror should be polished metal; even high quality, front-surfaced glass mirrors have been vaporized with high power densities. Special attention should be taken to distinguish the perpendicular reflected operating beam from a tangential beam image in the mirror. A tangential beam and a perpendicular beam have a similar appearance in the mirror but cut in different directions.

Other instruments such as retractors, scissors, clamps, needle holders, and forceps should be etched or blackened. This will decrease the chance of unintended reflection of the beam.

### Laparoscopy

Laparoscopy with the laser is the most time-consuming technique to learn, even when the surgeon has extended experience in intra-abdominal laser surgery. In addition, there must be a high degree of coordination between the surgeon and the laser panel operator so that the laser will be on standby when not being actively used inside the pelvic cavity. Therefore, laser laparoscopy should be performed only by a surgical team experienced in surgical laparoscopy and in the use of the laser at laparotomy.

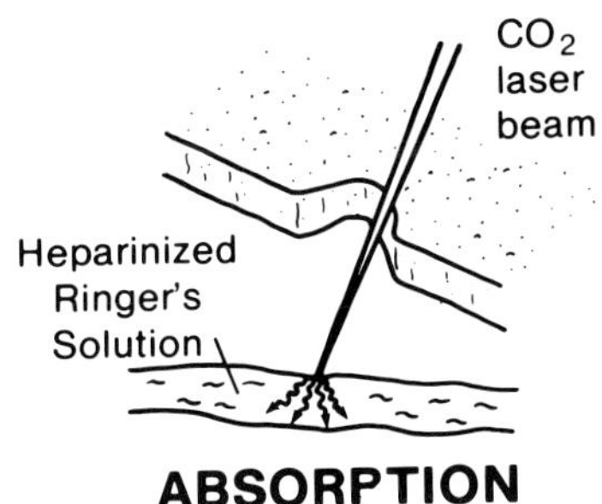


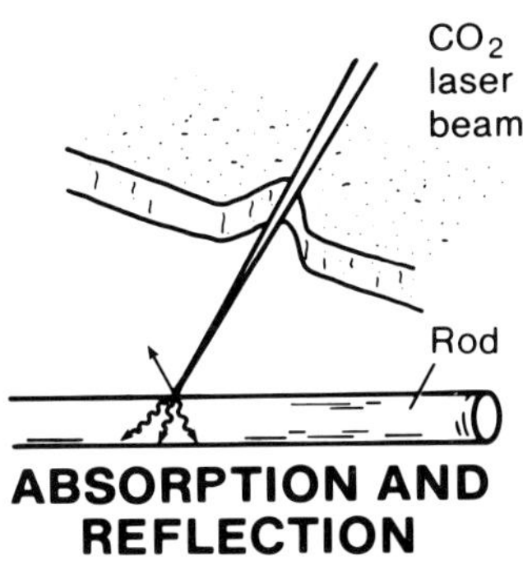


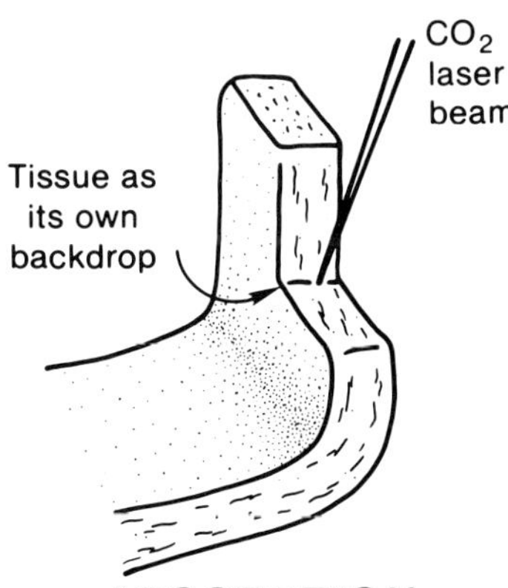


**FIG 3–2.**
The $CO_2$ laser is generally stopped with solutions, rods, or the tissue itself. Solutions and tissue absorb the beam in its entirety. Rods both absorb and reflect the beam. (From Martin DC (ed): *Intra-abdominal Laser Surgery,* ed 2, in preparation. Used by permission.)

Insufflation is maintained to assure adequate visualization. If there is any question of loss of visualization, the laser should be placed on standby while insufflation is reinstituted.

Currently, recirculating insufflators are available that maintain a constant pressure. In addition, the carbon plume is constantly being filtered. This increases the safety by maintaining a constant field of vision and decreases time clearing out the smoke plume. In addition, these insufflators can refill at 4 liters per minute when needed.

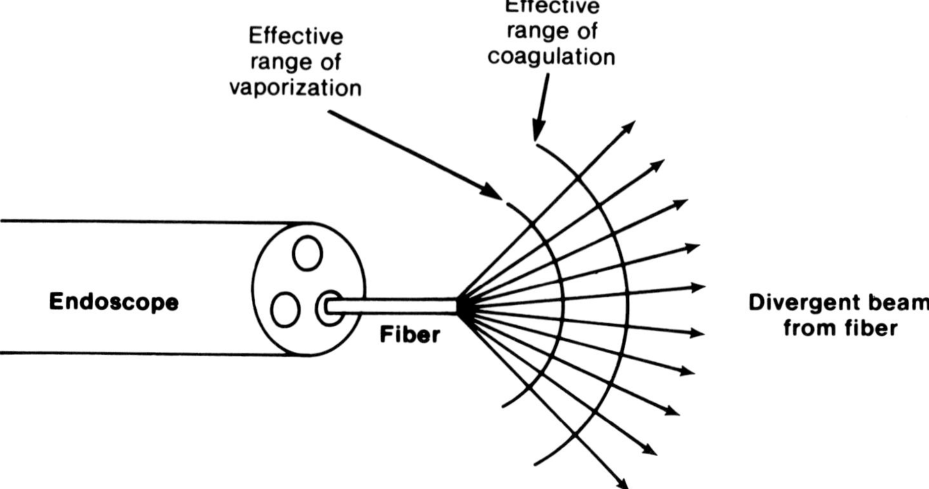


**FIG 3–3.**
Fiber-directed lasers diverge rapidly from the end of the fiber. With a high-enough power density, the initial zone is vaporization. At a distance from this is coagulation and past this point there is only heating. (From Martin DC (ed): *Intra-abdominal Laser Surgery,* ed 2, in preparation. Used by permission.)

The complications reported at laparoscopy have been those of operative laparoscopy in general and have included such minor problems as losing sponges in the abdomen, transient hypothermia, dissecting emphysema, and ileus. In addition, hemorrhage requiring transfusion and laparotomy has occurred, as has laparotomy for colostomy due to a bowel laceration. At least one death has been associated with cardiac arrest in the operating room.[3] The electrocardiogram is closely monitored to watch for cardiac arrhythmia secondary to a rise in $pCO_2$.[32] This rise may occur as a result of the use of 20 to 40 L of carbon dioxide gas for insufflation and smoke evacuation during laser laparoscopy. This amount of gas is used because it is necessary to replace the carbon dioxide within the abdomen continually.

The depth of coagulation or vaporization for a specific laser setting can vary, depending upon the alignment of the beam and the output of the machine. If biologic testing of the power density is needed, the peritoneal surface of the uterosacral ligament gives a reasonable test site. The ureter should be identified through the peritoneum, however, before vaporizing the uterosacral ligament.

When working in the upper pelvis, it is necessary to keep the deep pelvis flooded with a solution such as Ringer's. This flooding will protect the deep pelvic organs and the bowel. The potential for significant gastrointestinal complications, including peritonitis, colostomy, and death, exists in a fashion similar to that of cautery.[33] A generally minor concern of using flooding is the spill into the upper abdomen with volumes of 20 to 80 cc with the patient in modified Trendelenburg position (Fig 3–4). In the presence of infection or a spilled dermoid cyst, reverse modified Trendelenburg position is used, along with controlling the volume of irrigant in the pelvis. Constant irrigation and aspiration systems can be used to avoid the accumulation of irrigant when desirable.

Bleeding that cannot be controlled with the laser may occur.[1] Bipolar coagulation and knowledge of its use in these situations is needed. Laparotomy may be necessary, as with bleeding at any laparoscopy.

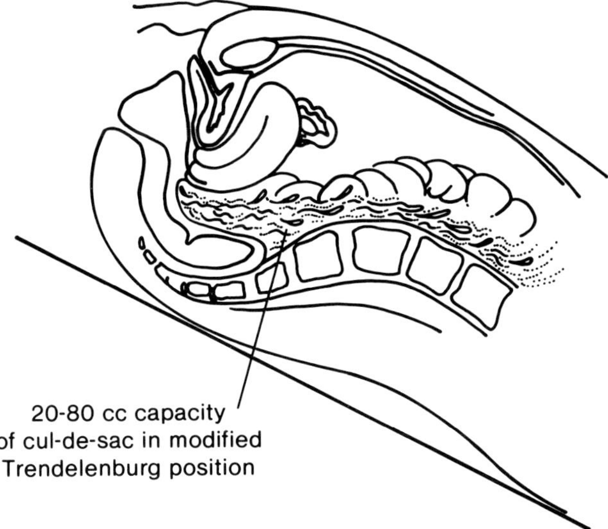


**FIG 3–4.**
In modified Trendelenburg position, the capacity of the cul-de-sac is around 20 to 80 cc. If the pelvis is contaminated by opening an abscess or dermoid, the tilt must be reversed so that the contents do not spill into the upper abdomen. (From Martin DC (ed): *Intra-abdominal Laser Surgery*, ed 2, in preparation. Used by permission.)

### Photovaporization of the Endometrium

The Nd:YAG laser has been used in a slow and studied fashion to systematically ablate the endometrial cavity and to incise adhesions and septa. Hypervolemic congestive heart failure is the most common worry in cardiac patients. This is similar to the problems associated with transurethral resection of the prostate and is accentuated by procedures lasting more than one hour. Careful monitoring of fluids is needed to avoid this.[34, 35] In addition, no-touch techniques of endometrial ablation decrease the disruption of the endometrial surface and decrease the potential for intravasation.[36] Also, current hysteroscopes are designed to decrease the time of surgery and to decrease the fluid load.[37] However, noncardiogenic pulmonary edema has also been associated with hysteroscopy when performed with 32% dextran 70 (Hyskon).[38]

Also, the potential for perforation of the uterus and bowel exists. Damage in this case can be the same as discussed in the previous section on laparoscopy.

## SUMMARY

Laser surgery has been performed for more than 15 years with an excellent safety record. In gynecology, morbidity has been low and fatalities rare. With proper education and preparation, this record of safety can be maintained in the future.

## REFERENCES

1. Baggish MS: Complications associated with carbon dioxide laser surgery in gynecology. *Am J Obstet Gynecol* 1981; 139:568–574.

2. Rogers P, Schellhas HF, Moss E: Hazards associated with the use of surgical lasers, in Rockwell J (ed): *Laser Safety in Surgery and Medicine* ed 4. Cincinnatti, Rockwell Associates, 1983, pp 61–81.
3. Martin DC, Diamond MP: Operative laparoscopy: Comparison of lasers with other techniques. *Curr Probbl Obstet Gynecol Fertil* 1986; 9:563–617.
4. Wulwick R, Brenner SH: Pneumothorax in association with laseroscopy. *Colpos Gynecol Laser Surg* 1987; 3:221–223.
5. TeLinde RW: Foreword, in Ridley JH (ed): *Gynecologic Surgery - Errors, Safeguards, Salvage.* Baltimore, Williams & Wilkins, 1981, p ix.
6. American National Standards Institute, Inc: *American National Standard for the Safe Use of Lasers in Health Care Facilities.* (ANSI Z136.3–1988) New York, American National Standards Institute, Inc, 1988.
7. Rockwell RJ: Laser safety and training: Reviewing risks and safety protocols, in Breedlove B and Schwartz D (eds): *Clinical Lasers: Expert Strategies for Practical and Profitable Management.* Atlanta, American Health Consultants, Inc, 1985, pp 39–56.
8. American National Standards Institute, Inc. *American National Standard for the Safe Use of Lasers.* (ANSI Z136.1–1986) New York, American National Standards Institute, Inc, 1986.
9. Schellhas HF: Safety aspects for carbon dioxide laser surgery, in Bellina JH (ed): *Gynecologic Laser Surgery.* New York, Plenum Press, 1981, pp 95–102.
10. Tsuzuki M: System approach for safety assurance in laser surgery, in Atsumi K, Nimsakul N (eds): *Proceedings of the Fourth Congress of the International Society for Laser Surgery.* Tokyo, Japanese Society for Laser Medicine, 1981, 2:16–17.
11. Fisher JC: $CO_2$ lasers for gynecologic surgery, how safe are they? *Contemp Ob/Gyn* 1983; 21:39–54.
12. Patel KF, Hicks JN: Prevention of fire hazards associated with the use of carbon dioxide laser. *Anesth Analg* 1981; 60:885–888.
13. Sliney D, Wolbarsht M: *Safety With Lasers and Other Optical Sources.* New York, Plenum Press, 1980.
14. Frank F, Halldorsson T, Manhart S, et al: Laser safety aspects for various Neodymium YAG laser applications, in Atsumi K, Nimsakul N (eds): *Proceedings of the Fourth Congress of the International Society for Laser Surgery.* Tokyo, Japanese Society for Laser Medicine, 1981, 2:12.
15. Kato K, Nagasawa A, Nishikawa K, et al.: Thermal changes of soft tissue with irradiation by $CO_2$, YAG and argon lasers, in Atsumi K, Nimsakul N (eds): *Proceedings of the Fourth Congress of the International Society for Laser Surgery.* Tokyo, Japanese Society for Laser Medicine, 1981, 22:17–20.
16. Konichi T, Iwasaki M, Sasako M, et al: Fundamental experiment on endoscopic laser photocoagulation, in Atsumi K, Nimsakul N (eds): *Proceedings of the Fourth Congress of the International Society for Laser Surgery.* Tokyo, Japanese Society for Laser Medicine, 1981, 5:1–4.
17. Gulacsik C, Auth DC, Silverstein FE: Ophthalmic hazards associated with laser endoscopy. *Applied Optics* 1979; 18:1816–1823.
18. Joffe SN, Schroder T: Lasers in general surgery. *Adv Surg* 1987; 20:125–154.
19. Mihashi S, Ueda S, Hirano M, et al: Some problems about condensates induced by $CO_2$ laser irradiation, in Atsumi K, Nimsakul N (eds): *Proceedings of the Fourth Congress of the International Society for Laser Surgery.* Tokyo, Japanese Society for Laser Medicine, 1981, 2:25–27.
20. Nezhat C, Winer WK, Nezhat F, et al: Smoke from laser surgery: Is there a health hazard? *Lasers Surg Med* 1987; 7:376–382.
21. Tomita Y, Mihashi S, Nagata K, et al: Mutagenicity of smoke condensates induced by $CO_2$ laser irradiation and electrocauterization. *Mutat Res* 1981; 89:145–149.
22. Baggish MS, Elbakry M: The effects of laser smoke on the lungs of rats. *Am J Obstet Gynecol* 1987; 1260–1265.
23. Garden JM, O'Banion MK, Shelnitz LS, et al: Papillomavirus in the vapor of carbon dioxide laser-treated verrucae. *JAMA* 1988; 259:1199–1202.

24. Hoye RC, Ketcham AS, Riggle GC: The airborne dissemination of viable tumor by high energy Neodymium laser. *Life Sci* 1967; 6:119.
25. Bellina JH, Sterjernholm RL, Kurpel JE: Analysis of plume emissions after papovavirus irradiation with carbon dioxide laser. *J Reprod Med* 1982; 27:268–270.
26. Mihashi S, Jako GJ, Nicze J, et al: Laser surgery in otolaryngology: Interaction of $CO_2$ laser in soft tissue. *Annals NY Acad Sci* 1976; 267:263–294.
27. Jako GJ: $CO_2$ laser in surgery for prophylaxis of HIV infection. (Letter to the Editor) *Lasers Surg Med* 1988; 8:139.
28. Baggish MS, Baltoyannis P, Sze E: Protection of the rat lung from the harmful effects of laser smoke. *Lasers Surg Med* 1988; 8:248–253.
29. Apfelberg DB, Mittelman H, Chabi B: Carcinogenic potential of in vitro carbon dioxide laser exposure of fibroblasts. *Obstet Gynecol* 1983; 61:403–496.
30. Martin DC, Hubert GD, VanderZwaag R, et al: Laparoscopic appearances of peritoneal endometriosis. *Fertil Steril* 1989; 51:63–67.
31. Daniell JF: $CO_2$ laser in infertility surgery. *J Reprod Med* 1983; 28:265–268.
32. Lim HS: Prevention and management of local and general anesthesia complications, in Hulka JF (ed): *1977 AAGL Complications Committee Report: The Prevention and Management of Laparoscopic Complications*. Irvine, Calif, American Association of Gynecologic Laparoscopists, 1977, pp 5–6.
33. Wheeless CR: Gastrointestinal injuries associated with laparoscopy, in Hulka JF (ed): *1977 AAGL Complications Committee Report: The Prevention and Management of Laparoscopic Complications*. Irvine, Calif, American Association of Gynecologic Laparoscopists, 1977, pp 16–19.
34. Goldrath MH, Fuller TA, Segal S: Laser photovaporization of endometrium for the treatment of menorrhagia. *Am J Obstet Gynecol* 1981; 140:18–19.
35. Lomano JM: Photocoagulation of the endometrium with the Nd:YAG laser for the treatment of menorrhagia. *J Reprod Med* 1986; 31:148–150.
36. Loffer FD: Hysteroscopic endometrial ablation with the Nd:YAG laser using a non-touch technique. *Obstet Gynecol* 1987; 69:679–682.
37. Baggish MS: New laser hysteroscope for neodymium YAG endometrial ablation. *Lasers Surg Med* 1988; 8:99–103.
38. Leake JF, Murphy AA, Zacur HA: Noncardiogenic pulmonary edema: A complication of operative hysteroscopy. *Fertil Steril* 1987; 48:497–499.

Chapter 4

# Human Papillomavirus-Associated Diseases of the Lower Genital Tract: Implications for the Laser Surgeon*

Richard Reid, M.D.

Human papillomaviruses (HPV) have been the Cinderella of medical research. Genital warts were recognized as having a venereal etiology by the ancient Greeks, yet condylomas received negligible medical attention for the next 2000 years. Papillomaviruses were experimentally transmitted at the turn of the century by vaccinating volunteers with cell-free extracts from human skin warts and genital condylomas.[1] Even though the principles of tumor virology were formulated during the 1930s by the experimental induction of squamous carcinomas with cottontail rabbit papillomaviruses,[2, 3] HPV remained unstudied for the next 80 years. With the wisdom of hindsight, this lack of scientific interest in HPV is astounding, especially since condylomas and flat skin warts are the only viral lesions that have been regularly reported to undergo malignant transformation in humans.

In 1974, zur Hausen nominated the human papillomavirus as a likely candidate for the role of a sexually transmitted carcinogen;[4] however, since papillomaviruses could not be propagated in cell culture, basic scientists of the day had no tools with which to study this hypothesis. Following the realization that most gynecologic HPV infections were subclinical, presenting as abnormal Papanicolaou smears rather than as patient-recognized warts,[5–7] interest among clinicians and pathologists was rekindled in the mid-1970s. In 1983, a matched, double-blind study showed that koilocytotic atypia were detectable at the margin of 95% of Wertheim hysterectomy specimens, as compared to 12.5% of hysterectomies performed for ovarian or endometrial carcinoma;[8] however, early attempts to detect HPV DNA within the cervical tumors by high stringency hybridization with existing HPV probes were negative.

The major advance came in 1974, when Durst et al., probed a bank of cervical cancer biopsies at *low* stringency and was fortunate enough to detect an unusually strong signal from a novel HPV DNA within one of these cancers.[9] This signal was subsequently ex-

*Portions of this chapter have been reproduced with permission from Reid R (ed): *Obstetrics and Gynecology Clinics of North America*. Philadelphia, WB Saunders Co, 1987.

tracted, cloned, verified as a papillomavirus, and then used as a radiolabeled probe. Hybridization with this new probe (now designated HPV-16) detected an identical signal within almost two-thirds of these cervical cancer specimens. Subsequent cloning of HPVs 18, 31, 33, 35, 39, 45, 51, 52, and 56 have increased the cumulative detection rates for high-rise HPV types to 90% or more.[10, 11]

Throughout the occidental world, there has been a significant increase in the occurrence of HPV-associated genital malignancies[12, 13] and the modal age at diagnosis has fallen by 1 to 2 decades.[14, 15] Hence, as the biological principles are becoming better understood, the therapeutic approach to sexually transmitted HPV infections is changing.

## BASIC VIROLOGY OF THE PAPILLOMAVIRUSES

### Taxonomy

Papillomaviruses are small, double-stranded DNA viruses. Because of superficial similarities in electronmicroscopic appearance and biologic properties, papillomaviruses were originally classified within the same family as polyomaviruses, this group being termed papovaviruses. However, papillomaviruses (genus A) have a larger chromosome (7,900 versus 5,200 base pairs), a larger virion capsid (55 versus 44 um), and a completely different genomic organiation.[16] For this reason, it is best to regard papillomaviruses as a distinct and unique family.

In reality, papillomaviruses represent a divergent group of evolutionarily related viruses that manifest qualitatively similar biological characteristics. All papillomaviruses exhibit a similar pattern of genetic organization, in that sequencing of the different types has shown preservation of broadly equivalent areas of protein coding potential (known as open reading frames or ORFs). But the actual nucleotide sequences within these ORFs are widely disparate,[16, 17] so that individual papillomaviruses show enormous differences in species specificity, site of predilection, and degree of oncogenicity.

Papillomaviruses are named according to species and subclassified into types according to nucleotide sequence. Within the same species, any new isolate that exhibits less than 50% homology with existing members (by solution hybridization) is designated as a new type and numbered in order of discovery. Human papillomaviruses comprise the largest group, with more than 60 known types. Other members of scientific importance include the cottontail rabbit, bovine, canine, ovine, equine, elk, and mastomys papillomaviridae.

### Virion Structure

Papillomavirus particles, whether isolated from infected rabbits, cattle, or humans, are remarkably similar in overall appearance. Virions consist of a central core of viral DNA enclosed within an outer capsid of viral protein. The viral capsid is composed of 72 subunits (capsomeres, which are arranged in a symmetrical, 20-sided (icosahedral) pattern that gives the individual virion an almost spherical shape on electronmicroscopy. The virion does not have an outer membrane such as is found in some other viruses (for example, human immunodeficiency virus). This fact may account for the low antigenicity of papillomavirus infections.

Biochemical analysis of the viral capsid has revealed two different families of structural protein: a major protein (molecular weight 54,000 daltons) and a minor protein (molecular weight 76,000 daltons).

## DNA Organization

All papillomavirus chromosomes are covalently closed, circular, double-stranded DNA molecules with a molecular length of about 7,900 base pairs and a molecular weight of about 5.2 × 16 daltons (about half a million times smaller than the genome of a human cell). Whether isolated from disrupted virions or extracted from transformed cells, the viral DNA is combined with histones (derived from the cellular pool of the natural host) to form a small chromosome.[16] Thus, viral DNA constitutes only 12% of the virion by weight.

When the nuclear proteins are stripped away, the viral DNA assumes a super-coiled shape (form I). Super-coiling is visible on electronmicroscopy and is also detectable at electrophoresis because of the relatively rapid mobility of these tight circular molecules. Cleavage of only one DNA strand by bacterial enzymes (restriction endonucleases) results in a relaxed circle (form II), while cleavage of both strands at a single site produces a linear molecule that migrates more slowly in electrophoresis gels (form III).

## Viral Genetic Function

As previously mentioned, alignment of sequenced papillomavirus DNAs revealed a highly conserved pattern of protein coding potential—the open reading frames (ORFs). In essence, each of these ORFs represents a viral gene. Virus-specified proteins apparently determine such characteristics as host range, tissue tropism, and the clinicopathologic consequences of infection.

Studies of the nonproductive interaction between bovine papillomaviruses and mouse fibroblasts have shown that the viral genome can be subdivided into three functional portions. Although it has not been experimentally demonstrated that the same relationship holds for HPV infection of epithelial cells, it is still valuable to examine human disease in relationship to this model (reviewed in references 16 and 17).

**The Upstream Regulatory Region.**—The upstream regulatory region (URR) is a non-coding segment, representing about 15% of the viral genome. This region contains the origin of DNA replication, several promoters (sequences needed to initiate viral RNA synthesis), and several enhancers (sequences that increase the rate of RNA transcription).

**The E (Early) Region.**—The E region is the longest segment, representing about 45% of the viral genome. This region contains at least six ORFs that code for proteins; these either induce cell transformation or control viral DNA replication. Individual ORFs are named according to their relative size. Therefore, the number assigned to a particular ORF bears no relationship to its actual location within the viral genome.

Functions of individual ORFs are as follows:

1. **E1, 2,** and **5** ORFs are primarily concerned with viral replication and with the maintenance of the episomal state.
2. **E6** and **7** ORFs appear to code for proteins involved in "malignant" transformation.
3. **E4** ORF produces several proteins that are found in relative abundance as parabasal cells differentiated into mature keratinocytes; it is thought that messages from this region might initiate the onset of koilocytotic changes.

**The L (Late) Region.**—The L region comprises about 40% of the viral genome and contains two ORFs that are essential to productive viral replication:

1. **L1** ORF encodes the major capsid protein (molecular weight 54,000 daltons). The L1 gene product is highly conserved among most animal and human papillomaviruses. Accordingly, antisera directed against disrupted, denatured HPV-1 capsid are used as cross-reactive, group-specific immunocytochemical reagents.[18] Unfortunately, only about 50% of genital condylomas produce detectable L1 protein, and this percentage declines with increasing degrees of neoplasia.[19, 20]
2. **L2** ORF encodes the minor capsid protein (molecular weight 76,000 daltons). The minor capsid protein is highly type-specific. For this reason, L2 proteins might serve as distinguishing targets for immunocytochemical typing of infected tissues. Within the intact virion capsid, however, type-specific epitopes of the L2 protein are shielded and probably could not form the basis for a vaccine.[21]

## CLINICAL GROUPS OF HUMAN PAPILLOMAVIRUSES

From the viewpoint of biologic properties, human papillomaviruses comprise three clinicopathologic groups: cutaneotropic viruses found in immunologically normal individuals, cutaneotropic viruses found in immunosuppressed patients, and mucosotropic viruses infecting the genital, oral, and respiratory mucosae.

### Cutaneous HPVs in the Immunocompetent Population

Viruses in this group always produce reproductive infections that, by definition, can never be carcinogenic. Viral type correlates with lesion location, clinical features, and histologic appearance:[16, 17]

1. HPV 1 and 4 produce plantar warts, HPV 1 being found preferentially in deep, painful lesions and HPV 4 in more superficial varieties.
2. HPV 2 is found in the common warts (verrucae vulgaris) acquired by most of the population during childhood, causing very keratotic lesions that primarily affect the dorsal skin of the upper or lower limbs.
3. HPV 3 occurs in flat warts (seen as minimally elevated red patches on the hands and face).
4. HPV 7 produces common warts in meat and animal handlers.

Such site specificity probably reflects the fact that cellular susceptibility to HPV infection depends on the types of keratin it produces during terminal differentiation, for there is a relatively constant relationship between viral type and lesion morphology. Nonetheless, occasional exceptions occur, such as reports of HPV 1 or 4 on common warts, and HPV 2 in plantar and genital warts.

### HPVs Affecting the Anogenital and Aerodigestive Mucosae

About 15 of the known HPV types are mucosotropic, infecting either anogenital skin or mucous membranes.[10, 11] These viruses are also associated with specific disease patterns:

1. HPV 6 and 11 are primarily responsible for two types of disease: papillomas of the upper airways and benign exophytic condylomas affecting the external genitalia, the lower third of the vagina, and the anal canal. Detection of HPV 6 or 11 in minor lesions of the transformation zone has fostered a mistaken belief that these types account for the majority of minor cervical atypia. In fact, HPV 6 or 11 probably causes only about 15% of the "flat condylomas" or mild dysplasias.[22]

2. HPV 16 is the viral type detected with greatest frequency in high-grade intraepithelial neoplasias and invasive cancers. Nonetheless, HPV 16 is also found in at least 10% of minor-grade cervical lesions. Moreover, in a high-risk British population, HPV 16 also was found in 40% of the subclinical lesions on the vulva and penis and in up to 10% of the condylomata acuminata.

3. HPV 18 shows a bimodal distribution pattern, being present in about 15% of invasive cervical cancers (especially aggressive adenocarcinomas of young women) and about 5% of minor-grade genital lesions.[10, 23, 24] HPV 18 is, however, significantly underrepresented in patients with only cervical intraepithelial neoplasia, suggesting this virus may produce lesions that progress too rapidly to be easily detected by mass-screening programs.

4. HPV 31, 33, 35, 51, 52, and 56 exhibit intermediate oncogenicity, with a predilection for the squamous cells of the cervix or vagina. The "thirties" viruses are overrepresented in cervical intrepithelial neoplasia (about 30%) and underrepresented in cervical cancer (about 10%).[24]

5. HPV 42, 43, and 44 are more recently isolated, benign viruses that seem to have the same disease associations as HPVs 6 and 11.

6. HPV 39 and 45 are a pair of recently isolated, apparently oncogenic HPVs. Disease patterns associated with these novel types have not been fully defined. Therefore, for the present, these two viruses are probably best grouped as being of intermediate risk.

### Cutaneous HPVs in Immunosuppressed Individuals

Almost half of the currently known HPV types have been isolated from the skin of immunosuppressed individuals,[16] the main source being patients who suffer from a rare autosomal recessive disease termed epidermodysplasia verraciformis (EV). This disease is characterized by multiple flat warts of non-genital skin, generally affecting patients with congenital impairment of their cellular immunity (Fig 4–1,A).[25] Unlike other warts, these flat lesions do not regress. Rather, lesions persist for life, spreading over the entire body. Experience has shown that 25% to 33% of the affected individuals will develop skin cancer, usually within sunlight-exposed areas (Fig 4–1,B).[26] Lag time between the appearance of flat warts and progression to squamous carcinoma averages about 25 years. Similar HPV types have also been isolated from warts in patients taking immunosuppressive drugs and in skin cancers occurring in renal allograft recipients.[27] Although more than 35 different HPV types have been isolated from skin lesions in immunocompromised patients, HPVs 5 and 8 are detected in 90% of malignancies.

## STAGES IN THE NATURAL HISTORY OF HPV INFECTION

### Inoculation

During intercourse with an infected consort, inoculation occurs at sites of microtrauma.[21] HPV virions are thought to penetrate to the basal layer and then shed their outer

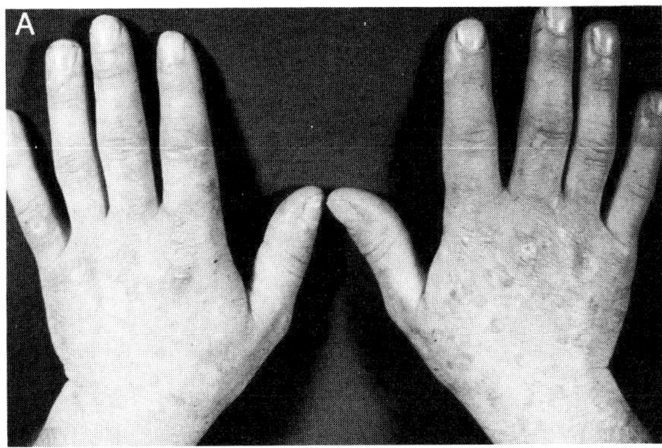


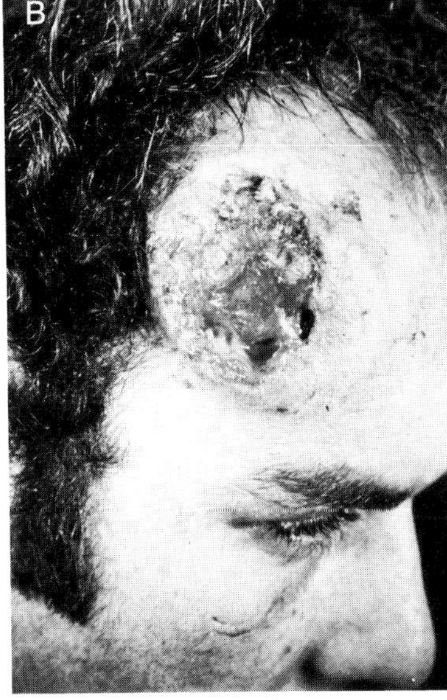


**FIG 4–1.**
**A,** multiple flat warts and reddish plaques on the hands and **B,** an ulcerated bowenoid carcinoma on the temporal area of a patient with epidermo-dysplasia verruciformis, who is infected with at least six HPV types. Only DNA of HPV 5 was detected in the cancer. From Nürnberger S, Pfister H: *Obstet Gynecol Clin North Am* 1987; 14:349–361. Used by permission.)

protein capsid. Somehow, the viral genome crosses the cell membrane and is then transported to the cell nucleus. Then the infecting genome is translated and transcribed, thereby producing various virus-specified proteins. Transforming proteins induce conductive host cell functions, while regulatory proteins control viral gene expression.

## Incubation Phase

Initially, the virus exists as a self-replicating extrachromosomal plasmid, termed an episome. Proteins specified by the early viral genes (especially E1, 2 and 5) result in an initial burst of episomal replications producing additional viral genomes, which will gradually transect neighboring cells. Because these episomal viral plasmids will replicate with each cell division, there is little dilution of viral copy numbers over the succeeding years. And, during an incubation period ranging from as little as 6 weeks to as long as 8 months, large areas of the anogenital epithelium are colonized by a "steady-state" latent HPV infection.[28]

## Active Expression Phase

Many exposed individuals will remain in long-term latent infection; however, in susceptible hosts, viral colonization can lead to active viral expression. Capture of the host cell results in pronounced alteration in cell growth in the basal layers, increased replication of the viral genome in the middle layers, and viral cytopathic effects in maturing cells. Such progression from episomal to productive viral replication depends upon the interplay of cell permissiveness, viral type, host susceptibility, and cofactor activity.

Although latent HPV infection is a diffuse, essentially regional phenomenon, active viral expression occurs only at particular foci. The distribution and extent of the resulting lesions is highly variable, producing a wide array of disease patterns in different patients.

Morphologically, active expression is characterized by rapid epithelial and capillary proliferation,[22] usually lasting for a period of 3 to 6 months (Fig 4–2,A). Epithelial proliferation results in acanthosis, hyperchomasia, and increased mitotic activity. With extensive vascular overgrowth, stromal projections may become visible to the unaided eye in the form of an exophytic papilloma. In contrast, if capillary growth is insufficient to produce a wart, the lesion will remain subclinical.[18] But the same characteristic epithelial changes can be recognized through the colposcope after the replication of 5% acetic acid (see Fig 4–2,A).[29]

Exophytic condylomas and subclinical papillomavirus infection (SPI) differ only at the macroscopic level. Histologically, these different clinical manifestations of HPV infection look the same, and there is evidence that both variants can be part of the continuum leading to CIN. Of course, the volume of diseased epithelium (and hence the size of any viral inoculum) within an exophytic condyloma is much greater than for a similar area of subclinical infection.

## Host Containment Phase

About three months after the emergence of any clinically apparent or subclinical lesions, a host immune response occurs.[28] Individuals with impaired T-lymphocyte function

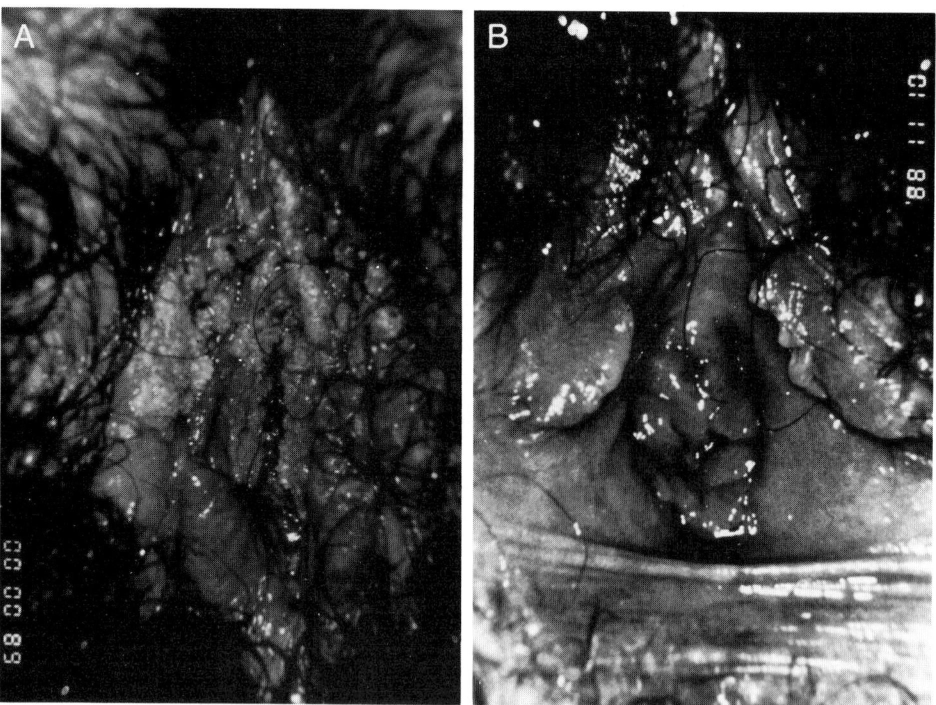


**FIG 4–2.**
**A,** condylomas of recent origin, showing multiple fresh lesions with a filiform, papillary morphology occurring simultaneously at several sites on the vulva. Intervening areas show a prominent acetowhite reaction, indicative of subclinical HPV infection in these areas. **B,** the same patient one month later, without any intervening therapy. These lesions regressed spontaneously while the patient was awaiting outpatient laser surgery.

do not manifest this containment stage,[30] suggesting that cellular immunity plays a major role in host defense against HPV infection. Although the antibody response sometimes seen in patients with regressed warts suggests that B-lymphocytes might also participate.[29]

Outcome from this point probably varies according to the sites involved:

1. External Condylomas. During this containment stage, external condylomas will undergo spontaneous regression in as many as 20% of infected individuals, marking the end of any clinically apparent episodes (Fig 4–2,B).[31] In another 60% of patients, localized destruction of just the obvious vulvar condylomas leads to a lasting clinical remission.[32] In the remaining 20%, HPV-induced lesions linger through the containment phase and prove refractory to standard office treatments. Control of these lesions often requires more extensive laser surgery,[33] and even antiviral adjuvant regimens.[34]

2. Cervical HPV Infections. Women with a history of koilocytotic atypia on a cervical smear are at increased risk of subsequently developing CIN 3 or invasive cancer.[35] Prospective follow-up suggests that about one-third of minor-grade lesions will evolve into CIN 3, about one-third will regress, and about one-third will persist unchanged for years (Fig 4–3). Within one 12-month period, Evans and Monaghan demonstrated progression to CIN 2 to 3 in 16% of histologically proven cervical SPI, including one case that developed into a microinvasive carcinoma.[36] This progressive potential has also been documented by Campion, et al., in a recent study that followed women with cytologic and colposcopic evidence of mild atypia.[37] Within a 2-year period, 26% progressed to CIN 3. Moreover, the spontaneous regression rate was very low (11%), and those women who did regress remained at high risk of future recurrence of their cervical disease. Significantly,

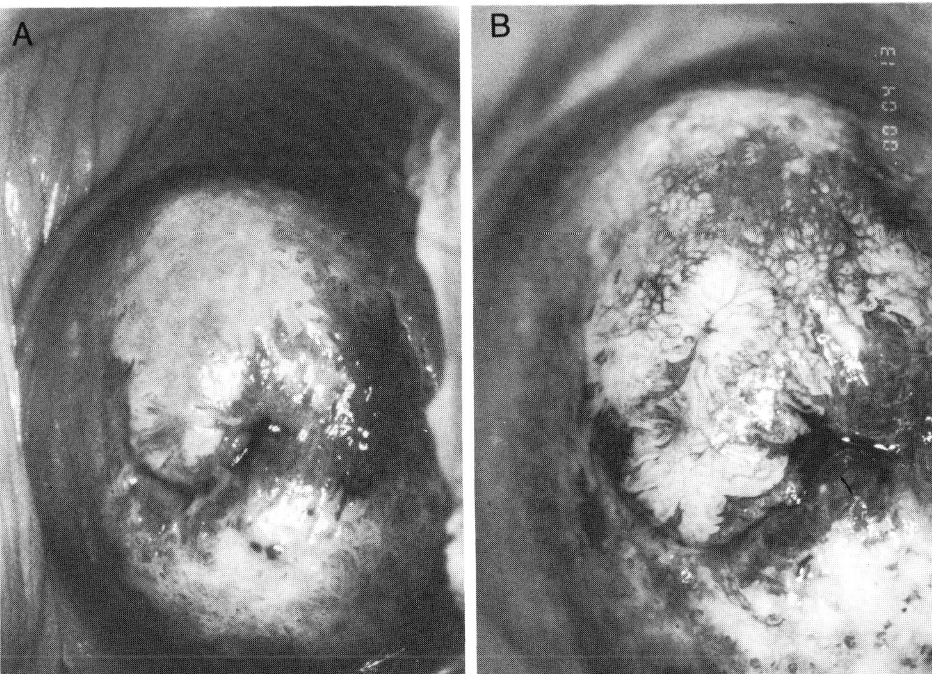


**FIG 4–3.**
**A,** minor grade cervical lesion found to contain HPV 16 at the time of recruitment into a longitudinal study, designed to follow such cases without treatment. **B,** a high-power view of the right anterior cervical lip, showing a focus of CIN 3 that emerged during a 6-month period of observation.

85% of those showing progression had cervical smears that tested positive for HPV 16 on filter hybridization at the time of entry into the study. These results were very similar to the earlier prospective study of Richart and Barron,[38] but the transit time to CIN 3 for this modern group of women was shorter.

### Late Phase

After about 9 months, patients diverge into two groups: those who remain in sustained clinical remission and those who relapse into continued active disease expression. Even though women in the first group no longer present with new condylomas, it is likely that latent HPV infection will persist within the anogenital epithelium.[39] Such "cured" patients may even remain contagious to other sex partners. In contrast, the second group of patients (who either remain in active disease expression or who "recur" after a lesion-free interval) represent the subset most likely to undergo neoplastic progression (Fig 4–4).[40]

## INDIVIDUAL DIFFERENCES IN DISEASE EXPRESSION

Among HPV-exposed individuals, progression to papilloma formation is probaby the exception, rather than the rule. Even so, the prevalence of venereal warts now approximates that of gonorrhea (0.5% in low-risk populations, rising to more than 5% in high-risk

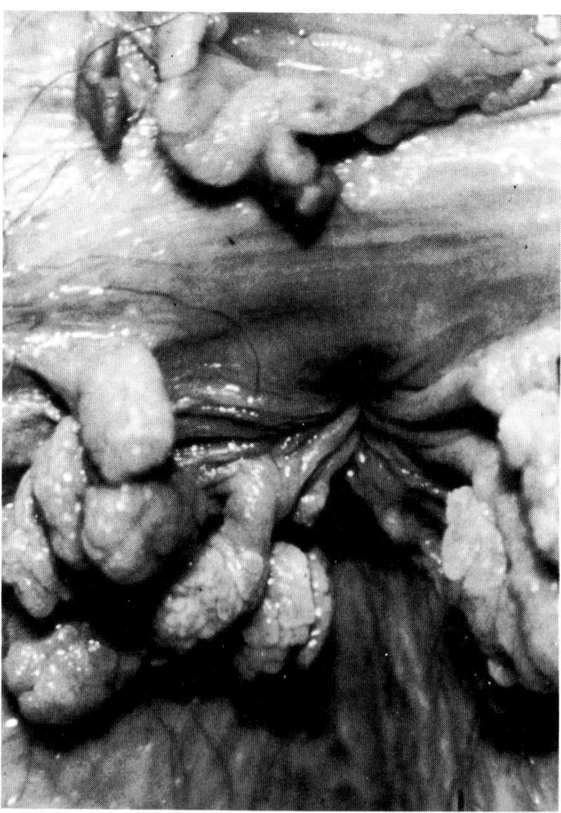

**FIG 4–4.**
Papular pedunculated perianal warts of four years' duration.

groups).[31] In addition to patients seeking medical attention because of external condyloma (one million privately insured Americans in 1984),[41, 42] Cytology Registries have reported morphologic signs of subclinical HPV infection in 2% to 5% of routine Papanicolaou smears.[43] Even more alarming, several recent studies have detected HPV DNA within 10% to 15% of smears taken from "normal" women.[44–46] Although colposcopic work-up will reveal high-grade neoplasia in a proportion of these women, it is clear that the majority of positive results represent latent HPV infections. The true significance of these observations is not yet known.

Why the clinical consequences of papillomaviral infection should be generalized in some patients, yet localized to differing anatomic sites in others, is a major puzzle. In a study of 160 women presenting with papillomavirus-associated diseases, HPV DNA was detected in 69% of the acetowhite epithelium surrounding the florid vulvar lesions, 40% of the "normal" vaginal mucosa, and 25% of unremarkable squamous metaplasia from just proximal to a high-grade CIN lesion.[10] These observations indicate that the presence of HPV genomic sequences is a necessary but insufficient cause for disease formation. Therefore, HPV-induced diseases of the anogenital tract are best regarded as chronic, regional infections. After episomal infection is established, cell-virus interaction must be regulated thereafter by local factors. Areas of overt disease seem to represent the focal breakdown of cellular control within a field of diffuse papillomaviral infection.[22]

To reconcile this iceberg concept with the realities of patient care, morphologic stigmata of HPV infection are best viewed as a cascade in which disease expression ranges from minimal to florid (Table 4–1).

## Chronic, Latent Papillomavirus Infections

In a strict sense, the concept of latency implies the presence of viral genomes within morphologically normal cells (Fig 4–5). The rare hereditary skin disorder, epidermodysplasia verruciformis, provides an important insight into the nature and extent of latent HPV infection.[26] Almost half of the currently known HPV types have been isolated from non-genital warts affecting immunosuppressed individuals. Because it is highly unlikely that these novel cutaneotropic viruses would persist in nature if they infected only immunocompromised hosts, normal individuals must serve as the reservoir for these rare viruses.

The detectability of HPV DNA in 10% to 15% of genital swabs collected from clinically normal women[44, 45] suggests that the anogenital mucosae are also susceptible to chronic, latent HPV infection by sexually transmitted HPVs. Moreover, a large proportion

**TABLE 4–1.**
Varing Levels of Disease Expression

| |
|---|
| Well-developed Papillomavirus infections: |
| Vegetative viral replication (benign condyloma and SPI*) |
| Non-productive viral infection (intraepithelial neoplasia and invasive cancer) |
| Low-grade Papillomavirus infections: |
| Normal cell phenotype ("true latency") |
| Minimal viral cytopathic effect (MEPI) |

*SPI = Subclinical papillomavirus infection.

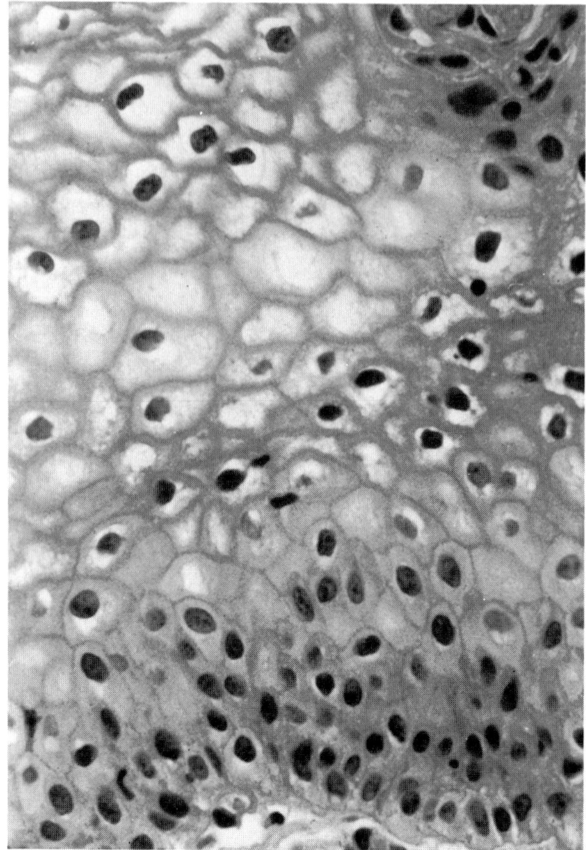

**FIG 4–5.**
A bland-appearing biopsy of essentially normal histology which proved positive for HPV types 16 and 18 by Southern blot hybridization. (From Reid R, Greenberg M, Jenson AB, et al: *Am J Obstet Gynecol* 1987; 156:212–222. Used by permission.)

of positive hybridization tests reveal HPV types not yet detected in biopsies from clinically significant disease (R. Reid, unpublished data). Therefore, it seems likely that many of the anogenital papillomaviruses may be ubiquitous saprophytes (analogous to those in EV), rather than sexually transmitted pathogens.

## Minimally Expressed Papillomavirus Infections

A common colposcopic sign in patients with HPV infection of the lower genital tract is the finding of a myriad of tiny acetowhite flecks highlighted against the flat pink vaginal mucosa. Each of these white dots corresponds to a pinpoint to parakeratotic epithelium capping a prominent intraepithelial capillary (Fig 4–6,A). Changes are subtle and diffuse, often being described as "reverse punctation" for lack of a better term.[47] Appearances are made more prominent by staining with quarter-strength Lugol's iodine. The well-glycogenated normal epithelium stains mahogany brown, whereas the parakeratotic flecks turn yellow.

Histologic findings are characterized by minimal basal hyperplasia, mild koilocytosis,

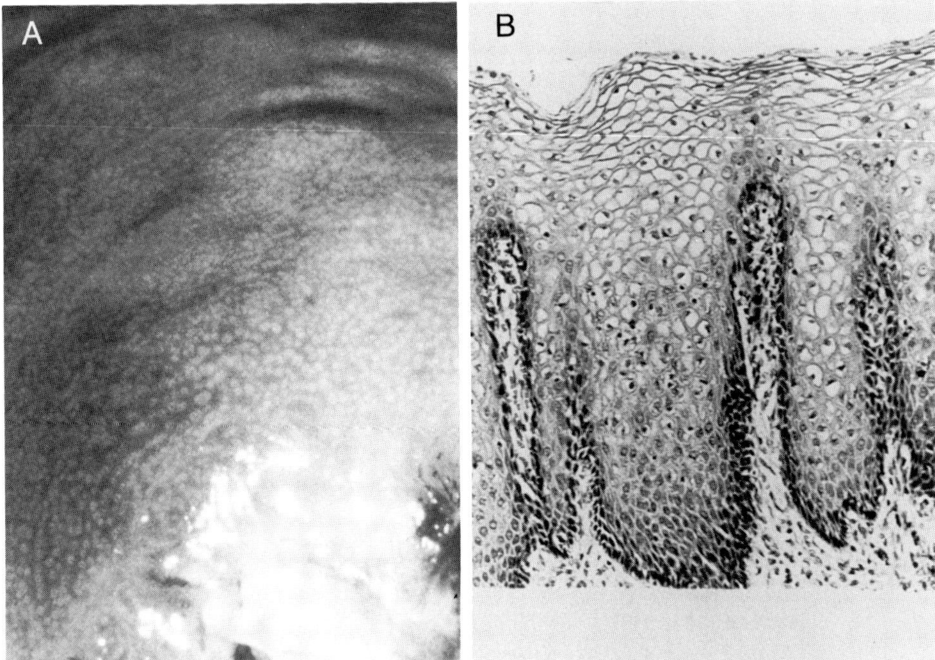


**FIG 4–6.**
**A,** subtle, diffuse surface elevations affecting the entire original squamous epithelium of the cervical portio. **B,** low-grade koilocytotic atypia, suggestive of minimally expressed papilloma virus infection.

variable dyskeratosis, and prominent intraepithelial capillaries (Fig 4–6,B). Pathologists not accustomed to reading such biopsies may report these changes either as condyloma or as normal. Strictly speaking, neither designation is correct. Despite essentially normal histology, HPV DNA was detectable in vaginal biopsies from almost half the women triaged for unequivocal CIN or invasive cervical cancer.[10] Therefore these changes are probably best seen as minimal HPV expression within latently infected tissues.

## Well-Developed Papillomavirus Infections

When pathologic sequelae do occur, there is enormous variability in the sites involved, the extent of the disease, lesion morphology, clinical course, therapeutic response, and the risk of neoplastic transformation.[22] Recommendations for management are complicated by the fact that virtually every patient presents a unique disease pattern. However, some insight is provided by an understanding of virologic principles.[16, 17, 48]

From the functional viewpoint, the viral genetic information is divided into early and late regions.[49] Genes from the early region establish viral control over the infected cell and initiate viral DNA replication, while genes from the late region are involved in capsid protein synthesis and virion assembly. Different types of cell virus interaction occur, depending upon the relative expression of these various genes.

**Productive Viral Replication.**—Episomal HPV infection remains latent in the basal cells but progresses to active expression in the parabasal layer (Fig 4–7,A,B).[10, 18, 50]

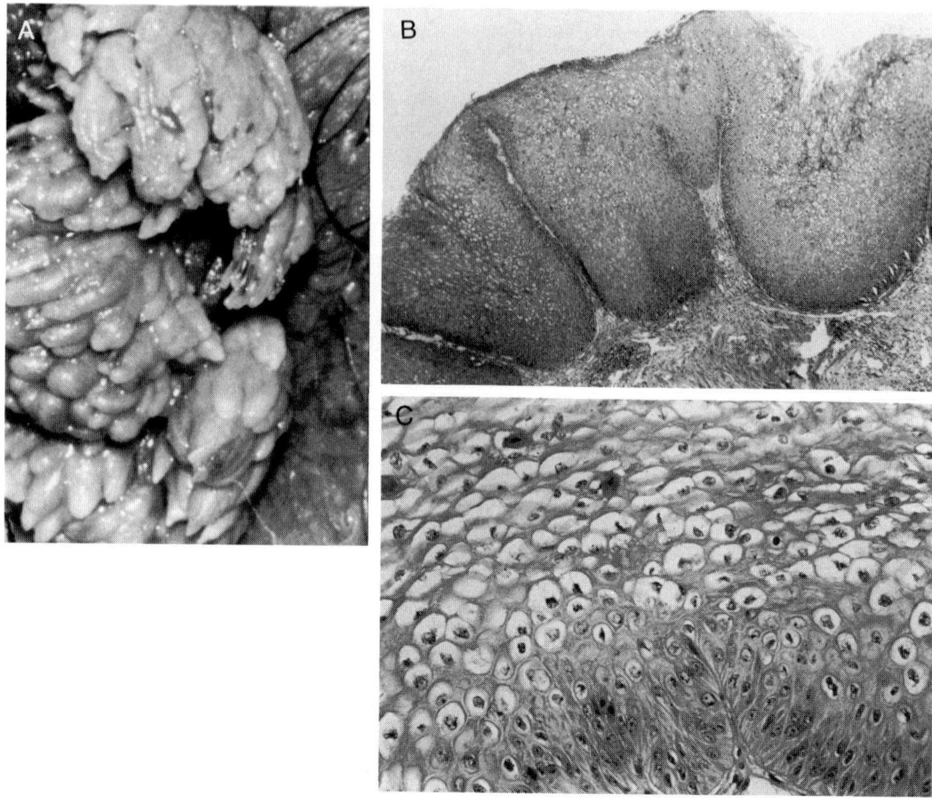

**FIG 4–7.**
**A,** prominent papillomatosis in a benign condyloma of recent onset. **B,** a low-power photomicrograph showing papillomatosis, acanthosis, and slight parakeratosis. **C,** a high-power view showing increased basal division activity, blending with prominent koilocytotic atypia in the maturing cells of the midepithelial layers.

Proteins encoded by the early genes act as mutogenic stimuli, causing increased division activity (acanthosis) and capillary overgrowth (papillomatosis). Continued DNA synthesis by parabasal and intermediate cells is seen microscopically as mild hyperchromatism, dyskaryosis, and delayed surface maturation (Fig 4–7,C). However, despite a degree of morphologic similarity to dysplasia, cells showing a vegetative infection still have a euploid DNA content (i.e., diploid or polyploid).[22] Viral DNA production averages 50 to 200 within each affected nucleus, with occasional "hot cells" containing up to ten copies.[50]

In the upper layers, the late events in the viral life cycle (those concerned with actual viral replication) produce a characteristic viral cytopathic effect. Such koilocytosis is characterized by degenerative clumping of host cell chromatin, nuclear collapse, and the formation of cytoplasmic vacuoles (Fig 4–8). Within a small proportion of these degenerating surface cells, large gene expression may proceed to the point of virion assembly (see Fig 4–8).

Since viral cytopathic effect occurs only in dying or dead cells, koilocytes can never undergo malignant transformation. Rather, such cytopathic effects represent the contagious stage in the HPV life cycle. Although vegetative infection is the hallmark of the low-risk HPV types, it is crucial to understand that high-risk HPVs will be detected in 10% to 15% of lesions showing only koilocytotic atypia.[22]

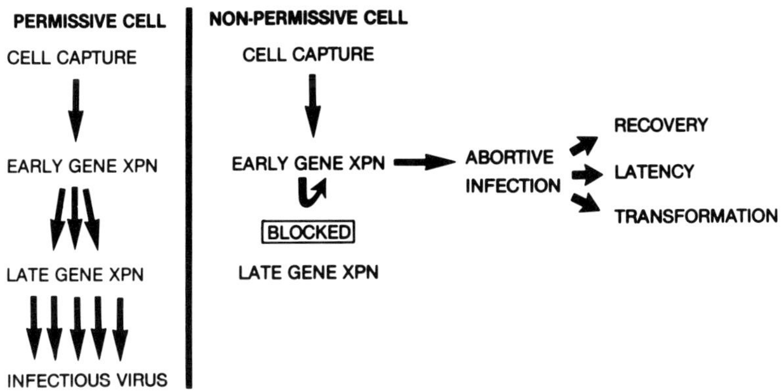


**FIG 4–8.**
A diagram of different types of cell virus interaction. (From Reid R: *Colpo Gynecol Laser Surg* 1984; 1:3–34. Used by permission.)

**Abortive Potentially Transforming Infections.**—The papillomaviruses are unique in that effective late viral expression is tied to the cellular events of squamous differentiation and keratinization.[49, 50] Because genital epithelia have a limited ability to keratinize, the viral replicative cycle does not always proceed to the point of virion production (see Fig 4–8).[50] Instead, cells may show an abortive type of cell virus interaction, wherein early gene activity is not counterbalanced by late gene expression (Fig 4–9).[51]

Certain high-risk papillomaviruses break the host cell chromosomes at random points,

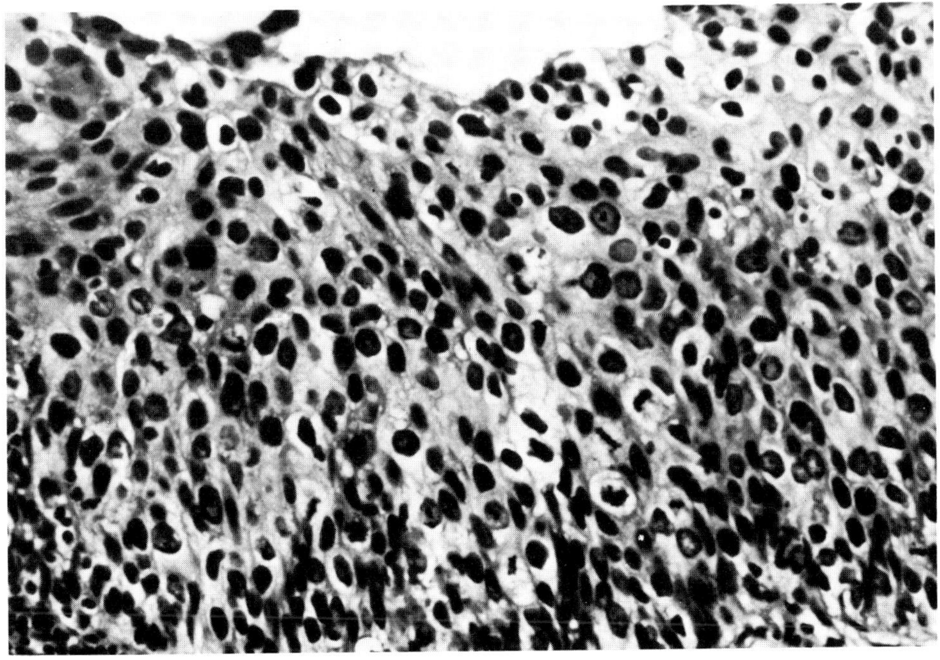

**FIG 4–9.**
A photomicrograph of a CIN 3 lesion. Despite the absence of any viral cytopathic effect, this lesion proved positive for HPV 16.

thereby splicing viral genes into the host genome.[52] Transcription of these genes promotes heightened division activity, which can continue throughout most of the epithelial thickness. Because these alien genes are joined to the host chromosomes by covalent bonds, integrated viral DNA will replicate with the host chromosomes during each subsequent cellular mitosis. The host cell will soon develop an aneuploid chromatin content and a dysplastic morphology will evolve.[22] Viral copy number much less than in vegetative infections, and late gene products are almost never seen. Therefore, nonproductively infected cells are not usually contagious but have taken several steps in the direction of malignant transformation.

## HPV AND GENITAL CANCER: CAUSAL OR CASUAL?

### Evidence Implicating HPV Infection

Specific HPV types are incriminated as the etiologic agent for a group of epithelial proliferations that may progress to anogenital malignancy.[53] The detection of HPV DNA within genital tumor tissues must be distinguished from various statistical associations between other sexually transmitted diseases and cervical, vulvar, and penile cancers. The relationship between HPV infection and malignancy is quite strict.[25] More than 90% of cancers contain oncogenic HPVs, and the same HPVs are detected in malignancies throughout the world, despite the heterogeneity of the genus. Archival cervical cancer specimens from the 1930s can also be shown to contain the same HPV types (DJ McCance, personal communication).

The precursor lesions of anogenital malignancies also harbor the same HPV types as detected in invasive cancers.[10, 23] Within premalignant tissue, the viral DNA exists as a free episome (i.e., a self-replicating, extrachromosomal, nuclear plasmid). In contrast, most of the viral DNA within invasive cancers is integrated into the host chromosomes (i.e., spliced into the host genome by covalent bonds, often in tandem arrays).[52, 54]

The persistence of viral DNA in malignant cells has also been shown by the detection of HPV DNA in cervical cancer-derived human cell lines. Seven of nine such cell lines contain HPV DNA, including HeLa cells (derived from an HPV 18–containing adenocarcinoma) and Ca-Ski cells (an HPV 16–containing squamous carcinoma).[55] RNA mapping has revealed transcription of E6 or E6* (a message shortened by interval splicing). In addition, an E7 protein has been identified in several cell lines.[56] Preliminary experiments indicate that continued expression of E6/E7 proteins may be required for maintenance of the transformed state.[57] The fact that a putative transforming segment is consistently transcribed argues strongly that specific HPV types play a role in the pathogenesis of human genital cancer. These observations are consistent with the operation of other oncogenic viruses in other animal systems.[25]

### The Possible Operation of Other Co-carcinogens

Notwithstanding the probable role of papillomaviruses, it seems likely that HPV infection alone is insufficient to induce a carcinoma in an immunocompetent host. This conclusion is suggested by the long lag time between initial infection and eventual malignant conversion and by the spontaneous regression of many primary lesions. The risk of a given type of HPV infection producing a carcinoma can be roughly estimated by comparing the prevalence of that type in the normal population versus its prevalence in HPV-positive cancers.[25] Such a preliminary calculation indicates that only about 1 in 100 HPV 16– or 18–infected women will develop cervical cancer. The risk of malignant progression by an intermediate-risk HPV type appears to be five- to tenfold times lower than for HPV 16.

Studies of the Shope papillomavirus system in rabbits have shown that carcinogenesis is influenced by the operation of additional etiologic agents.[2, 13] Malignant progression was facilitated by exposure to physical (ultraviolet light or x-rays) and chemical carcinogens (dietary components or hydrocarbons). In addition, chronic irritation or inflammation exerted a weaker, less specific effect.

Plausible cofactors within the lower genital tract include use of tobacco products, infection by other microbial agents, and immunosuppression. Heavy smoking is suspected as a risk factor,[58] and tobacco metabolites have been detected in cervical mucus.[59] Whether concomitant herpes virus infection could also act as a co-carcinogen is an open question.[58] Nonetheless, it is conceivable that concomitant herpetic infection might affect papillomavirus genes or cellular control genes, either of which could change viral expression.[60]

Both the prevalence of genital condylomas and the risk of developing carcinoma in situ are increased in immunosuppressed patients.[30] The increased prevalence and accelerated progression of HPV-induced cervical atypia in patients with impaired host immunity contrasts with findings in the Shope papillomavirus models, where corticosteroid administration did not influence malignant conversion.[2, 3]

### The Prospects of Vaccination

If HPV infection is indeed necessary for the induction of anogenital cancer, the prospect of controlling the disease by vaccination opens an exciting possibility.[21] In human medicine, healthy women cannot be deliberately infected with an oncogenic papillomavirus. For this reason, proof along the lines of the experiments conducted in the Shope papillomavirus system will never be possible. Rather, the best evidence of causality in humans would be the demonstration that vaccination of non-exposed individuals reduced the subsequent occurrence of anogenital malignancy. Aside from the question of cancer prophylaxis, the morbidity caused by condylomas and dysplasia (which are clearly HPV-induced) may be reason enough for a vaccination program.

Observations in spontaneously regressing skin warts are most noteworthy.[61] Histologic examination reveals strong mononuclear cell infiltrates. Electronmicroscopy has shown activated Langerhans cells and macrophage attacks on HPV-infected epidermal cells. These data indicate that wart cell–specific surface antigens are being detected by the cell-mediated immune system. Once started, regression of multiple warts is usually a systemic phenomenon, and the host thereafter remains immune to reinfection by that HPV type.[21]

Notwithstanding the host's potential to fight HPV infections, the immune response is often weak and slow. This failure could reflect low levels of HPV surface antigens, perhaps too low for immunologic detection. Therefore, in addition to preventing HPV infections, vaccination might also be able to enhance the immune rejection of the virus to infected cells.[21] Vaccination might also offer the prospect of immunotherapy for established disease. Since any vaccine should be based on specific, virus-coded, membrane-bound proteins, future research will need to identify and characterize such antigens.

## CLINICAL FEATURES OF PREINVASIVE VULVO-VAGINAL DISEASE

### Condylomata Acuminata

Exophytic condylomas usually present as soft, pink or whitish, vascular, sessile tumors with multiple, fine, fingerlike projections (see Fig 4–7,A). They occur primarily in moist areas, especially those exposed to coital friction. Thus, the most common sites are the posterior part of the introitus, the adjacent labia minora, throughout the vestibule, and on the perianal or anal skin (Fig 4–10). Less commonly, condylomas occur in the clitorial region (even under the clitoral hood) and may extend on to the mons pubis. In the nonmucosal areas, the condylomas may be more keratotic and less papilliferous, similar in appearance to the typical hand warts (verruca vulgarae).

Condylomata acuminata now represents one of the most common sexually transmitted diseases.[62] Contact tracing studies suggest that over 60% of exposed individuals will develop lesions after a variable incubation period.[28] The reported incidence of vulvar condylomata acuminata has greatly increased throughout the occidental world over the past 20 years. In the United Kingdom, the reported incidence has risen 10% per year,[61] and in the United States there has been a 460% increase over the last 15 years.[41, 42] Age incidence peaks between 16 and 25 years,[31] as does that of other sexually transmitted diseases.

The vast majority of exophytic condylomata acuminata are induced by HPV 6 (65%) or HPV 11 (20%). Most of the remainder will contain HPVs 42, 43, or 44.[10, 11] Mixed infections involving more than one genital HPV type are not uncommon. Importantly, HPV 16 or 18 will be detected in up to 10% of these common, benign genital proliferations.[22]

Progression from vulvar condylomas to vulvar cancer is well documented;[63] however, the relative risk is very low.[47] Rarely, large papillomas may show excessive growth with associated local invasion. Such slowly spreading, genital masses are termed giant condylomas of Buschke-Löwenstein or verrucous carcinomas. These lesions are usually induced by either HPV 6 or 11 and represent indolent malignancies that rarely metastasize.[64]

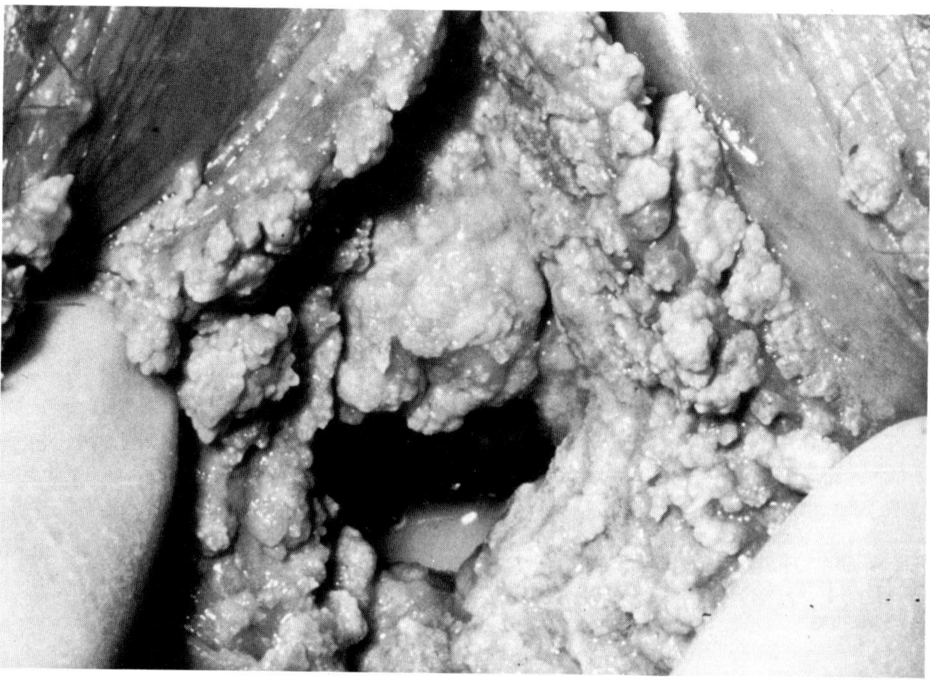

**FIG 4–10.**
Multiple, relatively uniform, filiform papillomas that principally affect the areas of coital friction.

## Maculo-Papular Lesions

HPV infection of the vulvar skin can also produce small (3 to 7 mm), smooth, flat papules (Fig 4–11,A)[65] or discolored, keratotic plaques (Fig 4–11,B). Lesions may be pigmented or non-pigmented, or, in dark-skinned women, associated with depigmentation. Maculo-papular lesions often occur in association with condylomata acuminata but may occur in the absence of other clinically apparent disease. Lesions are usually multiple, sometimes coalescing to produce a larger area of disease.

The histology of these papular lesions is quite variable, ranging from benign HPV infection to significant dysplasia.[47] More than 70% of vulvar and penile papules showing significant histologic atypia will be found to contain HPV 16 DNA.[66] For this reason, these inconspicuous lesions may represent an important male and female reservoir for oncogenic HPV types.

## Subclinical Papillomavirus Infections

Subclinical HPV infection is common in the vagina and the vulva. Vaginal lesions are present in one of these forms: elongated vaginal papillae, flat acetowhite epithelium, or reverse punctation.[47]

Vulvar SPI can be either micropapillary (Fig 4–12,A) or completely flat and therefore invisible without the aid of acetic acid smoking (Fig 4–12,B). The acetic acid subclinical vulvar lesions are sometimes symptomatic, producing chronic pruritis, burning, or postcoital pain.

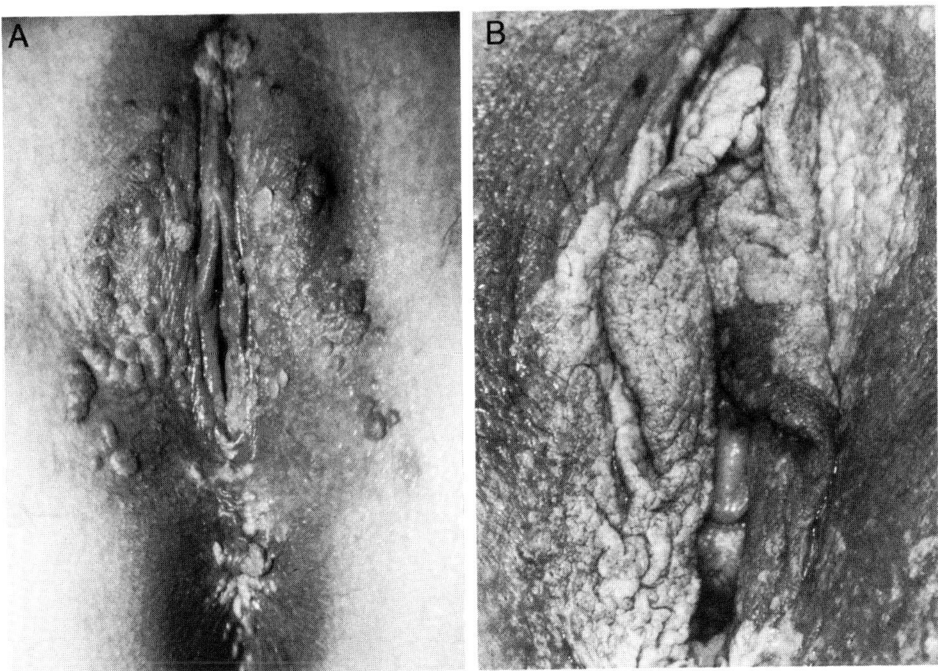


**FIG 4–11.**
**A,** pigmented papular lesions of the hair-bearing labial skin, which showed VIN 3 on directed biopsy. **B,** a discolored, surface-roughened plaque of VIN 3 affecting the labia minora and hairless skin of the interlabial sulci.

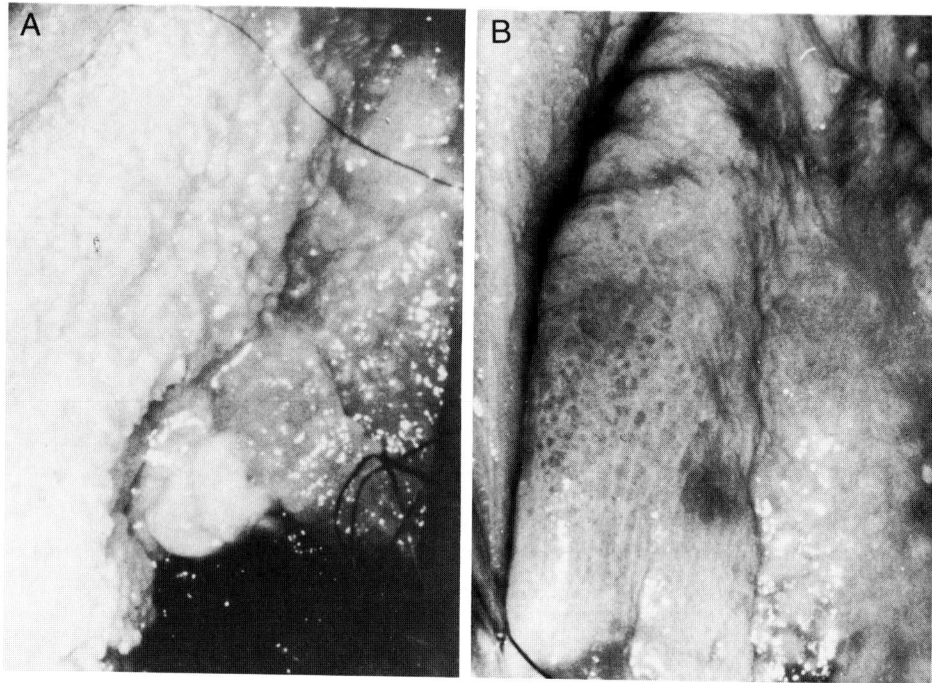


**FIG 4–12.**
Subclinical HPV infection of the vestibule. **A,** the micropapillary variant. **B,** the flat variant.

## CLINICAL FEATURES OF PREINVASIVE CERVICAL DISEASE

### Exophytic Condylomas

In 1921, Wharton described condyloma acuminatum of the cervix as one of the rarest of gynecologic disorders.[67] This observation was affirmed in 1948, when Suran and Meister added one case to only 15 others collected from the literature.[68] Although cervical papillomas are now seen with greater frequency, it is still clear that only a minority of HPV infections result in exophytic condylomas. In 1971, Oriel found macroscopic cervical condylomas in 6% of women presenting with vulvar warts.[28] Ten years later (and with the aid of the colposcope), Roy et al., reported seeing clinically apparent cervical lesions in 20% of HPV-infected women.[69]

Such lesions may affect either the cervical transformation zone (Fig 4–13,A) or the original squamous epithelium (Fig 4–13,B). In either case, most lesions will contain HPV 6 or 11, and accompanying papillomas of similar morphology will often be found on the vagina and vulva.[22, 47] Individual papillomas may be small or large, single or multiple, scattered or confluent.

Classic condylomas can usually be recognied with the naked eye with their color ranging from pink to white (depending upon epithelial thickness). Through the colposcope, most exophytic papillomas will be seen as an aggregate of small papillae, each with a vascular loop beneath the translucent surface epithelium (Fig 4–14). Application of acetic acid produces stark acetowhitening of the individual papillae, thereby causing a marked enhancement of the visual appearance. Alternatively, some exophytic papillomas present as flat or micropapillary plaques of leukoplakia (indicative of a keratotic surface that is recognizable prior to vinegar soaking) (Fig 4–15).

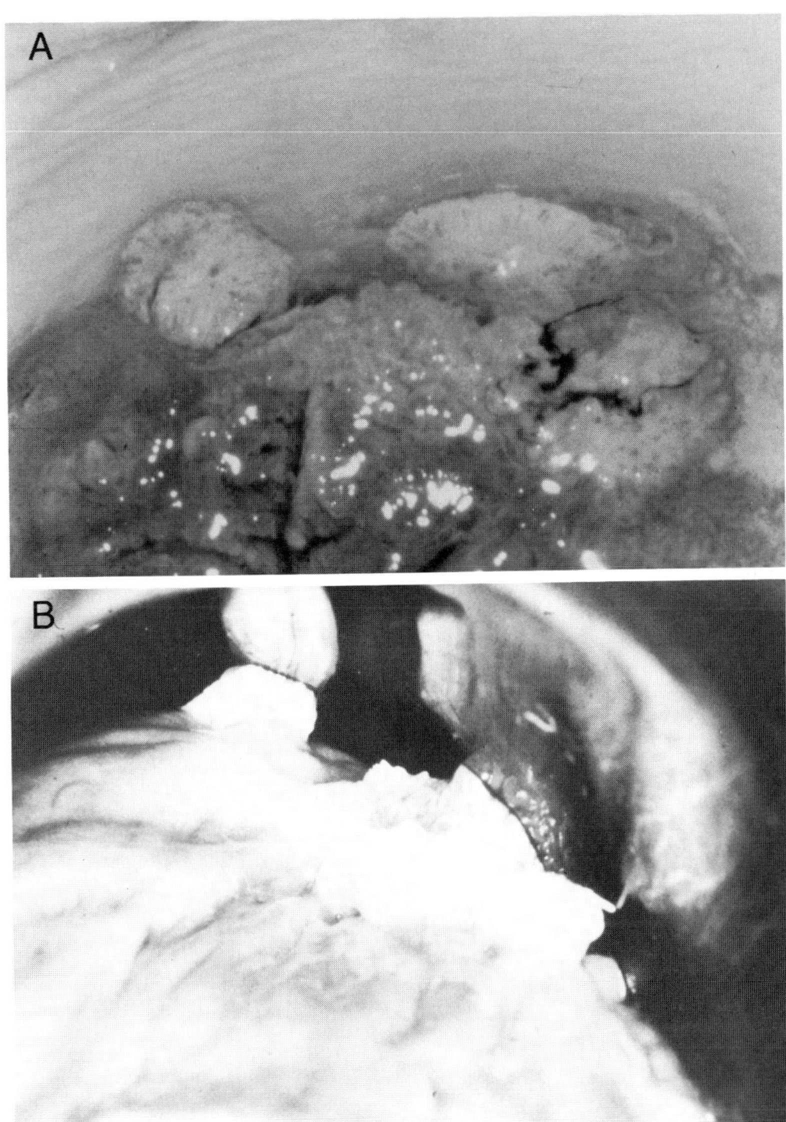


**FIG 4–13.**
**A,** filiform vascular condylomas growing on immature metaplastic tissue within the cervical transformation zone. **B,** papillary condylomas affecting the original squamous epithelium of the cervical portio.

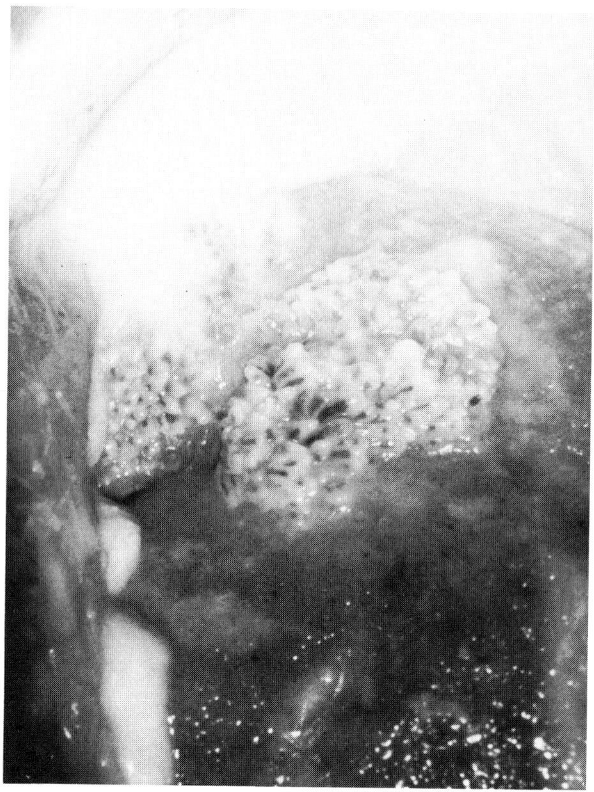

**FIG 4–14.**
A small condyloma seen at high colposcopic magnification showing the presence of central vascular cores surrounded by HPV-infected surface epithelium.

Most classic condylomas can be confidently recognized as benign; however, some lesions are sufficiently uncharacteristic as to raise a suspicion of cancer.[70] Angiogenesis within multiple papillae can produce coarse capillary loops, some of which have a horizontal orientation. Indeed, the resemblance to a neoplastic vascular pattern may be striking (Fig 4–16). However, with condylomas, vascular spacing and papillary growth often show a definite regularity, thereby allowing differentiation from invasive carcinoma. Obviously, if bizarre vessels are seen within an exophytic lesion, multiple biopsies are mandatory.

## Clinically Inapparent, Minor-Grade Lesions

Although cervical condylomas are relatively rare, subclinical HPV infection is astoundingly common. In the past, cervical HPV infections were overlooked because the lesions are entirely invisible to the unaided eye.[29] At that time, it was believed that HPV infections caused only papillomas of the vagina, vulva, and anus. Even when subclinical HPV infection was seen at colposcopy, these changes were usually dismissed as physiological variations or interpreted as mild dysplasia. However, clinical interest was rekindled in the mid-1970s, when HPV infection was recognized as the cause of many abnormal Papanicolaou smears.[5–7]

Given the divergent natural histories of specific disease patterns and the poor predic-

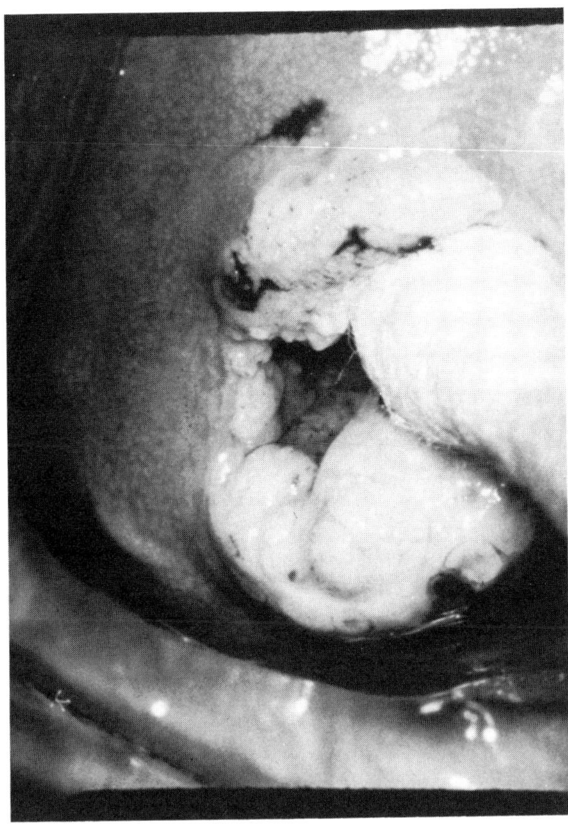

**FIG 4–15.**
A keratotic plaque replacing most of the cervical transformation zone, which showed the classical features of a benign condyloma on biopsy.

tive value of fine morphologic distinction within a general subset, there is no reason to grade premalignant lesions beyond a simple division into high grade (CIN 2 to 3) versus low grade (CIN 1 and flat condyloma). High-grade lesions represent an homologous population of aneuploid lesions, most of which are induced by oncogenic HPVs (Table 4–2). Expert gynecologic pathologists can reliably identify such epithelia as bona fide precursors. Unfortunately, the converse does not hold true.

**TABLE 4–2.**
Type-Specific Disease Association

| | Low Risk HPV Type | Medium Risk HPV Type | High Risk HPV Type | No HPV DNA Detected | Total |
|---|---|---|---|---|---|
| Exophytic cervical papilloma | 16 | 0 | 4 | 1 | 21 |
| Flat, minor grade acetowhitening | 24 | 4 | 14 | 4 | 46 |
| Flat, major grade acetowhitening | 11 | 15 | 31 | 5 | 62 |
| Invasive cervical cancer | 0 | 2 | 8 | 1 | 11 |
| Totals | 51 | 21 | 57 | 11 | 140 |

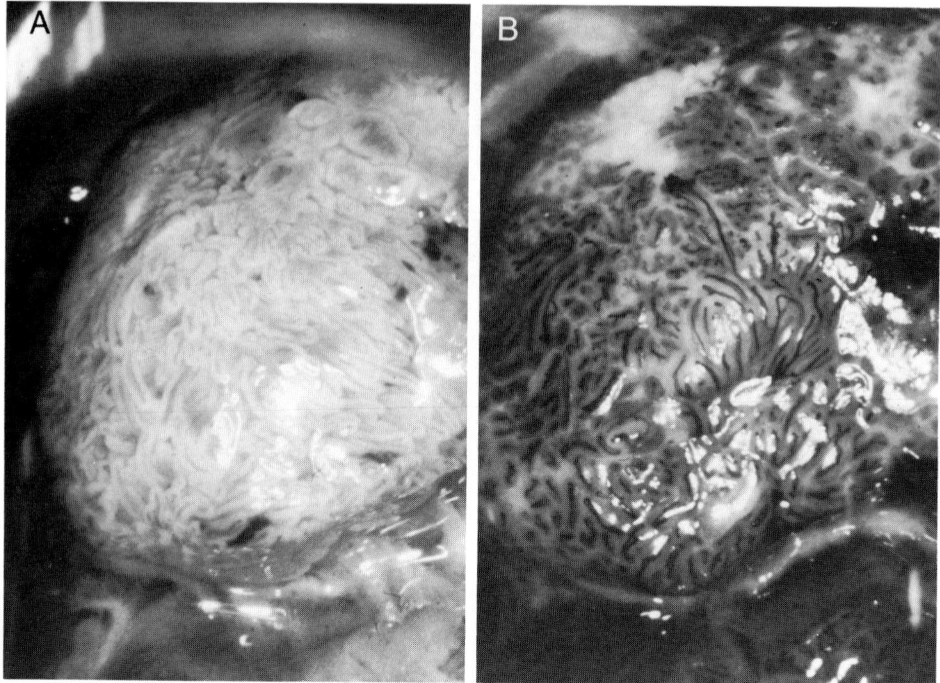


**FIG 4–16.**
**A,** a subtle, frond-like change to the anterior lip of the cervix that was barely recognizable prior to the application of acetic acid. **B,** vinegar soaking has produced a series of horizontal vascular patterns that strikingly resemble those seen in invasive cancers.

Low-grade lesions are a heterologous mixture of genuine precursors and benign HPV infections (see Table 4–2). Although it has been suggested that low-grade lesions containing oncogenic types can be recognized by the presence of atypical mitotic figures, this has not been our experience.[22, 71] In addition, a great deal of time and effort is wasted in trying to differentiate condyloma from mild dysplasia. Such attempts are meaningless, subjective, and nonreproducible. Rather, low-grade lesions are best approached as a population of known but uncommon, malignant potential. Unless virologic probes are used to differentiate high-risk from low-risk types, empiric destruction of the transformation zone remains the most cost-effective approach, irrespective of whether the lesion is reported as CIN 1 or as just koilocytotic atypia without accompanying dysplasia.[72]

From the colpocopic viewpoint, minor-grade lesions manifest themselves in one of two forms; some display micropapillae and fine vascular loops analogous to a miniature condyloma (Fig 4–17,A), while others present as flat plaques of acetowhite epithelium that broadly resemble high-grade CIN (Fig 4–17,B). For the less-experienced physician, colposcopic differentiation of flat, minor-grade lesions from flat, major-grade lesions is relatively difficult. Although this diagnosis will ultimately be made by histologic examination, a colposcopic impression is important in order to direct the biopsy to the areas of most significant disease.[73, 74]

On the cervix, minor-grade lesions are usually characterized by an indistinct degree of acetowhitening or a shiny, gray-white color. Most often, such lesions are distinguished by a shiny, gray discoloration, and a peripheral margin that displays either an angular, geographic shape (Fig 4–18) or a feathered edge (Fig 4–19). Capillary patterns are usu-

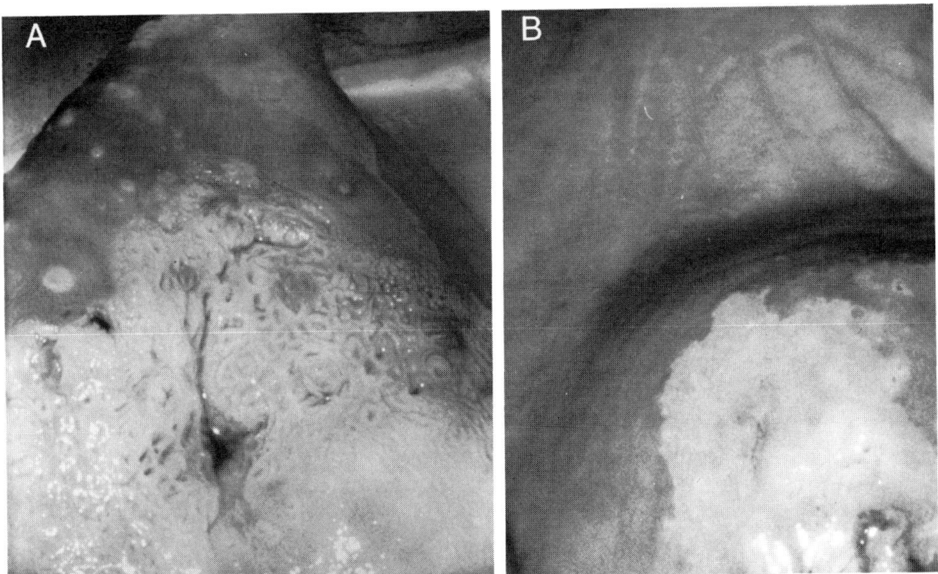


**FIG 4–17.**
Subclinical HPV infection of the cervix. **A,** the micropapillary variant. **B,** the flat variant.

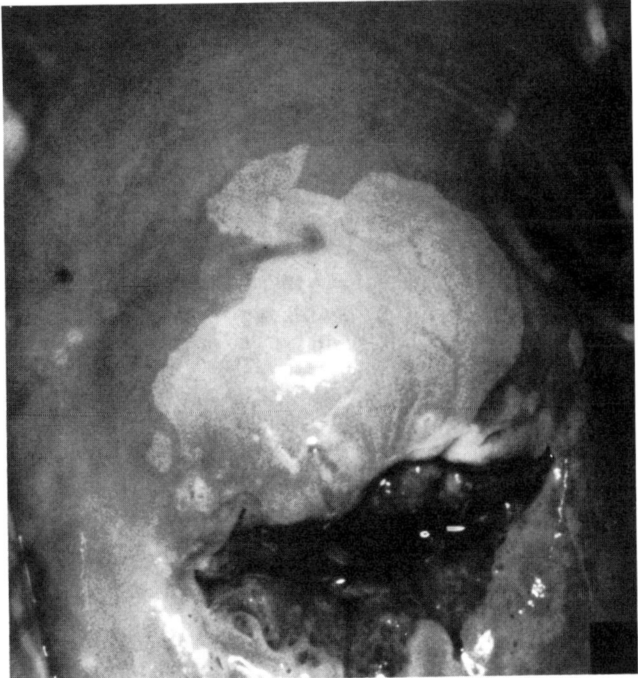

**FIG 4–18.**
A minor-grade cervical lesion showing a distinctly angular geographic shape.

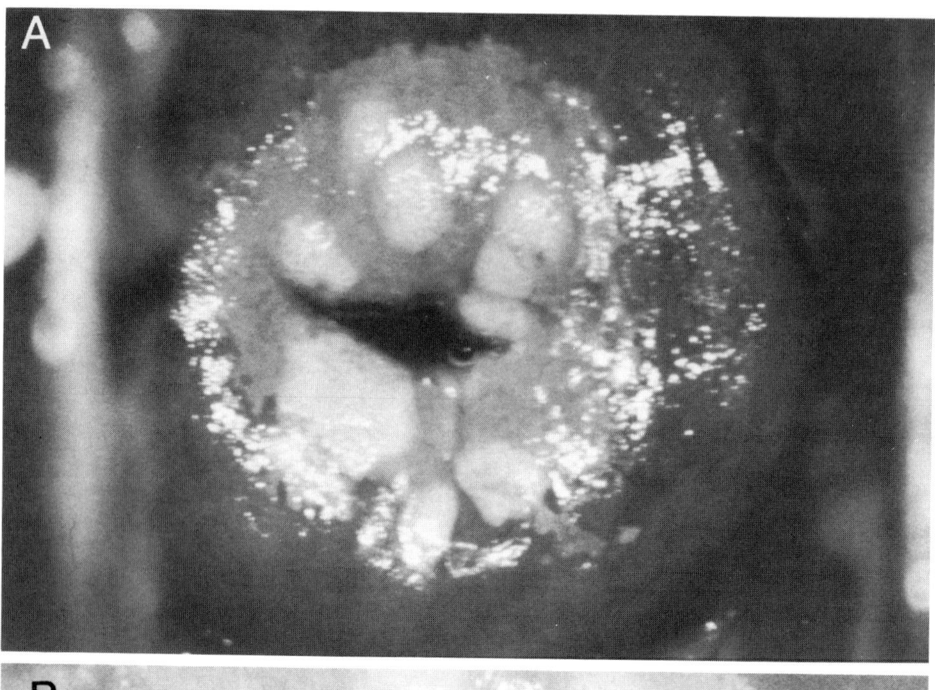


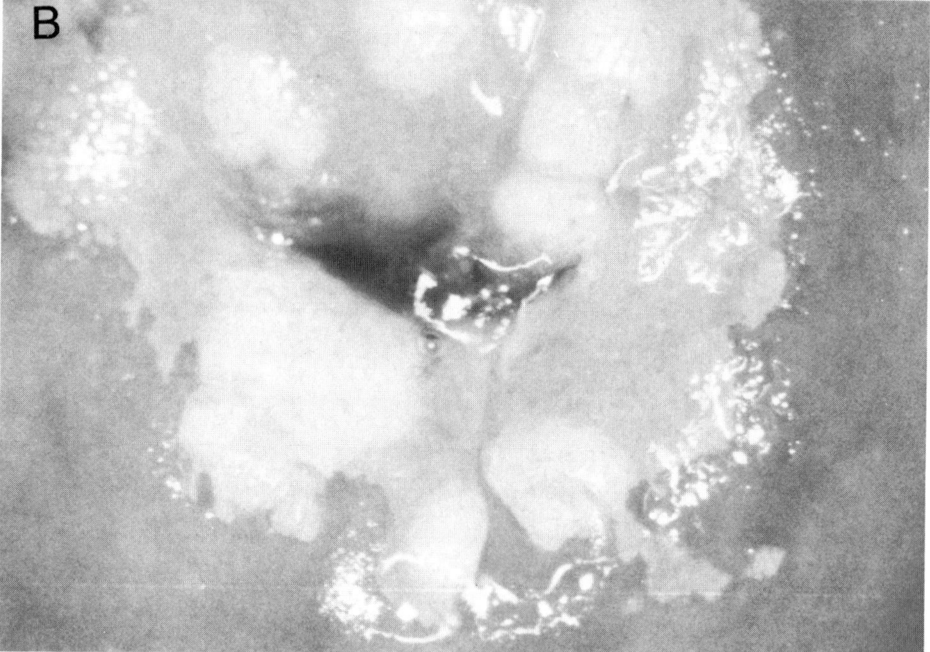


**FIG 4–19.**
A minor-grade lesion of the cervical transformation zone, presenting both exophytic condylomas and surrounding areas of subclinical papillomaviral infection. The condylomas have a shiny snow-white color. In contrast, the adjacent SPI has a gray-white appearance but is characterized by a feathered peripheral margin.

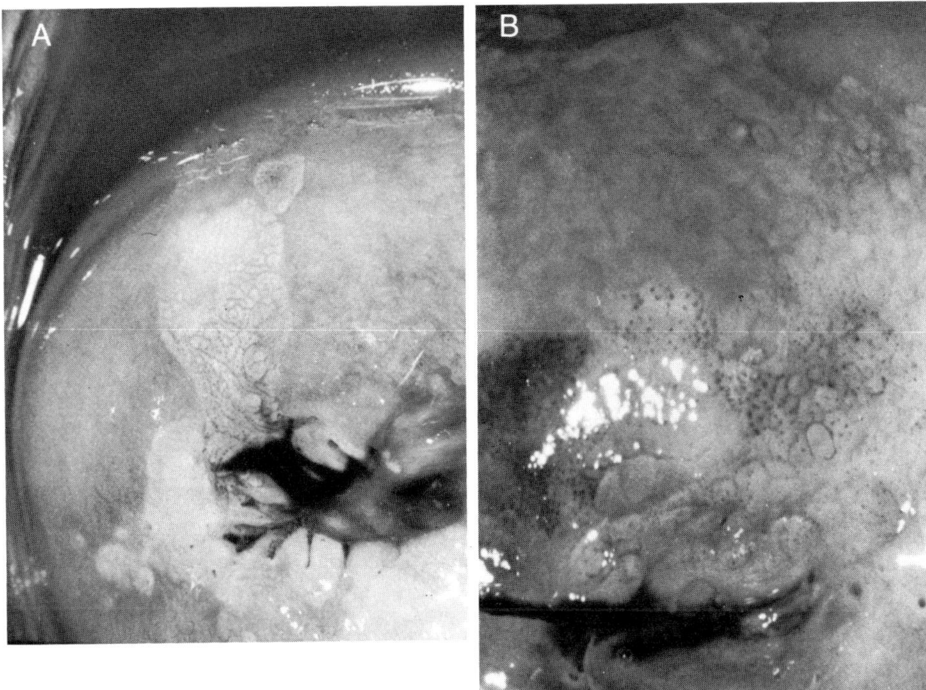


**FIG 4–20.**
Vascular patterns seen in minor-grade lesions. Although mosaic-like and punctate patterns are seen, the capillaries present within minor-grade lesions are distinguished by a uniform caliber and the lack of vascular dilation.

**TABLE 4–3.**
The Combined Colposcopic Index

| Colposcopic Sign | Zero Points | One Point | Two Points |
|---|---|---|---|
| Margin | Condylomatous or micropapillary contour. Indistinct acetowhitening. Flocculated or feathered margins. Angular, jagged lesions. Satellite lesions and acetowhitening that extends beyond transformation zone. | Regular lesions with smooth, straight outlines. | Rolled, peeling edges. Internal demarcations between areas of differing appearance. |
| Color | Shiny, snow-white color. Indistinct acetowhitening. | Intermediate shade (shiny gray). | Dull, oyster white. |
| Vessels | Fine-caliber vessels, poorly formed patterns. Condylomatous or micropapillary lesions. | Absent vessels. | Definite punctation or mosaicism. |
| Iodine | Positive iodine staining. Minor iodine negativity. | Partial iodine uptake. | Negative staining of significant lesion. |

Colposcopic score: 0–2 = SPI or CIN I; 3–5 = CIN 1–2; 6–8 = CIN 2–3 "aneuploid lesions".

ally present, often being so pronounced as to be confused with the mosaicism and punctation characteristic of CIN 2 and 3 (Fig 4–20); however, trivial vascular patterns are distinguished by their nondilated, uniform caliber. Horizontal vessels generally produce a loosely arranged mesh, reminiscent of a bizarre spider web (fine mosaic). Vertical capillaries are also characterized by a uniform vessel caliber throughout their course, forming a fine punctate stippling at the epithelial surface (fine punctation). Finally, staining with quarter-strength Lugol's iodine is another valuable aid to colposcopic diagnosis (Table 4–3).

## Clinically Inapparent, High-Grade Dysplasias

High-grade dysplasias are distinguished by a flat contour, a symmetric shape, a straight peripheral margin, and a dull oyster-white color. Since the squamocolumnar junction moves caudad with age, high-grade dysplasia often forms at the proximal edge of a pre-existing minor-grade lesion. For this reason, CIN 2 and 3 lesions are commonly signaled by an internal line of demarcation separating a central area of significant colposcopic atypia from a much larger peripheral field of minor-grade acetowhitening (Fig 4–21).

If colposcopy is done with normal saline, virtually every lesion will have a vascular pattern; however, when tissues are soaked with acetic acid, the majority of CIN 3 lesions

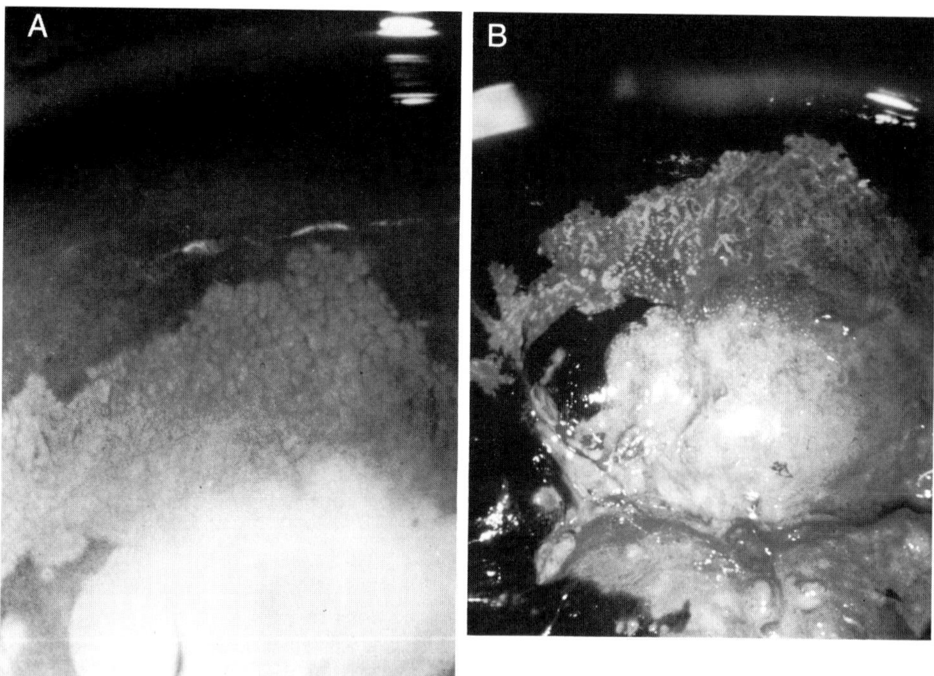


**FIG 4–21.**
**A,** two different grades of CIN. The peripheral area of CIN is characterized by a feathered peripheral margin, a shiny gray color and the presence of a fine mosaic pattern. Centrally, the focus of CIN 3 is distinguished by an internal demarcation between the minor-grade peripheral lesion and the central high- grade lesion (characterized by a dull oyster-white color and the absence of any surface capillaries). **B,** Lugol's iodine stain of the same lesion, showing that the internal demarcation remains visible. The peripheral lesion shows a partial uptake of iodine and the central area stained a characteristic mustard-yellow. (From Reid R, Stanhope CR, Herschman BR, et al: *Am J Obstet Gynecol* 1984; 149:815–823. Used by permission.)

are characterized by an absence of any vascular patterns (Fig 4–22), because of the constriction of these narrow vessels by the vinegar-induced swelling of the dysplastic epithelium. However, with increasing degree of premalignant change, these dilated capillaries become too robust for constriction by such epithelial swelling. Therefore, any vascular pattern found in a CIN 2–3 lesion will be coarse and dilated (see Table 4–3). Vertically oriented vessels are seen as an array of randomly directed, irregularly coiled, corkscrew-like structures (Fig 4–23). Likewise, dilatation of thin, uniform caliber, horizontal vessels will manifest as prominent, dilated channels separating the surface epithelium into a series of individual blocks (Fig 4–24). With increasing severity, combinations of punctation and mosaic structures often intermingle.

In very severe lesions, neovascularization results in the formation of horizontal vessels that demonstrate gross variation in caliber and course, and that show bizarre irregular branching patterns (Fig 4–25).[70] Those atypical vessels must be distinguished from punctation or mosaicism. Although characteristic of invasive cancer, atypical vessels are also seen in a proportion of preinvasive lesions (especially in CIN 3 bordering overt carcinoma).

## LABORATORY DIAGNOSIS OF HPV INFECTION

Human papillomaviruses are not readily detectable by the laboratory procedures used to diagnose most viral infections. No serologic tests are available, and the virus cannot be recovered through tissue culture. However, there are three direct methods of HPV detec-

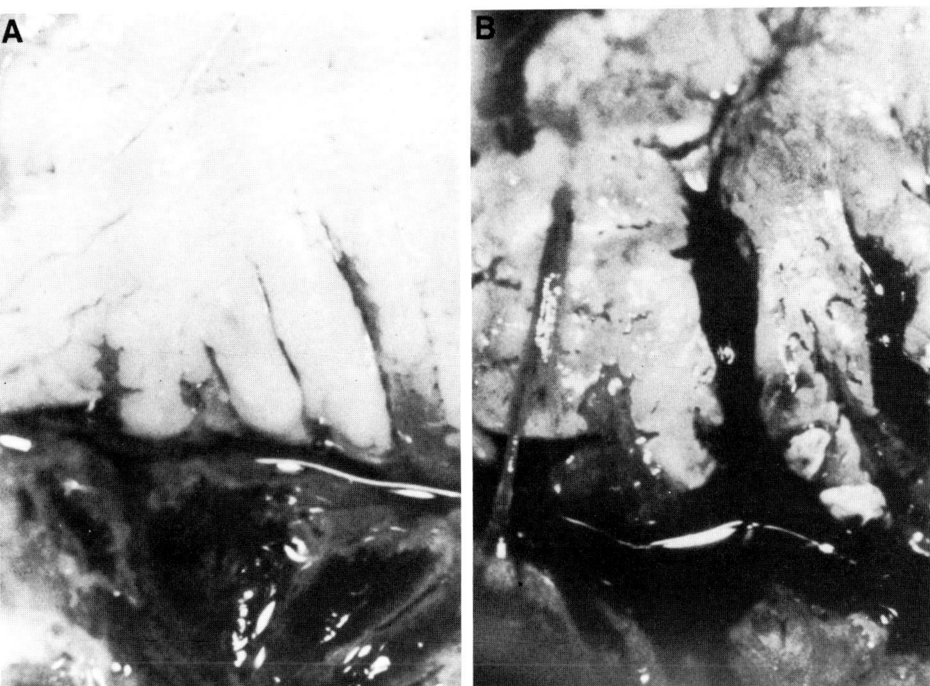


**FIG 4–22.**
**A,** high-grade cervical lesion characterized by a dull oyster-white color and the absence of surface vessels. **B,** An iodine staining of the same lesion showing the characteristic mustard-yellow discoloration.

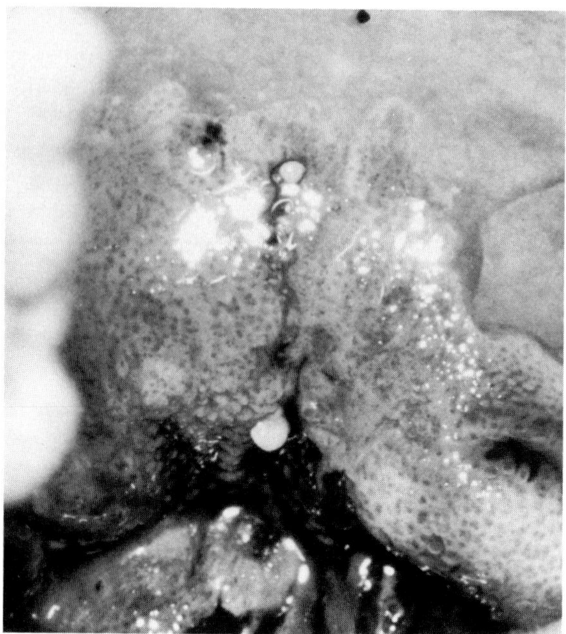

**FIG 4–23.**
A high-grade lesion with straight peripheral margins and the presence of coarse punctation throughout.

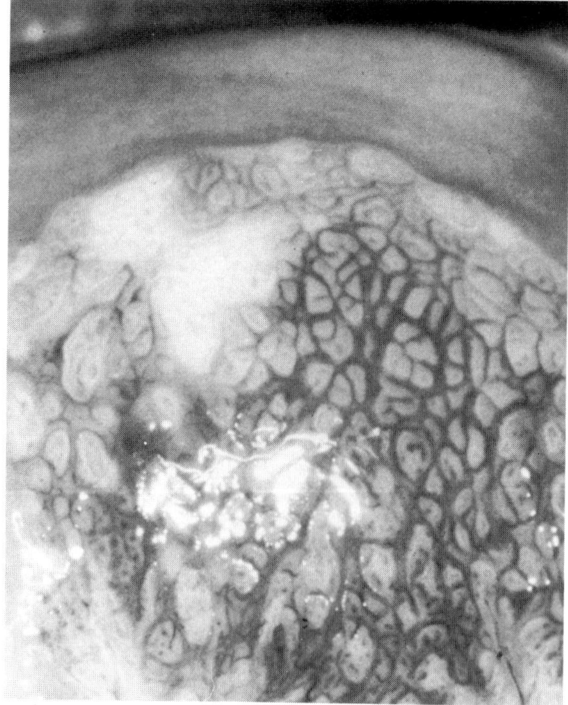

**FIG 4–24.**
A high-grade lesion showing a straight peripheral margin, dull white color, and a coarse mosaic pattern that occupies the entire anterior cervical lip.

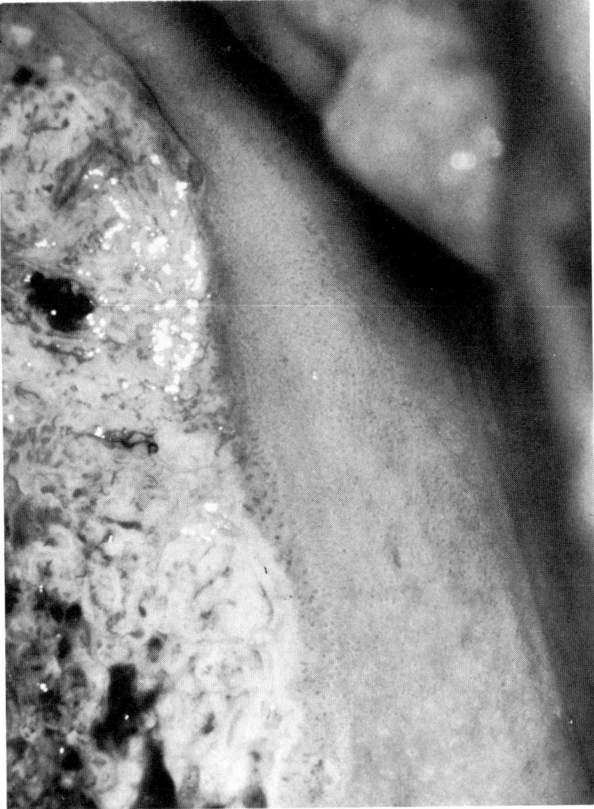

**FIG 4–25.**
Numerous horizontal vessels indicating the presence of early microinvasion.

tion: visualization of 55-nm particles by transmission electromicroscopy, immunocytochemical staining for viral structural proteins, and nucleic acid hybridization of viral DNA or RNA. Electromicroscopy[29] and immunocytochemistry[18, 19] are insensitive and impractical. Because virion assembly or capsid antigen production occur in only a small proportion of reproductive infections, such methods can do little more than confirm the relationship between HPV expression and obvious koilocytotic atypia.[21] Moreover, neither electronmicroscopy nor immunocytochemistry can differentiate one viral type from another.

Progress in this area of medicine has stemmed from a molecular biological technique called nucleic acid hybridization, which relies upon the re-annealing of a single-strand–labeled nucleic acid probe and any single-strand HPV DNA or RNA molecules within the sample. Hybridization tests are the only methods capable of detecting HPV genomes within neoplastic tissues and distinguishing between specific HPV types. These tests fall into one of two basic varieties: blot hybridization, in which the target is extracted cellular DNA fixed to a nylon filter; and in situ hybridization, in which the targets are HPV-infected nuclei within a standard, paraffin-fixed histologic section (Table 4–4). Specific methods are described below.[48]

## Southern Blot Hybridization

Although the Southern blot remains the gold standard against which other nucleic acid hybridization tests are compared, this method is expensive and laborious, and must

**TABLE 4–4.**
Different Patterns of Cell: Virus Interaction

| | Vegetative | Nonproductive |
|---|---|---|
| Viral genetic expression | Balanced transcription of early and late viral genes | Unopposed early gene transcription (especially E6 and E7) |
| Basic tissue effects | Basal proliferation, progressing to viral cytopathic effect in mid and upper layers | Increased division activity, acanthosis and reduced surface maturation |
| Dysplastic change | Absent or low grade | Mild to severe |
| Viral copy number | 50 to 200 copies per cell | 10 to 20 copies per cell |
| Physical state of viral genome | Episomal | May be integrated |
| Cellular genotype | Euploid (diploid or polyploid) | Often aneuploid |
| Clinical significance | Potentially infectious, but never premalignant | Rarely contagious, but potentially premalignant |
| Type-specific association | All HPV types (low greater than medium and high) | Predominantly high and medium risk HPVs |

be performed by highly qualified molecular biologists, rather than by laboratory technicians. Therefore, the main applications of Southern blots are for research and in quality control (Fig 4–26).

## Filter In Situ Hybridization

Filter in situ hybridization (FISH) is a now outmoded simplification of the Southern blot, in which cytological samples were applied directly to a target filter. Although simple and rapid, the FISH test had two fatal flaws. First, because of the irregular distribution of cellular material on the target filter, positive results often produced blotches, which were very hard to distinguish from artifact. Second, because the viral nucleic acids remained intermingled with cellular debris and mucus, false-positive results were common (Fig 4–27,A).

## Dot Blot Hybridization

The dot blot is a rapid, inexpensive method in which the target DNA is quickly purified prior to the hybridization stage. Properly performed, dot blots have about the same sensitivity and specificity as the Southern blot. Because samples are analyzed in batches and because the test can be done by a technician rather than a scientist, dot blot hybridization is sufficiently cost effective for routine clinical use. The biggest limitation of the dot blot is that this test cannot be done at low stringency to probe for related (rather than homologous) HPV types (Fig 4–27,B).

## In Situ Hybridization

In situ hybridization analyzes histological sections that have been glued to specially prepared glass slides. Because the target viral nucleic acids remain within the cell nuclei,

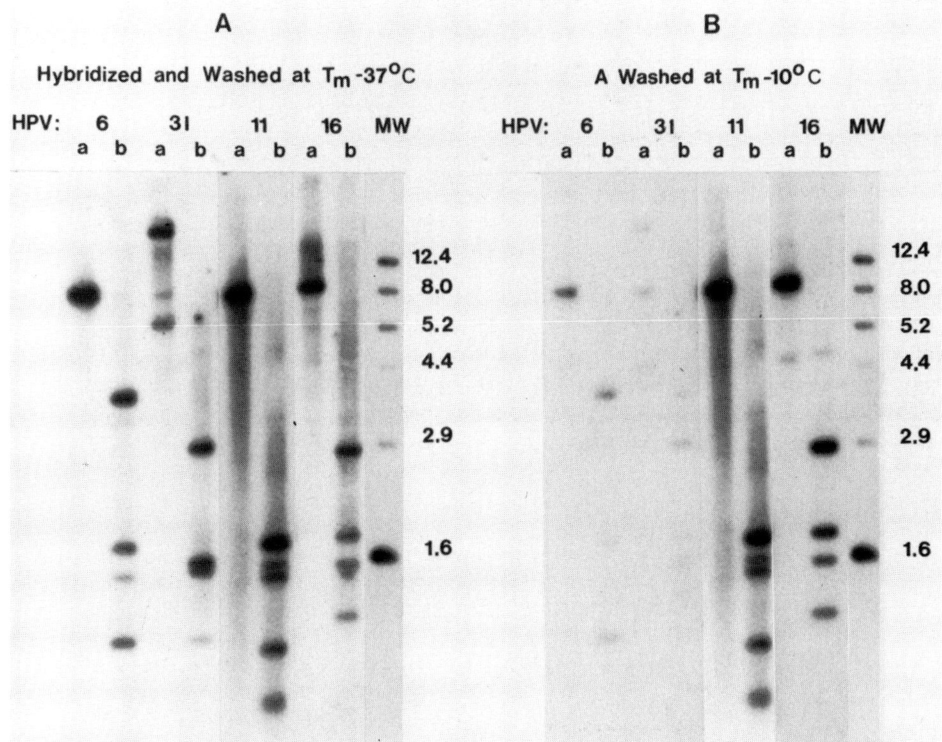


**FIG 4–26.**
**A,** two Southern blot analyses of the same four biopsies. Shows the effect of hybridization with probes HPV 11 and 16 at low stringency, such that the HPV 6 and 11 probes recognize areas of partial homology between the HPV 6 and 31 genomes. **B,** the hybridization was repeated at high stringency and significant bands are seen only within the 11 and 16 lanes because hybridization conditions will only allow hybrid formation between segments of high nucleotide homology. (From Lorincz AT: *Obstet Gynecol Clin North Am* 1987; 14:451–469. Used by permission.)

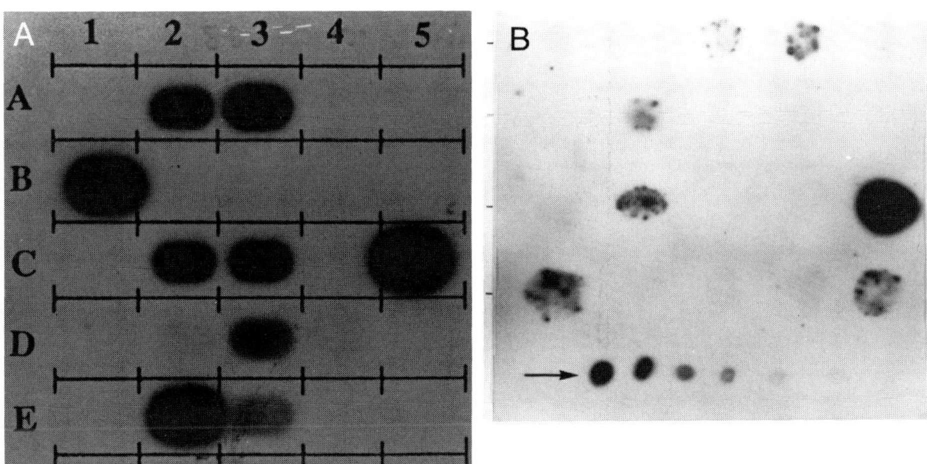


**FIG 4–27.**
**A,** a dot blot showing how easy these "clean" uniform dots are to interpret. **B,** a FISH blot showing how blotchy photographic shadows can be difficult to interpret.

test results are interpreted through the microscope by a qualified histopathologist (Fig 4–28). Herein lies both the strength and weakness of in situ hybridization. On the one hand, positive results provide information about the distribution of any HPV DNA within the affected tissue. However, because hybridization is done upon the whole cell (rather than upon extracted, purified cellular DNA), this method is plagued by insensitivity and a risk of false-positive results. Such problems are minimized by using RNA (rather than DNA) probes.[50]

### Polymerase Chain Reaction (PCR)

This is an exciting new method in which oligonucleotide primers and DNA polymerase are used to amplify characteristic portions of the target viral genomes.[75] Amplification to the order of $10^5$ is possible, but meticulous precautions must be taken against contamination so as not to generate spurious results.

## THERAPEUTIC PRINCIPLES

Notwithstanding the etiologic relationship between the sexually transmitted HPV infections and lower genital tract neoplasia, clinicians must remember that the occurrence of

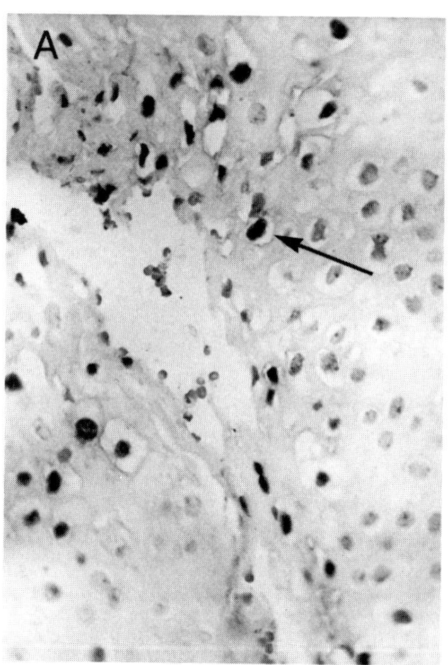


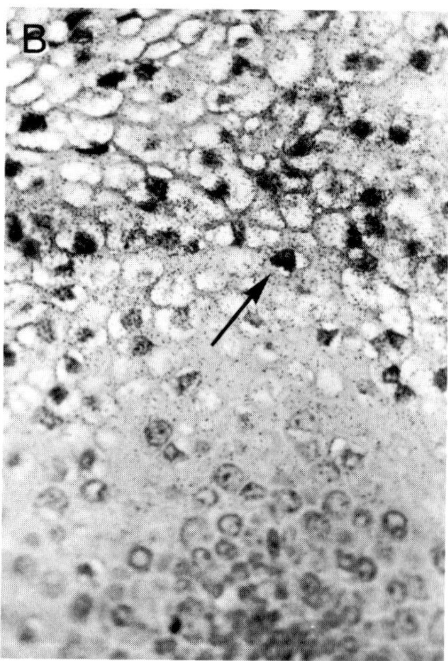


**FIG 4–28.**
In situ hybridization of a condyloma acuminatum with $^{35}S$ and biotin-labeled HPV 11 DNA shown under ×400 magnification. The tissue was sectioned on a microtome, and serial sections were taken for hybridization with various probes. **A,** $^{35}S$-labeled HPV 11 probe hybridized to a tissue section. Positive cells are indicated by the concentration of silver grains over the nuclei of many cells. Other cells exhibiting no silver grains presumably contain too few copies of viral DNA to generate positive signals. **B,** biotin-labeled HPV 11 probe hybridized to another section of the same lesion. Detection was by the alkaline phosphatase method. Cells containing HPV 11 DNA are indicated by the darkly staining nuclei. The *arrows* in both panels show cells positive for HPV DNA. Subsequent hybridizations of sections from these lesions with HPV 16 probes did not give any signals. (From Lorincz AT: *Obstet Gynecol Clin North Am* 1987; 14:451–469. Used by permission.)

carcinomas is both rare and predictable. Moreover, although oncogenic HPVs generally induce a "field infection," neoplastic sequelae within the stable squamous epithelia of the vagina and vulva are perhaps 100-fold less common than the risk of malignant progression within the metaplastic epithelium of the cervical transformation zone.[76, 77] For this reason, principles of management differ according to the anatomic sites affected. It clearly would be inappropriate to destroy the entire anogenital epithelium in every patient with an abnormal smear. Rather, the therapeutic objective is to ablate the transformation zone by the most conservative method possible and thereafter follow the patient for life. The treatment of most HPV-associated lesions of the vulva and vagina is undertaken primarily for sexually transmitted disease control, rather than as a prophylaxis against eventual gynecologic malignancy.

## Preinvasive Cervical Disease (High Grade and Low Grade)

The protocol for safe outpatient therapy of patients with abnormal cervical cytologic findings has three essential requirements.[72] First, the gynecologist must ensure that the "malignant cells" reported by the cytopathologist did not come from an actual cancer. Therefore, colposcopists must be sure of their ability to recognize any areas of invasive cancer present within the visible portion of the transformation zone. Second, the diagnostic conization is reserved for situations that extend out of colposcopic range and for patients in whom there is a genuine suspicion of occult invasive cancer. Provided that the new squamocolumnar junction is visible and the canal has been adequately assessed, final diagnosis can be safely inferred from the histologic findings in an adequate number of target biopsies. Third, provided that results from the target biopsies explain the changes reported by the cytopathologist, treatment is planned according to lesion topography rather than histologic grade. Therapy for carcinoma in situ is the same as that for mild dysplasia, with the majority of lesions being treated by destruction of the transformation zone under colposcopic control. In the small remainder of women requiring diagnostic conization, every effort is made to site the margins such that the operation will also be therapeutic.

The rationale of transformation zone ablation is best understood in terms of the "seed + soil" analogy, the seed being the HPV infection and the soil being the transformation zone. Since there are no conventional therapeutic measures for eradicating the seeds, treatment strategies revolve around efficient destruction of the soil.

Because tissue that is frozen to death is just as dead as tissue that is electrocuted, irradiated, or cut to death, it seems fatuous to argue that one modality would be significantly more effective than another.[77] In short, it is the mechanic, not the tool that is important. Poor success rates usually reflect errors of judgement—particularly failure to recognize the true extent of the disease. Hence, effective therapy depends more upon the physician's understanding of the transformation zone than upon the physical modality employed.[78]

Cervical neoplasia develops at the new squamocolumnar junction as this field of squamous metaplasia marches caudad with time. Conceptually, defining the proximal margin of the transformation zone is easy—it is the most cephalad extension of any squamous metaplasia (i.e., the proximal margin of the transformation zone is the point at which the reserve cell hyperplasia abuts a concentric ring of unaltered columnar epithelium).[79] Based upon their analysis of a series of autopsy specimens, Coppleson, Pixley, and Reid called this histologically definable margin the "new squamocolumnar junction".[70, 80] Thus, using the term in the way that it was originally intended, the transformation zone would be defined as a field of metaplastic epithelium lying between the original and new squamocolumnar junctions.

However, through common usage, "new squamocolumnar junction" has come to mean

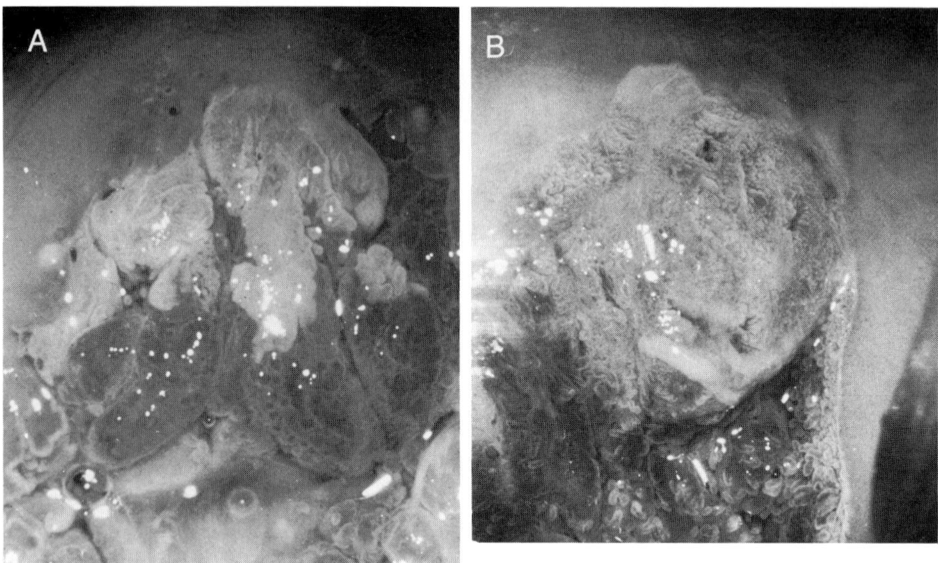


**FIG 4–29.**
**A,** an emerging area of squamous atypia seen at the new squamocolumnar junction. **B,** a "skip" area of acetowhitening near the external os. This represents a focus of adenocarcinoma in situ that is separated from and proximal to the new squamocolumnar junction.

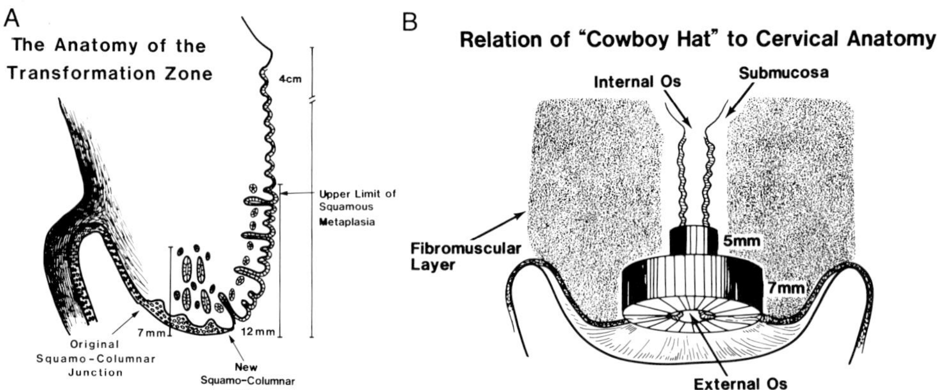


**FIG 4–30.**
**A,** the true anatomy of the transformation zone. The original squamocolumnar junction represents an embryologic boundary between an upgrowth of vaginal ectoderm and downgrowth of endocervical mesoderm. The original squamocolumnar junction denotes the distal margin of the transformation zone but its location in adults is camouflaged by the proximal migration of squamous metaplasia. The advancing edge of this new squamous epithelium is readily recognized through the colposcope. Many colposcopists erroneously believe that this new junction is the upper limit of the transformation zone. In reality, the new junction represents only a boundary between mature and immature metaplasia. The proximal border of the transformation zone is the upper limit of squamous metaplasia (the point at which immature squamous metaplasia abuts a circumferential ring of unaltered columnar epithelium). **B,** a diagram showing the volume of tissue that should be destroyed during transformation zone ablation. The peripheral disc has a vertical height of 7 mm and a lateral diameter that is set by the width of the lesion to be destroyed. The central cylinder has a lateral diameter of 1 cm (wide enough to encompass the cervical crypts of the canal epithelium) and a vertical height of 10 to 20 mm (high enough to reach the upper limit of squamous metaplasia). (From Reid R: *Obstet Gynecol Clin North Am* 1987; 14:513–535. Used by permission.)

a line visible through the colposcope (rather than through the light microscope). This colposcopic line describes the junction between mature cornified metaplastic squamous epithelium and less mature, non-cornified areas of reserve cell proliferation (see Fig 4–28). When disease expression assumes a squamous morphology, the advancing edge of this field of CIN will correspond to this colposcopic squamocolumnar junction (Fig 4–29,A). In contrast, should the HPV-infected progenitor cells express an adenocarcinomatous morphology, then the colposcopic squamocolumnar junction will represent the caudal border of any glandular atypia (Fig 4–29,B). An appreciation of what this colposcopic landmark really means (and what it does not mean) is the single most important element in the safe management of abnormal smears (Fig 4–30,A).[72, 77]

To ensure removal of all HPV-infected squamous metaplasia, it is preferable to destroy the transformation zone in a "cowboy hat" configuration,[78] rather than as a flat cylinder (Fig 4–30,B). The validity of this viewpoint is borne out by several observations. First, those who initially used the $CO_2$ laser to destroy just focal areas of acetowhite epithelium, rather than the entire transformation zone, reported failure rates approaching 50% by the second year of follow-up.[81] Second, surgeons who routinely treat the epithelium of the lower centimeter of the cervical canal have a primary success rate that is 10% to 15% higher than those who set the colposcopic new squamocolumnar junction as their upper limit of destruction.[77, 78] Third, treatment failures most commonly arise as an area of HPV-infected metaplasia within "rosebuds" of everted columnar epithelium near the external os.[82] Fourth, papillomaviral types 16 and 18 have been detected within biopsies of morphologically normal squamous metaplasia, taken just proximal to the colposcopic squamocolumnar junction in women with CIN 3.[10]

## Benign Vulvo-Vaginal Condylomas

Within just one decade, the carbon dioxide ($CO_2$) laser has become the modality of choice for treating anogenital condylomas; however, it should be emphasized that the great majority of patients can and should be managed by simpler therapies. Although sexually transmitted HPV infections are remarkably common, disease expression appears to be the exception rather than the rule. When disease expression does occur, differences in host susceptibility produce enormous variability in clinical outcome. Therefore, the use of the $CO_2$ laser for vaginal and vulvar disease must be approached with restraint.

Aggressiveness of treatment must be counterbalanced against the degree of disease expression in the individual patient. Because the majority of minor-grade acetowhite epithelia do not develop into either overt condylomas or dysplastic lesions, there are no grounds for treating such low-grade viral stigmata. Indeed, benign, asymptomatic, subclinical lesions of the vulva or vagina were detected in more than one-third of 1,200 Michigan women surveyed for the prevalence of HPV infection (R. Reid, unpublished data).

Even when disease expression does occur, exophytic condylomas represent just the "tip of the iceberg." Soaking with 3% to 6% acetic acid will usually produce prominent acetowhitening of skin that had appeared normal to naked eye examination (see Figs 4–2,A and 4–13). Nonetheless, clinical experience has taught that about 80% to 85% of patients will be cured by the destruction of just the macroscopically apparent papillomas.[32] If a caustic agent is to be used, 85% tricholoracetic acid is safer than 20% podophyllin resin.[83, 84] Likewise, if a destructive modality is preferred, either electrocautery or laser vaporization is more effective than cryosurgery.[85]

The 15% to 20% of women with extensive, refractory, or dysplastic lesions do present a management problem. Despite the unique physical properties of the $CO_2$ laser, using this instrument as a "spot welder" does nothing to solve the problem of the surrounding subclinical infection. Not surprisingly, a randomized trial comparing laser "spot welding" with electrodiathermy reported control rates of only 9 of 21 in the laser group and 8 of 22 in the diathermy group.[86] In contrast, using the laser to destroy all areas of colposcopically detectable papillomavirus infection produced remission in 156 (97%) of the 160 most difficult patients referred to the first author between 1983 and 1987.[87] In short, best results hinge upon wide, shallow ablation of the entire field of HPV infection, rather than upon deep destruction of resistant lesions.

## Vulvar Intraepithelial Neoplasia

Over the last decade, there has been a dramatic increase in the prevalence of vulvar intraepithelial neoplasia (VIN) in young women, particularly of the multifocal "bowenoid" variety.[14] Treatment of VIN is controversial, with recommendations ranging from wide excision to skinning vulvectomy. Although the treatment originally proposed for carcinoma in situ of the vulva was wide local excision, fears that the disease was preinvasive led to the widespread use of simple vulvectomy.[88] However, most documented instances of invasion have occurred in immunosuppressed or elderly women;[89] in young patients, the risk of malignant progression is insufficient to justify such multilating surgery. But recurrences following simple vulvectomy are common (Fig 4–31). Wide excision of small foci of VIN

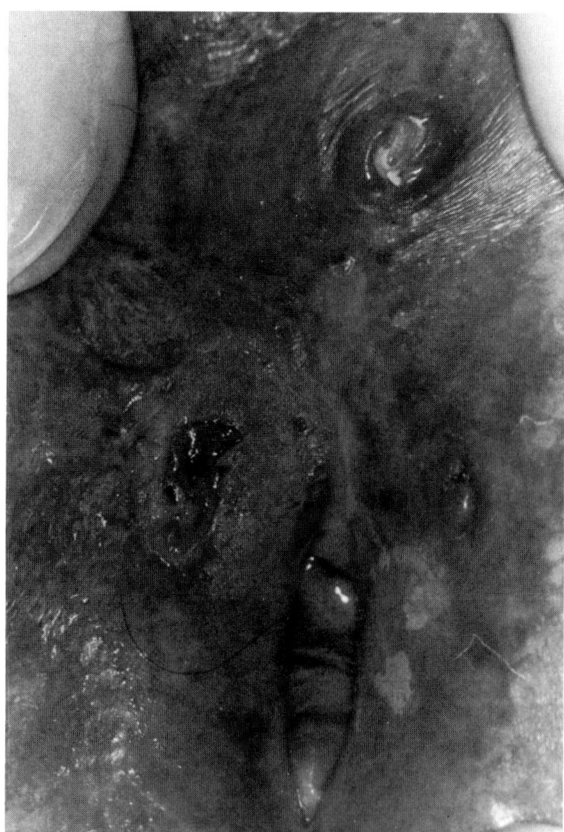

**FIG 4–31.**
Recurrence of VIN 3 at the margin of a previous simple vulvectomy.

yields excellent results, but multifocal or extensive lesions are difficult to treat by this method. In the past the only reasonable alternative was skinning vulvectomy with grafting.[90] Although a definite improvement over conventional vulvectomy, cosmetic and functional results are unpredictable. Fortunately, by providing an effective but nonmutilating treatment, the $CO_2$ laser offers an escape from this dilemma.

## Vaginal Intraepithelial Neoplasia

Vaginal intraepithelial neoplasia (VAIN) has also been seen with increasing frequency over the last decade. In contrast to premalignant changes of the vulva, VAIN has a well-defined potential for malignant progression. Indeed, about one-third of the invasive cancers following therapy for cervical neoplasia have occurred in the original squamous epithelium of the vaginal vault.[72] Because HPV-associated neoplasia within the lower genital tract does not affect tissues proximal to the upper limit of squamous metaplasia, removal of normal endometrium adds nothing to prophylaxis. In other words, not only does hysterectomy provide incomplete protection against subsequent cancer, but the operation complicates matters by burying islands of HPV-infected squamous epithelium beneath the scar.

Although the $CO_2$ laser is ideal for treating vaginal lesions when the uterus remains in situ, VAIN following hysterectomy often requires excision of the vault scar. In a series of 23 British women managed by laser vaporization of recurrent VAIN, Woodman et al. report that only six patients remained free of disease at 30 months after treatment.[91] Of the 21 women in whom VAIN 2-3 involved the vault scar, 3 developed invasive cancer in islands of buried vaginal epithelium. For this reason, ablation should be reserved for disease foci that can be seen in their entirety.

The basic objectives in the management of vulvar, vaginal, and perianal intraepithelial neoplasia (VIN, VAIN and PAIN) are:

1. To exclude occult cancer. When there is any suspicion of invasion, the pathologist must be provided with more than just a punch biopsy. Complex vaginal lesions, especially those involving the cuff of a prior hysterectomy, may need cold-knife excision and closure (as for an enterocele repair). In contrast, there is no place for "simple vulvectomy" when faced with complex external lesions. Rather the choice lies between wide excision and closure with rhomboid flaps (preferred method) versus "skinning vulvectomy" with split skin grafting (less satisfactory).

Invasion of less than 1 mm can be safely managed by observation alone. However, "superficially invasive" cancers of greater than 1 mm in depth carry a risk of potentially lethal nodal metastasis. Therefore, conservative therapy in this group means non-mutilative removal of the primary lesion, coupled with ipsilateral inguino-femoral lymphadenectomy.

2. To remove the preinvasive clones by the safest and most conservative method applicable to that individual. Most significant VIN and VAIN lesions are too mutlifocal for satisfactory treatment by wide excision. Laser ablation (using the principles explained below) is generally the best option, either alone or in combination with wide excision.

3. To prevent reactivation of the adjacent reservoir of subclinical and latent HPV infection. Clinical experience with local therapy for vaginal and vulvar lesions has shown that such patients are prone to diffuse recurrence during the succeeding years. The two strategies that help forestall such recurrences are the destruction of the adjacent areas of colposcopic acetowhitening and the use of an adjuvant agent in the postoperative period.

Unfortunately, topical 5-fluorouracil (5-FU) has not proven to be a statistically significant adjuvant (R. Reid, unpublished data). In contrast, topical 5-FU used to tolerance (usually twice weekly) is a very effective method for the office rescue of impending post-laser failure.

Preliminary experience with adjuvant systemic interferon has been very promising (R. Reid, unpublished data), and it is likely that this regimen may become a routine part of the management of difficult lower genital tract neoplasia.

## Idiopathic Vulvodynia

An illness possibly related to human papillomavirus and characterized by itching or burning of the vulva, plus intense tenderness around the vaginal opening, was recognized by gynecologists during the last 2 decades of the nineteenth century.[92] For mysterious reasons, this disease then disappeared from our society for the next 70 years, but since 1975, there has been a dramatic increase in the number of women who present with complaints of idiopathic vulvodynia.[93]

Indeed, suspected etiologic associations are similar in both variants of the vulvodynia syndrome. About 70% of affected women have a red-haired complexion and very sun-sensitive skin (R. Reid, unpublished data). In addition, morphologic findings (both through the colposcope and the light microscope) are suggestive of a low-grade HPV infection. As evidenced by the prominent vascular changes accompanying condylomas and intraepithelial neoplasia, HPV infection has a well-defined capacity for producing both epithelial and vascular proliferation. Although attempts to detect HPV DNA (by Southern blot hybridization) have been unsuccessful, there remain many as yet unclassified HPV types which do not hybridize with the existing panel of probes. Analysis with polymerase chain reaction

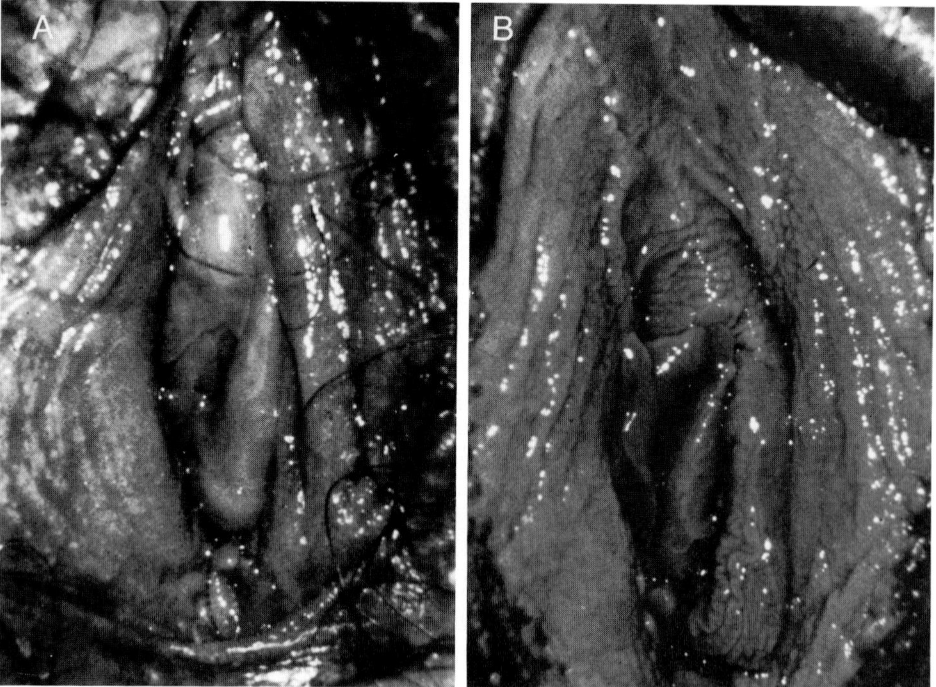


**FIG 4–32.**
A field of irritative acetowhite epithelium corresponding to the mildest component of the vulvodynia changes. **A,** before acetic acid. **B,** after acetic acid.

techniques will be necessary to answer this question. Until these data are available, the exact role of HPV infection will remain uncertain. Nonetheless, the most plausible hypothesis presently available is that vulvodynia represents a hypersensitivity syndrome, seemingly triggered by some as yet uncharacterized papillomaviruses of low pathogenic potential in women of susceptible skin type.

Physical examination has shown that this syndrome has three components:[94]

1. An irritative acetowhite reaction of the vulvar epithelium, seemingly attributable to chronic HPV infection (Fig 4–32). This irritative acetowhitening always involves the mucosa of the vestibule but also extends to the minimally keratinized, hairless skin of the interlabial grooves, clitoris, and perineum in about 50% of women.
2. Painful inflammation of the minor vestibular glands (embryologic remnants of the endothelial portion of the cloaca, which persists as shallow clefts located in the hymenal sulcus). In severe cases, this inflammation also involves the other structures derived from cloacal endothelium, namely, Skene's complex (shallow glands adjacent to the external urethral meatus) and the ducts of Bartholin's gland (two small orifices located just proximal to the mucocutaneous junction on the posteromedial surface of the labia minora) (Fig 4–33).
3. A vascular ectasia affecting the blood vessels of the entire connective tissue of the vulvar vestibule. Although most foci of painful erythema affect stroma that are immedi-

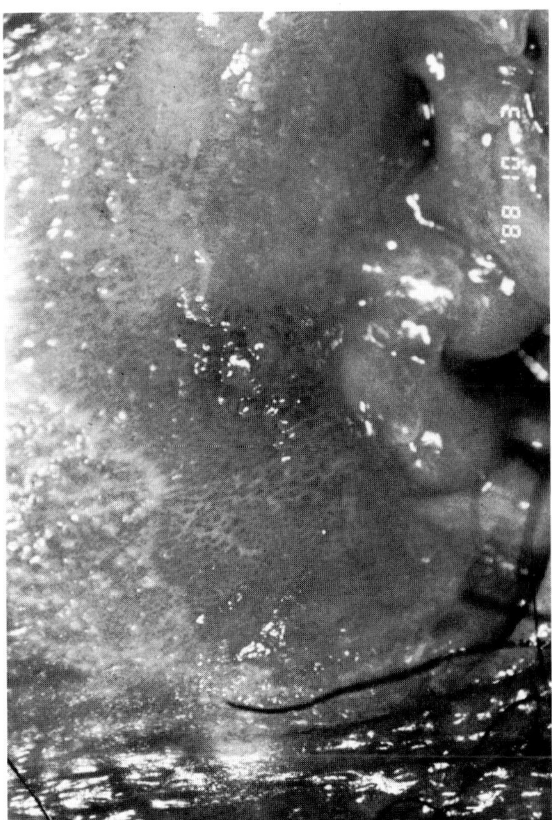

**FIG 4–33.**
Painful vestibular erythema, principally surrounding the minor vestibular and Skene's glands.

ately adjacent to vestibular gland epithelium, equally painful lesions can occur at other sites, as hyperemic telangiectatic vessels radiate to adjacent parts of the vestibule (Fig 4–34). These ectopic areas of painful erythema have proven to be more difficult to treat than initiating foci (those that surround the vestibular gland elements). In particular, such foci are aggravated (rather than relieved) by attempts at $CO_2$ laser photovaporization.

These three components are often associated, the first representing an earlier and milder manifestation and the other two denoting a more severe form of the syndrome. Although the surface papillomaviral infection will often respond to topical 5-fluorouracil cream, the inflammation surrounding the minor vestibular glands is refractory to anti-inflammatory medication, including topical or injected steroids. The standard therapy has been an operation described by Woodruff,[95] in which the posterior three-quarters of the hymenal ring (including the minor vestibular glands) is excised and the defect closed by downward advancement of the posterior vaginal wall.

Woodruff's procedure is unsatisfactory for three reasons.[93] First, excision of the minor vestibular glands cannot cure chronic burning discomfort that is caused by lateral extension of the HPV infection to involve the interlabial grooves or perineum. Second, even when hymenal resection is successful, the cosmetic results are somewhat dismaying. Although it is accepted that a cosmetic deformity may be preferable to a functional inability

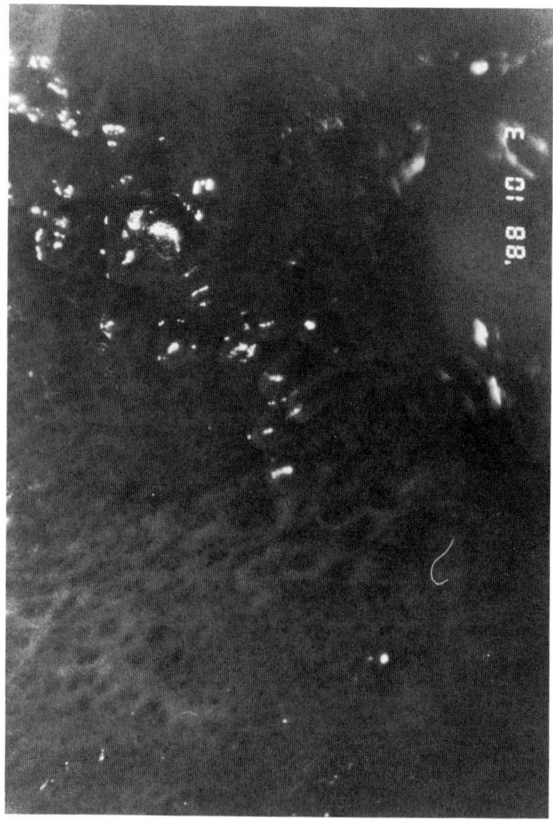

**FIG 4–34.**
Vascular ectasia affecting the dermis of the central vulva (rather than just the surrounding inflamed vestibular epithelium).

to have coitus, it is also clear that hymenal resection should be a treatment of last resort, rather than an initial surgical approach. Third, the success rate for hymenal resection is only about 50%. Moreover, the scarring induced by trying to approximate vaginal mucosa to perineal skin can exacerbate any incipient inflammation in the stroma surrounding Skene's and Bartholin's glands, sometimes resulting in a marked worsening of symptoms (Fig 4–35,A). Ectopic foci of painful erythema following previous surgery have usually proven difficult to treat.

Faced with patients who returned with postoperative inflammation of Skene's and Bartholin's glands, the first author has resorted to a wide re-excision of the original scar, plus an en block dissection of the periurethral tissue, Bartholin's ducts, and Bartholin's glands (Fig 4–35,A–C). Although generally successful, such surgery was technically difficult and produced just as much vulvo-vaginal deformity as Woodruff's operation (Fig 4–35,D).

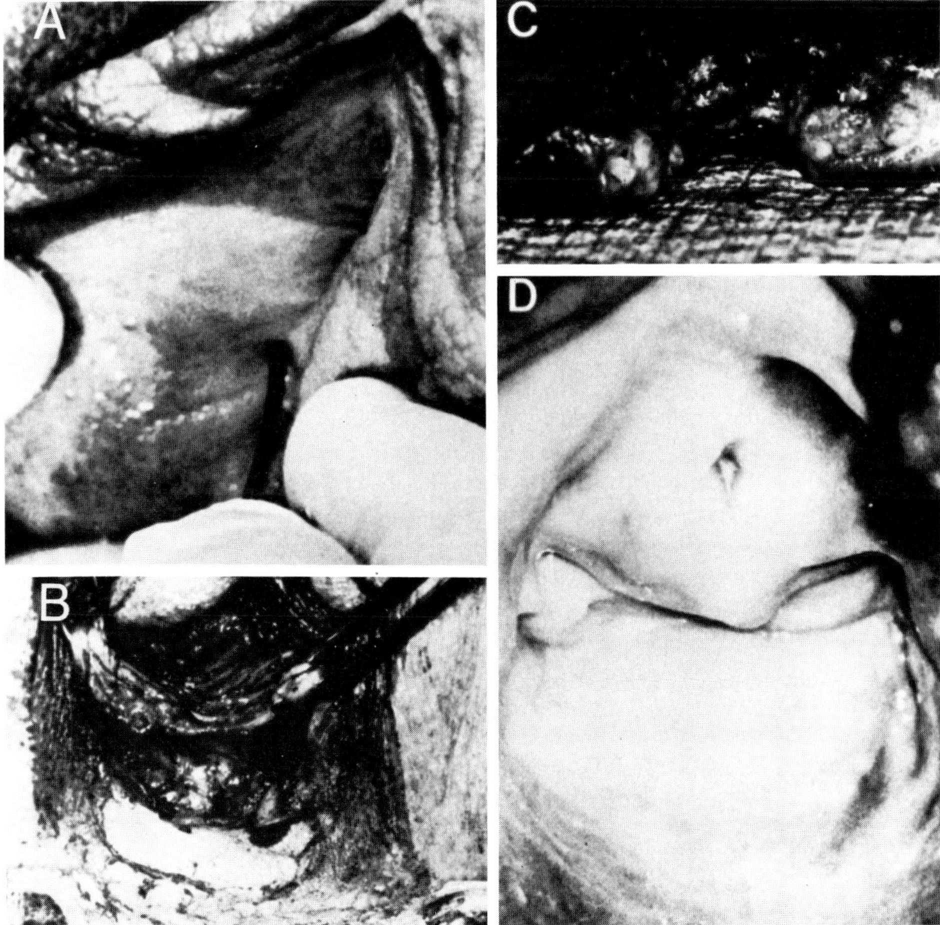


**FIG 4–35.**
**A,** cannulating a vestibular gland with a sialogram catheter prior to staining with 1% toluidine blue. Dissection confirmed that this structure was the duct of the right Bartholin's gland. **B,** en bloc dissection removed all the areas of toluidine blue staining. **C,** transected operative specimen showing deep downward extension of both the minor and major vestibular glands. **D,** end result showing removal of the hymenal ring and approximation of the vaginal mucosa to the perineal skin. (From Reid R, Greenberg M, Daoud Y, et al: *J Reprod Med 1988; 33:523–532. Used by permission.)*

Moreover, excising so much inflamed mucosa sacrifices a large portion of the vestibular epithelium.

We are currently investigating the use of both visible light and $CO_2$ lasers to achieve the same surgical objectives while avoiding disfigurement. Good results have been obtained from superficial $CO_2$ laser photovaporization of the irritative acetowhite epithelium and deep $CO_2$ laser photovaporization of inflamed vestibular glands. However, use of the $CO_2$ laser alone can trigger foci of ectopic erythema because of telangiectatic overgrowth of stromal blood vessels within the healing dermis (Plate 1,A). In the past some of these complications were cured by argon laser photocoagulation of these hyperemic vessels (Plate 1,B); however, because of the relatively poor affinity of blue-green light for oxyhemoglobin, use of the argon laser carries a risk of severe burning. Our present protocol employs a flash-pumped dye laser to produce selective photothermolysis of these target blood vessels.

## WHAT ADVANTAGES DOES THE $CO_2$ LASER OFFER?

Laser usage has expanded enormously over the last decade, particularly in treatments of the male and female genital tracts. Results are generally reported in glowing terms, and there is a widespread belief that surgical success is essentially guaranteed by the technical sophistication of the $CO_2$ laser. Unhappily, but not unexpectedly, such beliefs are ill-founded.

Certainly, because of the affinity of water for mid-infrared radiation, optical energy from the $CO_2$ laser has several unique surgical properties:[78] (1) diseased tissues can be vaporized under precise visual control; (2) heat propagation to adjacent tissue can be minimal; (3) microorganisms at the site will be automatically destroyed; and (4) vessels smaller than 0.5 mm will be thermally sealed. Unfortunately, these surgical advantages are easily dissipated by unskilled use.

The $CO_2$ laser resembles the hot cautery, the electrodiathermy, and the cryosurgical probe in that all are instruments of thermal destruction. With conventional devices, lateral heat propagation declines down a slow, linear gradient. Before the healing response can begin, adjacent tissues must recover from the ill-effects of a diffuse conduction burn or frostbite. In contrast, with skilled use of the laser, thermal injury to adjacent tissues can be confined within a very narrow and sharply defined band.

Unfortunately, it is not sufficiently appreciated that, unless strategies are employed to restrict heat conduction to adjacent tissues during photovaporization, the laser will produce the same kind of conduction burn as a hot cautery (Fig 4–36).[96] Several strategies for safe and effective laser surgery are outlined (these are explained in detail in reference 78).

### Strategies to Limit Lateral Heat Conduction

**Rapid Superpulse.**—Rapid superpulse is a major advance in laser technology and has two important features. First, laser energy is delivered in a series of high energy pulses, each with a peak power some 5 to 7 times higher than the output attainable in the continuous wave mode. Second, by keeping the pulse repetition rate low (below 300 pulses per second, 300 hertz), the surgeon allows enough time for thermal relaxation (wherein extra heat is radiated back into the air rather than being dispersed by conduction to adjacent tissues). Therefore, whenever possible, the laser should be used in the rapid superpulse temporal mode.

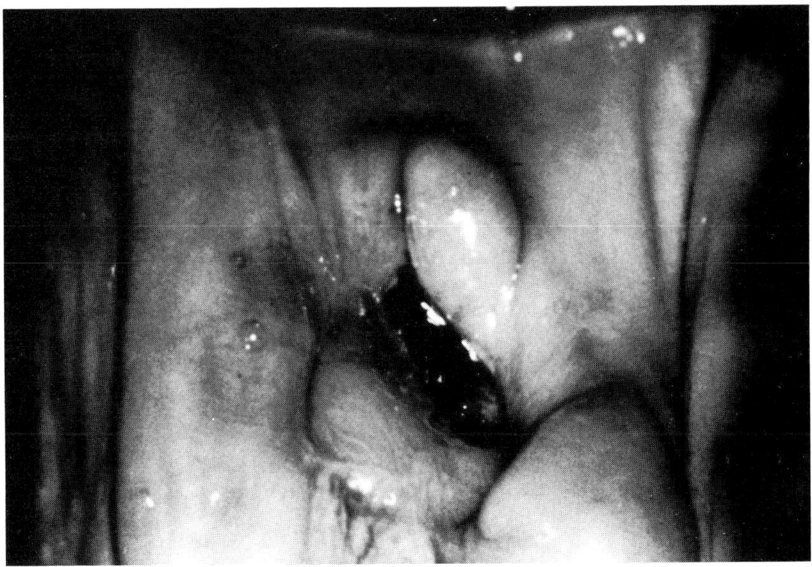

**FIG 4–36.**
A cervix that has been almost destroyed by unskilled low-power laser "ablative conization."

**High Power Outputs.**—To minimize the duration of any lateral heat conduction, the necessary energy dose should be delivered in the shortest possible time. Especially when using continuous wave, much better tissue effects will be obtained from high powers (80 to 100 watts) than from lower powers (less than 40 watts) with a spot size of 1.5 mm.

**Maintaining Average Power Density Above Carbonization Levels.**—Irrespective of power settings and temporal mode, average power density within the focal spot must be kept above the carbonization threshold (1000 watts/cm$^2$). Aside from causing excessive thermal damage, such slow rates of vaporization can cause steam formation within underlying blood vessels (the "popcorn effect"), thereby aerosolizing viable tissue fragments into the laser plume.[97, 98]

## Strategies to Aid Surgical Control

Surgeons must not try to control a laser by simply turning the power output down to a low setting, for low power outputs and low power densities will cause excessive thermal damage to adjacent tissues. Moreover, this is an ineffective strategy. Instead, the surgeon must utilize the physical principles that determine tissue interaction within the focal spot.

**Choice of a Comfortable Power Density.**—Power output (wattage emitted from the laser tube as it generates a "raw beam") is a quality-related variable, not a surgical control variable. Specifically, the *faster* the rate of energy supply, the *shorter* the duration of surgery. Hence, high power outputs will reduce the duration of any heat conduction to the skin appendages. This is crucial to vulvar surgery, because epithelial regeneration from the non-injured appendages is important for satisfactory healing. Surgeons who do extensive vulvar laser surgery at low powers (less than 40 watts of continuous wave) are in great danger of producing a third-degree burn.

Power density (effective power within the focused beam) is a surgical control strategy.

Provided that the surgeon keeps power density greater than 750 W/cm$^2$ (the level needed to avoid carbonization), then changing the power density will have no effect on the degree of non-specific thermal injury in the adjacent tissues.

The first author typically uses a power density of about 1,500 W/cm$^2$. But, as explained under the beam geometry section, the spot size is simply adjusted by turning the microslad until a comfortable point of defocus is reached. This point would have a spot size of about 1.5 mm for 40 watts and about 2.5 mm for 100 watts.

Speed of vaporization (and the speed at which the joystick or handpiece must be moved) depends upon the power density within the focal spot rather than upon the power output from the laser tube. Therefore, spot size must be titrated against power output to produce an operating speed comfortable to the individual surgeon.

**Choosing an Appropriate Beam Geometry.**—The energy profile of a laser beam is usually Gaussian (cone shaped). With this shape, the concept of an average power density does not mean very much. Surgeons must learn to think of beam geometry rather than spot size. Because the total energy within the focal spot remains constant for any given power setting, beam geometry will vary with the degree of focus. Because crater shape is a mirror image of the energy profile within the focal spot, thermal incision requires a tightly focused spot, while ablation always requires the beam to be defocused to a hemispherical geometry.

**Gated Pulsing Techniques.**—In delicate surgical situations, it is especially hazardous to turn the power down, because the increased thermal damage will nullify any potential advantage provided by the laser. Instead, the beam should be delivered in a series of 1/10- or 1/20-second bursts (usually by setting a mechanical timer on the laser console). This strategy allows ample surgical reaction time between each burst, thereby facilitating the use of high-power outputs for even the most intricate part of the operation.

## Other Surgical Strategies

As in other forms of surgery, success depends upon both sound theoretic principles and skilled operative technique. Besides selecting optimal physical parameters for each operation, the surgeon must also employ specific surgical strategies to ensure dexterous beam delivery, to minimize heat injury to adjacent tissues, to obtain hemostasis, to facilitate exposure, to delinate treatment margins, and to confine the depth of thermal denaturation to the desired level. The application of these principles to $CO_2$ laser surgery within the lower genital tract are fully discussed in reference 78. Only the techniques of depth control are reviewed in this chapter.

## Depth Control During Cervical and Vaginal Laser Surgery

Based upon measurements of the average depth of the cervical crypts,[99] most gynecologists destroy the transformation zone to a depth of 7 mm. The cylindrical nature of the resulting defect and the relatively large dimensions of the intended crater make it quite easy to control the depth of cervical ablation by actual measurement (see Fig 4–30,B).

Because there are no epithelial crypts beneath the original squamous epithelium, vaginal lesions should be destroyed only to the level of the lamina propria (less than 1 mm). The most reliable method of depth control is to laser until submucosal stromal fibers can be seen through the operating microscope.[100] In patients who present with positive Papanicolaou smears after hysterectomy, thought should be given to excising the top of the vagina to exclude occult invasion beneath the vault scar.[101] Of course, VAIN that does not involve the vault scar can be safely managed by laser ablation.[100]

## Depth Control During Vulvar Laser Surgery

Satisfactory healing of vulvar wounds depends upon the preservation of the skin appendages, a task that is too delicate to trust to crude measurement. The surgeon must learn to control depth according to the visual characteristics at the sites of impact.

From the surgical viewpoint, tissue destruction occurs through two distinct mechanisms: immediate photovaporization and delayed coagulation necrosis.[102] The depth of the photovaporization crater depends upon hand-eye control. In contrast, the thickness of the zone of coagulation necrosis is quite variable, depending upon laser settings. Surgeons who use *suboptimal* laser settings must understand that necrotic tissue on the wound surface will look normal at the time of surgery, only to separate as an eschar after activation of the host inflammatory response (i.e., when using low-powered continuous wave, any structures visible within the crater base will have already suffered irreversible thermal coagulation and will be sloughed off by the succeeding week). In contrast, with *optimal* settings, visual appearances correspond closely to the actual depth of destruction.

The art of expert $CO_2$ laser surgery is to judge crater depth such that the zone of thermal necrosis (rather than the zone of photovaporization) lies at the intended depth of penetration. Visual orientation is preserved by continuously wiping away the surface char.

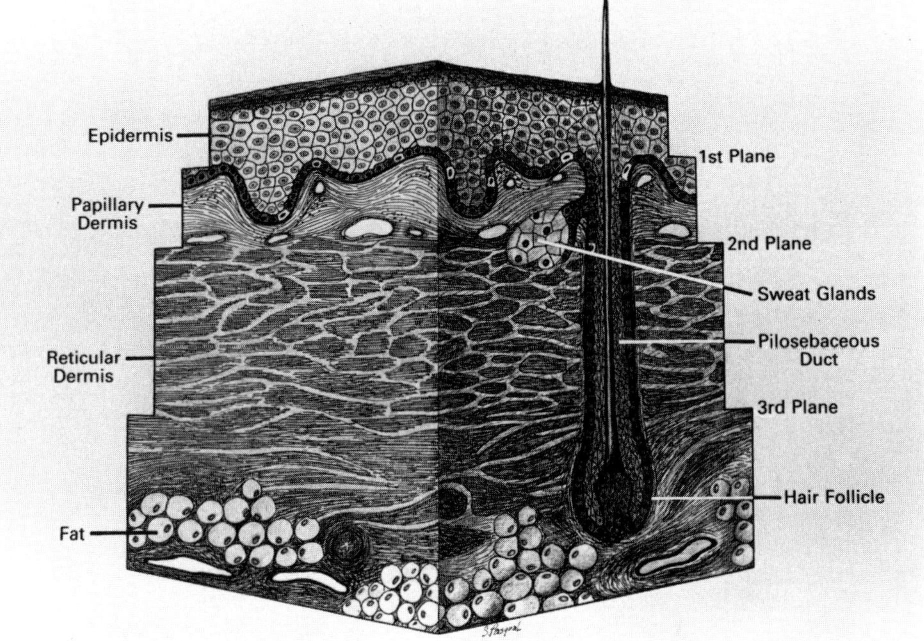


**FIG 4–37.**
A diagram depicting the first three surgical planes. Reading from surface to base, the points of reference for each plane are indicated as stepwise expansions. The first surgical plane corresponds to the basement membrane, the second to the papillary dermis, and the third to the midreticular dermis. (From Reid R: *Am J Obstet Gynecol* 1985; 152:505. Used by permission.)

Depth of destruction is inferred from anatomic landmarks in the crater base.[103] By means of this technique, four characteristic surgical planes[104] are identifiable (Fig 4–37).

**The First Surgical Plane.**—Destruction to the first plane removes only the surface epithelium to the level of the basement membrane. This plane is reached by limiting the laser crater to within the prickle cell layer. Penetration to the proper depth is accomplished by rapid oscillation of the micromanipulator, such that the helium:neon spot describes a roughly parallel series of lines. When done correctly, each pass of the laser beam will reveal bubbles of silver opalescence beneath the charred surface squames (Plate 2,A), and the maneuver will be accompanied by a distinctive crackling sound. Inadvertent penetration of the basement membrane is signaled by the loss of these two characteristic signs.

Lasing to the prickle cell layer shears the basal cells from the basement membrane, thereby producing a plane of cleavage. These detached basal cells are easily removed by wiping with moistened gauze, thus exposing the smooth, intact surface of the papillary dermis (Plate 2,B). Such wounds heal completely within 5 to 14 days, depending upon the temporal mode and power settings. The cosmetic appearance and functional qualities of the healed wound are entirely indistinguishable from normal vulvar skin.

**The Second Surgical Plane.**—Destruction to the second surgical plane will also remove the papillary dermis (the loose network of fine collagen and elastin fibers lying between the dermal papillae). This plane is reached by a similar set of rapid oscillations, moving the beam so quickly that the laser scorches (rather than craters) the exposed corium. When done correctly, the scorched surface should show a finely roughened contour and a yellowish color, somewhat reminiscent of a chamois cloth (Plate 3,A). This

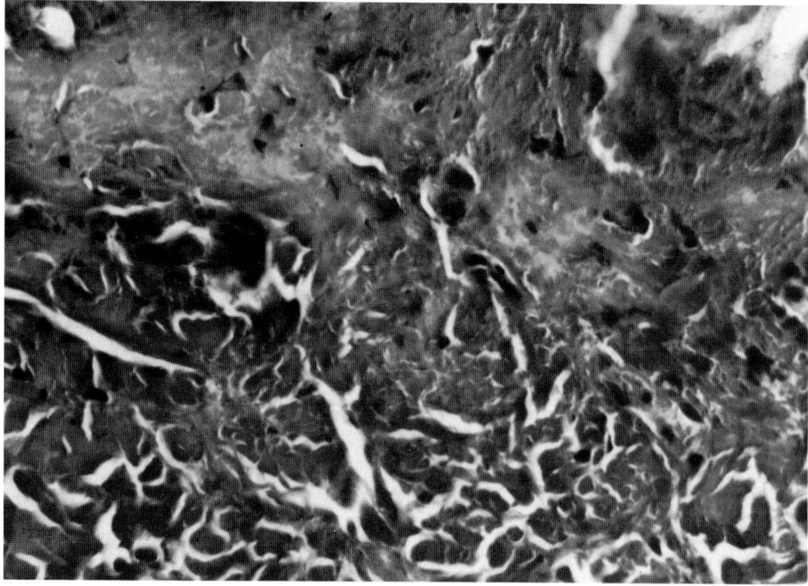

**FIG 4–38.**
The papillary dermis shows coagulation necrosis (top), but the reticular dermis is unaffected (bottom). (From Reid R, Elfont E, Zirkin R, et al: *Am J Obstet Gynecol* 1984; 152:268. Used by permission.)

clinical appearance indicates that the zone of coagulation necrosis will lie within the papillary dermis, with negligible thermal injury to the underlying reticular dermis (Fig 4–38). The second plane is the preferred level of ablation for extensive condylomas and symptomatic subclinical HPV infections. Such wounds heal rapidly and produce an end result indistinguishable from normal skin.

**The Third Surgical Plane.**—Vulvar intraepithelial neoplasia often extends into the pilosebaceous ducts (Fig 4–39). Involvement is generally limited to the superficial portions of the ducts, making laser ablation to the midreticular level (the third surgical plane) an ideal treatment in most instances. Nonetheless, intended depth of destruction should be individualized by examining representative histologic sections. Foci of deep pilar extension are rare; however, any areas of deep pilar extension must be managed by surgical excision, reserving the laser for the ablation of the adjoining superficial disease.

Destruction of the third surgical plane removes the epidermis, the upper portions of the pilosebaceous ducts, and a part of the reticular dermis. Ablation to the midreticular layer uncovers coarse collagen bundles that can be seen through the operating microscope as gray-white fibers resembling water-logged cotton threads (Plate 4,A). Wiping away the surface char will then reveal a pattern of starkly white collagen plates, interspersed by a horizontally oriented network of deep dermal vessels (Plate 4,B).

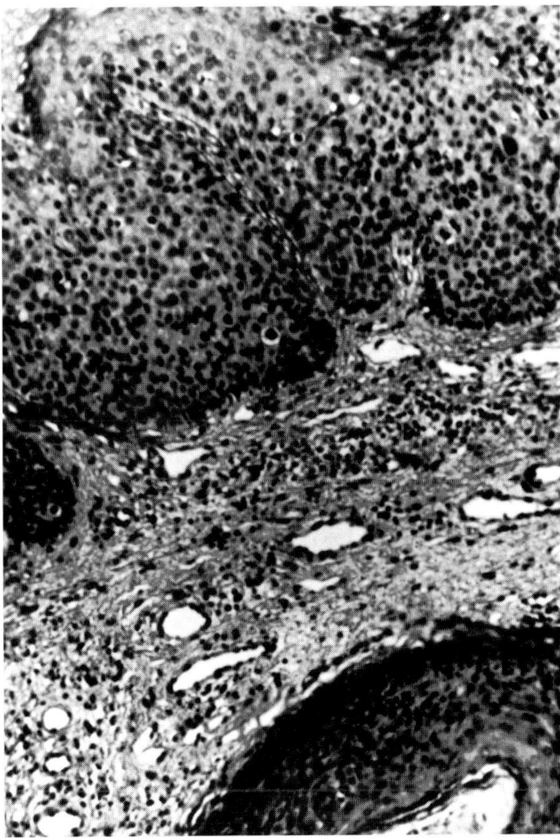

**FIG 4–39.**
A photomicrograph showing dysplastic cells replacing both the surface epithelium and the lining of a pilosebaceous duct.

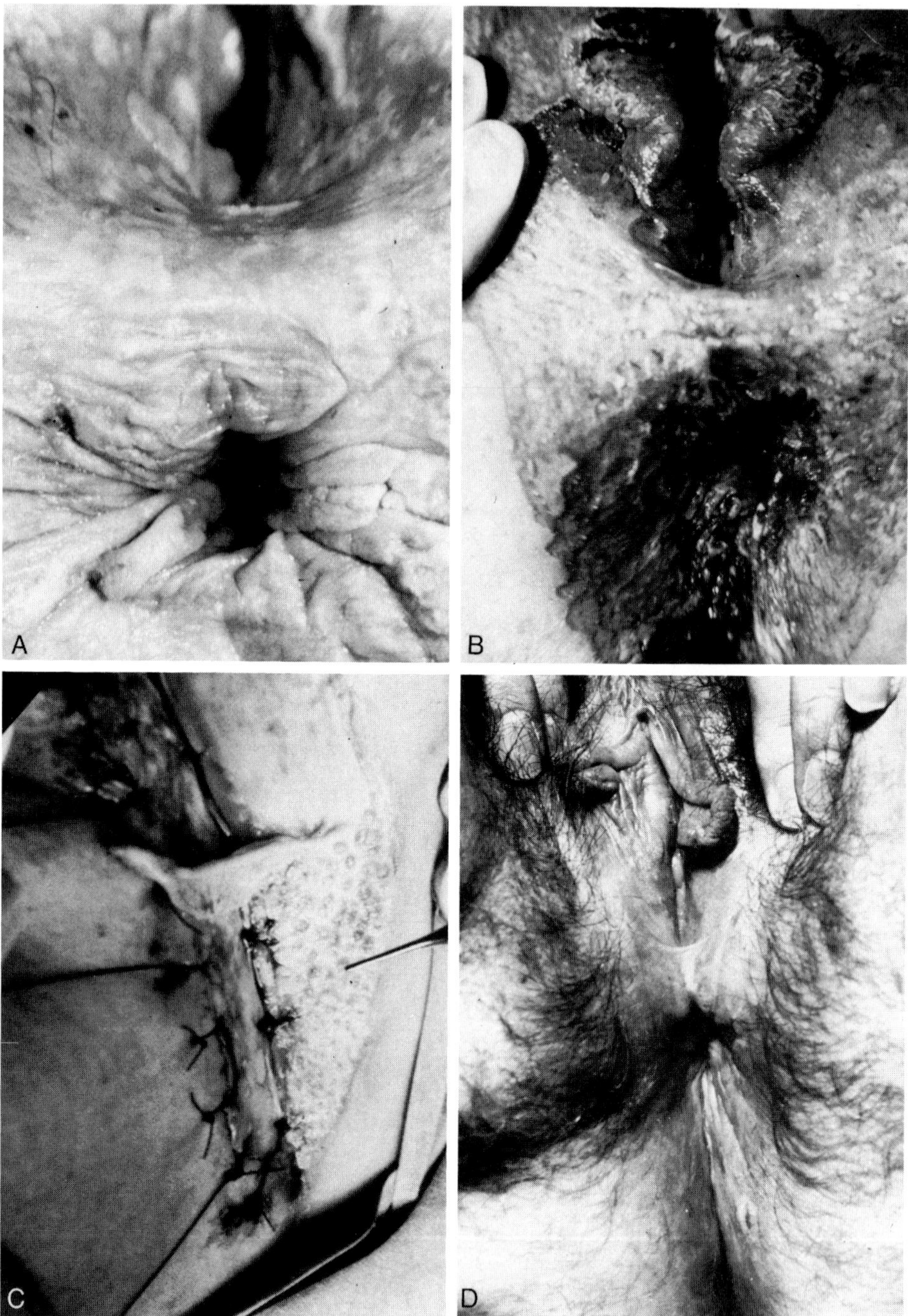


**FIG 4–40.**
The fourth surgical plane. **A,** an area of refractory perianal dysplasia that has failed three prior superficial laser vaporizations. **B,** vaporization of the perianal skin of the fourth plane. Each of the craters represents a site at which a skin appendage was destroyed, whereas the intervening areas represent viable collagen bundles within the deep part of the reticular dermis. **C,** the same area 10 days later, showing the extent of dermal regeneration at the time of skin grafting. **D,** the final result. (From Reid R: *Obstet Gynecol Clin North Am* 1987; 14:532. Used by permission.)

The third plane is reached by lasing the exposed corium with slow, deliberate movements of the beam. The speed of the cut is coordinated to the visual recognition of collagen bundles within the crater base. Moving the beam too rapidly will not expose these fibers, and moving the beam too slowly will uncover skin appendages within the deep reticular dermis. Such hair follicles and sweat glands are readily visible through the operating microscope, being seen as tiny refractile granules that resemble grains of sand. The rationale for limiting destruction to the third surgical plane is to allow the epithelium to regenerate from the keratinocytes within these skin appendages. Exposing these structures within the crater base signals the creation of a third-degree burn in that area. Thus, the third surgical plane represents the deepest level from which optimal healing will occur.

**The Fourth Surgical Plane.**—Under rare circumstances, it may be necessary to produce a deliberate third-degree burn to destroy abnormal keratinocytes within the hair follicles or sweat glands. Because of its precision, the $CO_2$ laser can destroy the adnexal epithelium while still preserving a layer of collagen fibers within the deep reticular dermis. Dermal regeneration produces a much better bed for skin grafting than either subcutaneous fat or granulation tissue. Hence, cosmetic and functional results are vastly superior to those attainable by skinning vulvectomy (Fig 4–40).

Although the physical principles governing the safe delivery of coherent radiation are well established, these rules are broken as often as they are followed. Of course, simply observing correct physical principles does not guarantee a successful outcome. Strategies are also required to ensure dexterous beam delivery and to oppose thermal injury to adjacent tissue. As in other forms of surgery, the gynecologist must learn how to control bleeding, to gain exposure, to delineate geographic margins, and to control the depth of destruction.

When these lessons are assimilated, $CO_2$ laser treatment of HPV-associated disease within the male or female genital tract will yield excellent success rates. Wounds will heal rapidly and the final result will be indistinguishable from untreated tissue. Patients who fail their initial therapy will usually respond to retreatment, especially if a preoperative antiviral regimen is prescribed.

## REFERENCES

1. Ciuffo G: Innesto positive con filtrado di verrucae volgare. *Giorn Ital Mal Venereol* 1907; 48:12–17.
2. Rous P, Beard JW: The progression to carcinoma of virus induced rabbit papilloma (Shope). *J Exp Med* 1944; 79:511–537.
3. Syverton JT: The pathogenesis of the rabbit papilloma-to-carcinoma sequence. *Ann NY Acad Sci* 1952; 54:1126.
4. zur Hausen H: Condylomata acuminata and human genital cancer. *Cancer Res* 1976; 36:794.
5. Purola E, Savia E: Cytology of gynecologic condyloma acuminatum. *Acta Cytol* 1977; 21:26.
6. Meisels A, Fortin R: Condylomatous lesions of the cervix and vagina. I. Cytologic patterns. *Acta Cytol* 1976; 20:505.
7. Laverty CR, Russell P, Hills E: The significance of non-condylomatous wart virus infection of the cervical transformation zone. A review with discussion of two cases. *Acta Cytol* 1978; 22:195.
8. Reid R, Stanhope CR, Herschman BR, et al: Genital warts and cervical cancer. I. Evidence of an association between subclinical papillomavirus infection and cervical malignancy. *Cancer* 1982; 50:377–387.

9. Durst M, Gissman L, Ikenberg H, et al: A new type of papillomaviral DNA from a cervical carcinoma and its prevalence in cancer biopsies from different geographic regions. *Proc Natl Acad Sci USA* 1983; 80:3812.
10. Reid R, Greenberg M, Jenson AB, et al: Sexually transmitted papillomaviral infections. I. The anatomic distribution and pathologic grade of neoplastic lesions associated with different viral types. *Am J Obstet Gynecol* 1987; 156:212–222.
11. Lorincz AT, Temple GF, Kurman RJ, et al: Oncogenic associations of specific human papillomavirus types with cervical neoplasia. *JNCI* 1987; 79:671–672.
12. Draper DJ, Cook GA: Changing patterns of cervical cancer roles. *Br Med J* 1983; 287:5109–5112.
13. Beral V, Booth M: Predictions of cervical cancer incidence and mortality in England and Wales. *Lancet* 1986; i:495.
14. Campion MJ, Singer A: Vulvar intraepithelial neoplasia: A clinical review. *Genitourin Med* 1987; 63:147–152.
15. Carmichael JA, Clarice DH, Moher D, et al: Cervical carcinoma in women aged 34 and younger. *Am J Obstet Gynecol* 1986; 154:264–269.
16. Broker TR: Structure and genetic expressions of papillomaviruses. *Obstet Gynecol Clin North Am* 1987; 14:329–348.
17. Reid R, Campion MJ: The biology and significance of human papillomavirus infections in the genital tract. *Yale J Biol Med* 1988; 61:307–325.
18. Jenson AB, Kurman RJ, Lancaster WD: Tissue effects of and host response to human papillomavirus infection. *Obstet Gynecol Clin North Am* 1987; 14:397–406.
19. Kurman RJ, Jenson AB, Lancaster WD: Papillomavirus infection of the cervix. II. Relationship to intraepithelial neoplasia based on the presence of specific viral structural proteins. *Am J Surg Pathol* 1983; 7:39.
20. Reid R, Crum CP, Herschman BR, et al: Genital warts and cervical cancer. III. Subclinical papillomaviral infection and cervical neoplasia are linked by a spectrum of continuous morphologic and biologic change. *Cancer* 1984; 53:943–953.
21. Lancaster WD, Jenson AB: Human papillomavirus infection and anogenital neoplasias: Speculations for the future. *Obstet Gynecol Clin North Am* 1987; 14:601–609.
22. Reid R: Human papillomaviral infection. The key to rational triage of cervical neoplasia. *Obstet Gynecol Clin North Am* 1987; 14:407–429.
23. Kurman RJ, Schiffman MH, Lancaster WD, et al: Human papillomavirus 18 in cervical cancer: A possible factor in rapid progression. *Am J Obstet Gynecol* 1988; 159:293–296.
24. Laverty CR, Stoler MA (In Preparation).
25. Pfister H: Relationship of papillomaviruses to anogenital cancer. *Obstet Gynecol Clin North Am* 1987; 14:349–361.
26. Jablonska S, Orth G: Epidermodysplasia verruciformis. *Clin Dermatol* 1985; 3:83–96.
27. Orth G: Detection of human papillomavirus type 5 DNA in skin cancers of an immunosuppressed renal allograft recipient. *Lancet* 1983; ii:422–424.
28. Oriel JD: Natural history of genital warts. *Br J Vener Dis* 1971; 47:1.
29. Reid R, Laverty CR, Coppleson M, et al: Noncondylomatous cervical wart virus infection. *Obstet Gynecol* 1980; 55:476–483.
30. Sillman FH, Sedlis A: Anogenital papillomavirus infection and neoplasia in immunodeficient women. *Obstet Gynecol Clin North Am* 1987; 14:537–558.
31. Chuang T, Perry HO, Kurland LT, et al: Condyloma acuminatum in Rochester, Minnesota, 1950–78. I. *Arch Dermatol* 1984; 120:469–475.
32. Bunney MH: *Viral Warts: Their Biology and Treatment*. New York, Oxford University Press, 1982.
33. Reid R: Superficial laser vulvectomy. I. The efficacy of extended superficial ablation for refractory and very extensive condylomas. *Am J Obstet Gynecol* 1985; 151:1047–1052.
34. Krebs HB: The use of topical 5-fluorouracil in the treatment of genital condylomas. *Obstet Gynecol Clin North Am* 1987; 14:559–568.

35. Mitchell H, Drake M, Medley G: Prospective evaluation of risk of cervical cancer after cytological evidence of human papillomavirus infection. *Lancet* 1986; i:573–575.
36. Evans AS, Monaghan JM: Spontaneous resolution of cervical warty dysplasia: The relevance of clinical and nuclear DNA features: A prospective study. *Br J Obstet Gynaecol* 1985; 92:165–169.
37. Campion MJ, McCance DJ, Cuzick J, et al: Progressive potential of mild cervical atypia: Prospective cytological and virological study. *Lancet* 1986; ii:237–249.
38. Richart RM, Barron BA: A follow-up study of patients with cervical neoplasia. *Am J Obstet Gynecol* 1969; 105:386–393.
39. Ferenczy A, Mitao M, Nagai N, et al: Latent papillomavirus and recurring warts. *N Engl J Med* 1985; 313:784–788.
40. zur Hausen H: Human papillomaviruses and their possible role in squamous cell carcinomas. *Curr Top Microbiol Immunol* 1977; 78:1–30.
41. Leads from the MMWR. Condylomas acuminata: United States 1966–81. *JAMA* 1983; 250:336.
42. Becker TM, Stone KM, Alexander ER: Genital human papillomavirus infection. A growing concern. *Obstet Gynecol Clin North Am* 1987; 14:389–396.
43. Meisels A, Morin C: Human papillomavirus and cancer of the uterine cervix. *Gynecol Oncol* 1981; 12:S111–S112.
44. Lorincz A, Temple G, Patterson JA, et al: Correlation of cellular atypia and HPV DNA sequences in exfoliated cells of the uterine cervix. *Obstet Gynecol* 1986; 68:508–512.
45. DeVilliers EM, Wagner D, Schneider A, et al: Human papillomavirus infection in women with and without cytologic signs of neoplasia. *Lancet* 1987; 2:703–706.
46. Reid R, Greenberg M, Lorincz A, et al: How common is cervical human papillomavirus infection? Presented at the Nineteenth Annual Meeting of the Society of Gynecologic Oncologists, Miami, Florida, February 1988.
47. Campion MJ: Clinical manifestations and natural history of genital human papillomavirus infection. *Obstet Gynecol Clin North Am* 1987; 14:363–388.
48. Lorincz AT: Detection of human papillomavirus infection by nucleic acid hybridization. *Obstet Gynecol Clin North Am* 1987; 14:451–469.
49. Reid R: Papillomavirus and cervical neoplasia. Modern implications and future prospects. *Colpo Gynecol Laser Surg* 1984; 1:3–34.
50. Stoler MH, Broker TR: In situ hybridization detection of human papillomavirus DNA and messenger RNA in genital condylomas and a cervical carcinoma. *Hum Pathol* 1986; 17:1250–1258.
51. Broker TR, Botchan M: Papillomaviruses: Retrospectives and prospectives. *Cancer Cells* 1986; 4:17–36.
52. Schwarz EH, Freese UK, Gissman L: Structure and transcription of HPV sequences in cervical cancer cells. *Nature* 1985; 314:111–114.
53. Kreider JW, Howett MK, Wolfe SA, et al: Morphological transformation in vivo of human uterine cervix with papillomavirus from condylomata acuminata. *Nature* 1985; 317:639.
54. Wettstein FO, Stevens JG: Variable-sized free episomes of Shope papillomavirus DNA are present in all non-virus-producing neoplasms and integrated episomes are detected in some. *Proc Natl Acad Sci USA* 1982; 79:790–794.
55. Yee C, Krishman-Hewlett I, Baker CC, et al: Presence and expression of human papilloma virus sequences in human cervical carcinoma cell lines. *Am J Pathol* 1985; 119:361–366.
56. Matlashewski G, Schneider J, Banks L, et al: Human papillomavirus type 16 DNA cooperates with activated ras in transforming primary cells. *EMBO J* 1987; 6:1741–1746.
57. Figge J, Smith TF: Cell-division sequence motif (L). *Nature* 1988; 334:109.
58. Vonka V, Kanka J, Jelinek J, et al: Prospective study on the relationship between cervical neoplasia and herpes simplex type-2 virus. I. Epidemiological characteristics. *Int J Cancer* 1984; 33:49.
59. Sasson IM, Haley NJ, Hoffman D, et al: Cigarette smoking and neoplasia of the uterine cervix: Smoke constituents in cervical mucus. *N Engl J Med* 1985; 312:315.

60. zur Hausen H: Herpes simplex virus in human genital cancer. *Int Rev Exp Pathol* 1983; 25:307.
61. Pfister H: Biology and biochemistry of papillomaviruses. *Rev Physiol Biochem Pharmacol* 1984; 99:111.
62. Sexually transmitted diseases: Extract from Annual Report of the Chief Medical Officer of the Department of Health and Social Security for the year 1983. *Genitourin Med* 1985; 61:204–207.
63. Rhatigan RM, Saffos RO: Condyloma acuminatum and squamous carcinoma of the vulva. *South Med J* 1977; 70:591.
64. Rastkar G, Okagaki T, Twiggs LB, et al: Early invasive and in situ warty carcinoma of the vulva. *Am J Obstet Gynecol* 1982; 143:814–820.
65. Gross G, Hagedorn M, Ikenberg H, et al: Bowenoid papulosis: Presence of human papillomavirus (HPV) structural antigens and HPV 16-related DNA sequences. *Arch Dermatol* 1985; 121:858–863.
66. Ikenberg H, Gissman L, Gross G, et al: Human papillomavirus type 16 DNA in genital Bowen's disease and in bowenoid papulosis. *Int J Cancer* 1983; 32:563–565.
67. Wharton LR: Rare tumors of the cervix of the uterus—condyloma and granuloma. *Surg Gynecol Obstet* 1921; 33:145.
68. Suran RR, Meister PC: Papilloma of the cervix uteri in pregnancy. *Am J Obstet Gynecol* 1948; 55:342.
69. Roy M, Meisels A, Fortier M, et al: Vaginal condylomata: A human papillomavirus infection. *Clin Obstet Gynecol* 1981; 24:461.
70. Coppleson M: Colposcopic features of papillomaviral infection and premalignancy in female lower genital tract. *Obstet Gynecol Clin North Am* 1987; 14:451–469.
71. Jenkins DJ, Tay SK, Campion MJ, et al: Histological and immunocytochemical study of cervical intraepithelial neoplasia associated with HPV 6 and HPV 16 infections. *J Clin Pathol* 1986; 39:1177–1180.
72. Reid R: Preinvasive neoplasia of the vagina and vulva, in Berek J, Hacker N (eds): *Practical Gynecologic Oncology*. Baltimore, Md, Williams & Wilkins, 1989, 195–239.
73. Reid R, Stanhope CR, Herschman BR, et al: Genital warts and cervical cancer. IV. A colposcopic index for differentiating subclinical papillomaviral infection from cervical intraepithelial neoplasia. *Am J Obstet Gynecol* 1984; 149:815–823.
74. Reid R, Scalzi P: Genital warts and cervical cancer. VII. An improved colposcopic index for differentiating benign papillomaviral infections from high grade cervical intraepithelial neoplasia. *Am J Obstet Gynecol* 1985; 153:611–618.
75. Shibata DK, Arnheim N, Martin WJ: Detection of human papillomavirus in paraffin embedded tissue using the polymerase chain reaction. *J Exp Med* 1988; 167:255–230.
76. Reid R; Symposium on cervical neoplasia. V. Carbon dioxide laser ablation. *Colpo Gynecol Laser Surg* 1985; 1:291–297.
77. Reid R, Atkinson K, Chanen W, et al: Symposium on cervical neoplasia. VI. Differing views. *Colpo Gynecol Laser Surg* 1985; 1:299–306.
78. Reid R: Physical and surgical principles governing expertise with the carbon dioxide laser. *Obstet Gynecol Clin North Am* 1987; 14:513–535.
79. Coppleson M: Cervical intraepithelial neoplasia: Clinical features and management, in Coppleson M (ed): *Gynecologic Oncology. Fundamental Principles and Clinical Practice*. Edinburgh, Churchill Livingstone, 1981, pp 404–433.
80. Coppleson M, Pixley EC, Reid BL: *Colposcopy: A Scientific and Practical Approach to the Cervix, Vagina and Vulva in Health and Disease*, ed 3. Springfield, Ill, Charles C. Thomas, 1986.
81. Burke L: The use of the carbon dioxide laser in the therapy of cervical intraepithelial neoplasia. *Am J Obstet Gynecol* 1982; 144:337.
82. Dorsey JH: Recurrent cervical and intraepithelial neoplasia (CIN) and the endocervical button. *Colpo Gynecol Laser Surg* 1984; 1:221–226.

83. Schwartz DB, Greenberg MD, Daoud Y, et al: The management of genital condylomas in pregnant women. *Obstet Gynecol Clin North Am* 1987; 14:589–599.
84. Rosemberg SK, Greenberg MD, Reid R: Sexually transmitted papillomaviral infection in men. *Obstet Gynecol Clin North Am* 1987; 14:495–512.
85. Simmons PD, Langlet F: Cryotherapy versus electrocautery in the treatment of genital warts. *Br J Vener Dis* 1981; 57:273–274.
86. Duus BR, Philipsen T, Christensen JD, et al: Refractory condyloma acuminata: A controlled clinical trial of carbon dioxide laser versus conventional surgical treatment. *Genitourin Med* 1985; 61:59–61.
87. Reid R, Greenberg MD, Daoud Y, et al: Superficial laser vulvectomy. IV. Strengths and limitations of aggressive surgical destruction. Proceedings of VII UCLA Symposium on Papillomaviruses. Taos, New Mexico, March 11–18, 1989.
88. Friedrich EG: Intraepithelial neoplasia of the vulva, In Coppleson M (ed): *Gynecologic Oncology. Fundamental Principles and Clinical Practice*. London, Churchill Livingstone, 1981, 303–344.
89. Buscema J, Woodruff JD, Parmley TH, et al: Carcinoma in situ of the vulva. *Obstet Gynecol* 1980; 55:225–230.
90. Rutledge F, Sinclair M: Treatment of intraepithelial carcinoma of the vulva by skin excision and graft. *Am J Obstet Gynecol* 1968; 102:806–815.
91. Woodman C, Jordan A, Wade-Evans T: The management of vaginal intraepithelial neoplasia after hysterectomy. *Br J Obstet Gynecol* 1984; 91:707.
92. Skene AJC: *Treatise on the Diseases of Women*. New York, D Appleton, 1889.
93. Friedrich EG, Jr: Vulvar vestibulitis syndrome. *J Reprod Med* 1987; 32:110.
94. Reid R, Greenberg MD, Daoud Y, et al: Colposcopic findings in women with vulvar pain syndromes. A preliminary report. *J Reprod Med* 1988; 33:523–532.
95. Woodruff JD, Parmley TH: Infection of the minor vestibular gland. *Obstet Gynecol* 1983; 62:609.
96. Reid R, Elson L, Absten G: A practical guide to laser safety. *Colpo Gynecol Laser Surg* 1986; 2:121–132.
97. Garden JM, O'Banion MK, Shelnitz LS, et al: Papillomaviruses in the vapor of carbon dioxide laser-treated verrucae. *JAMA* 1988; 26:1199–1202.
98. Baggish MS, Elbakry M: The effect of laser smoke on the lungs of rats. *Am J Obstet Gynecol* 1987; 156:1260–1265.
99. Anderson MC, Hartley RB: Cervical crypt involvement by intraepithelial neoplasia. *Obstet Gynecol* 1980; 55:546.
100. Dorsey JF, Baggish MS: Multifocal vaginal intraepithelial neoplasia with uterus in situ, in Sharp F, Jordan A (eds): *Gynaecological Laser Surgery*. Ithaca, New York, Perinatology Press, 1985, pp 173–179.
101. Sharp F, Jordan A (eds): *Gynaecological Laser Surgery*. Ithaca, New York, Perinatology Press, 1985.
102. Fuller TA: Laser tissue interaction: The influence of power density, in Baggish EM (ed): *Basic and Advanced Laser Surgery and Gynecology*. New York, Appleton-Century-Crofts, 1985, 51–60.
103. Reid R, Elfont EA, Zirkin RM, et al: Superficial laser vulvectomy. II. The anatomic and biophysical principles permitting accurate control over the depth of dermal destruction with the carbon dioxide laser. *Am J Obstet Gynecol* 1985; 152:261–271.
104. Reid R: Superficial laser vulvectomy. III. A new surgical technique for appendage-conserving ablation of refractory condylomas and vulvar intraepithelial neoplasia. *Am J Obstet Gynecol* 1985; 152:504–509.

Chapter 5

# Laser Therapy of the Vulva and Vagina

V. Cecil Wright, M.D.

Surgeons are traditionally trained to operate on the vulva in the appropriate tissue planes. However, with the new technology, finer dissection and more surgical precision are now possible. With the carbon dioxide laser, gynecologists can operate in the exact histological depth where a particular disease is located and spare more normal tissue. As a result, we are now re-evaluating some established procedures, such as cervical conization and simple vulvectomy, and comparing them with more precise and less radical laser procedures.

## VULVAR INTRAEPITHELIAL NEOPLASIA

Today vulvar intraepithelial neoplasia (VIN) is being identified more commonly in the young, reproductive-aged woman. Because many of these women have a history of vulvar viral infections, particularly involving the human papilloma virus, this has led investigators to suspect a cause and effect relationship.[1-4] VIN can develop on any area of the vulva, however, the majority of the lesions are on the non-hair-bearing parts. As many as 50% of the cases involve multifocal sites, many of which are confluent.[5]

Treatment by simple excision, simple vulvectomy, skinning vulvectomy, cryosurgery, and topical 5-fluorouracil have been disappointing.[5-8] Recurrence rates are also disappointing, comprising about 30% of cases after local excision and simple vulvectomy, and 39% of cases in which it is found at the margin after skinning vulvectomy. As many as 48% of the cases of multifocal disease recur.[5-8] Topical 5-fluorouracil is frequently too irritating for patients to complete the 4- to 6-week regimen.[8] Cryosurgery appears to offer little, and repeated surgical procedures often produce unsatisfactory and mutilating results.

### Lesion Locations

To best understand the topography and surgical approach to vulvar intraepithelial neoplasia, it is helpful to divide the vulva into hairy and non-hairy areas. The non-hairy areas include the clitoris, labia minora, inner surfaces of the labia majora, and the immediate perianal area. The hairy areas occur lateral, anterior, and posterior to these areas.

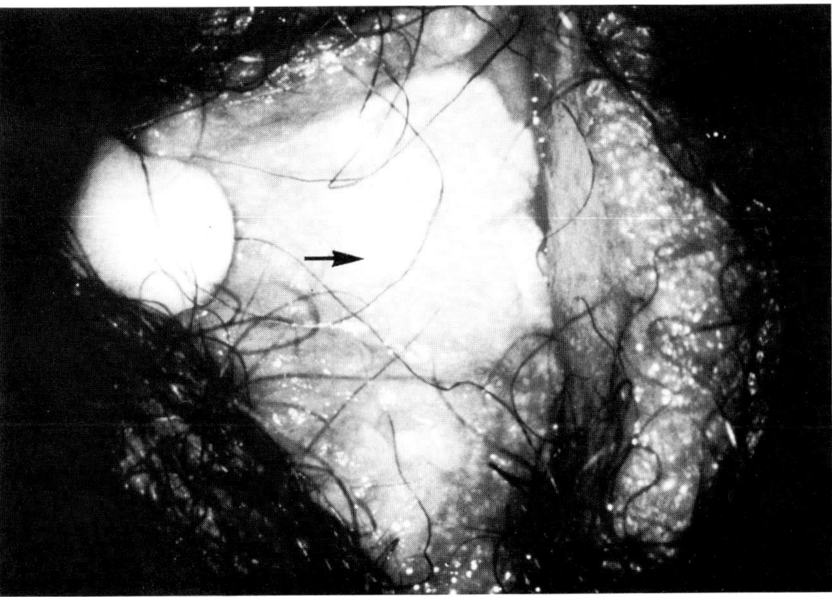

**FIG 5–1.**
This colpophotograph depicts a dense white lesion occupying the posterior two-thirds of the inner surface of the labia major (a non-hairy area). Biopsy confirmed VIN III disease. (From Wright VC, Lickrish GM (eds): *Basic and Advanced Colposcopy: A Practical Handbook.* Houston, Biomedical Communications, Inc, in press. Used by permission.)

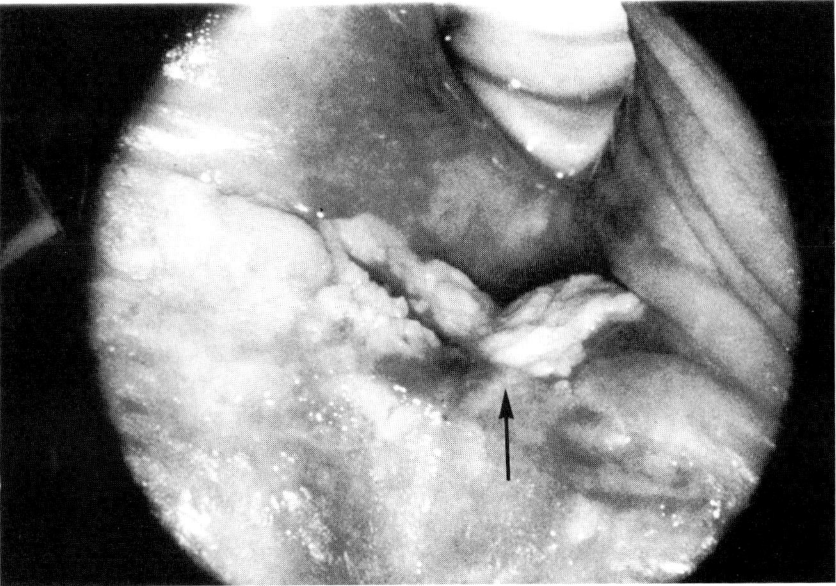

**FIG 5–2.**
VIN III lesions are frequently located at the posterior fourchette-perineal area. This is a typical well-demarcated, elevated lesion. The dense whiteness frequently reflects keratin, which is visible even before acetic acid application.

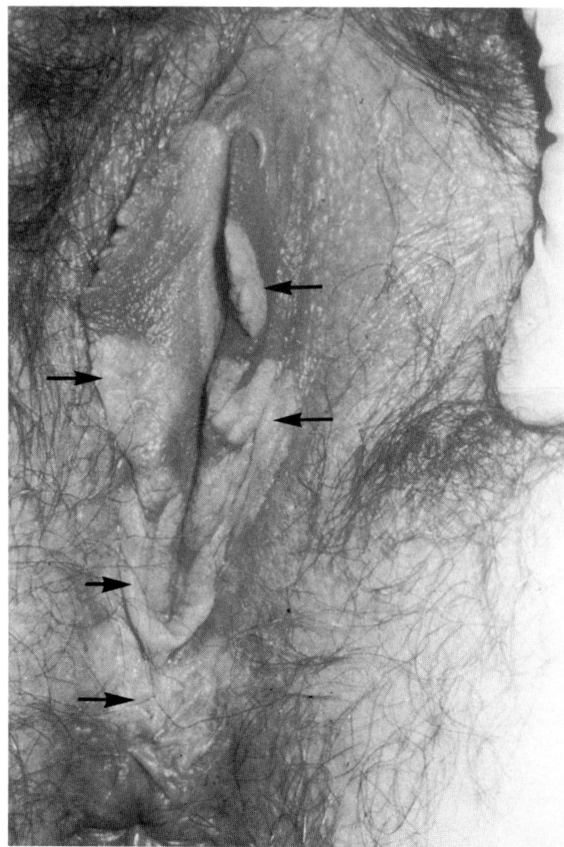

**FIG 5–3.**
Multifocal VIN can involve any site on the vulva (hairy or non-hairy). These white areas of VIN occupy mostly the non-hairy areas. Posteriorly, extension occurs to the perineum, a hairy area. (From Wright VC, Lickrish GM (eds): *Basic and Advanced Colposcopy: A Practical Handbook.* Houston, Biomedical Communications, Inc, in press. Used by permission.)

Approximately 75% to 85% of the VIN lesions occupy the non-hairy areas exclusively.[9] Among the non-hairy areas, the most common site of disease is the posterior two-thirds of the vulva (Fig 5–1). Lesions frequently extend onto the posterior fourchette and perineum (Fig 5–2). Although the majority of VIN cases demonstrate single lesions, as many as 30% to 40% are multifocal (Fig 5–3). Isolated areas of VIN in the hairy areas

**TABLE 5–1.**
Anatomical Distribution of VIN III (Severe Dysplasia and Carcinoma In Situ)

| Location | Number | Percent |
|---|---|---|
| Multifocal | 12 | 21.4 |
| Upper one-third only | 7 | 12.5 |
| Upper two-thirds only | 1 | 1.8 |
| Middle one-third only | 1 | 1.8 |
| Post one-third only | 23 | 41.1 |
| Post two-thirds only | 12 | 21.4 |
| Totals | 56 | 100.0 |

**TABLE 5–2.**
Distribution of VIN III According to Hairy and Non-hairy Areas

| Type Area | Number | Percent |
|---|---|---|
| Hairy areas only | 1 | 1.8 |
| Non-hairy areas only | 44 | 78.6 |
| Hairy and non-hairy areas | 11 | 19.6 |
| Total | 56 | 100.0 |

occur rarely. Table 5–1 demonstrates the anatomical distribution of VIN III (severe dysplasia, carcinoma in situ, or both) in 56 consecutive patients referred to the Abnormal Pap Smear Clinic at St. Joseph's Hospital, London, Ontario, during 1981 to 1987. The most common presentation involved the posterior one-third or two-thirds of the vulva (62.5% of cases). The VIN extended to the posterior fourchette with or without inclusion of the perineum in 41.1% of the cases. The clitoris and perianal areas were both involved in 7.1% of the cases.

Table 5–2 illustrates the VIN III distribution according to the hairy and non-hairy areas. The non-hairy areas accounted for 78.6% of the cases. It is unusual to find VIN III as an isolated lesion in the hairy area. Lesions found in the hairy areas usually represent a contiguous extension or reflect multifocal disease.

In the hairy sites, 7 of 12 cases (58.3%) had hair shaft extension of disease. The

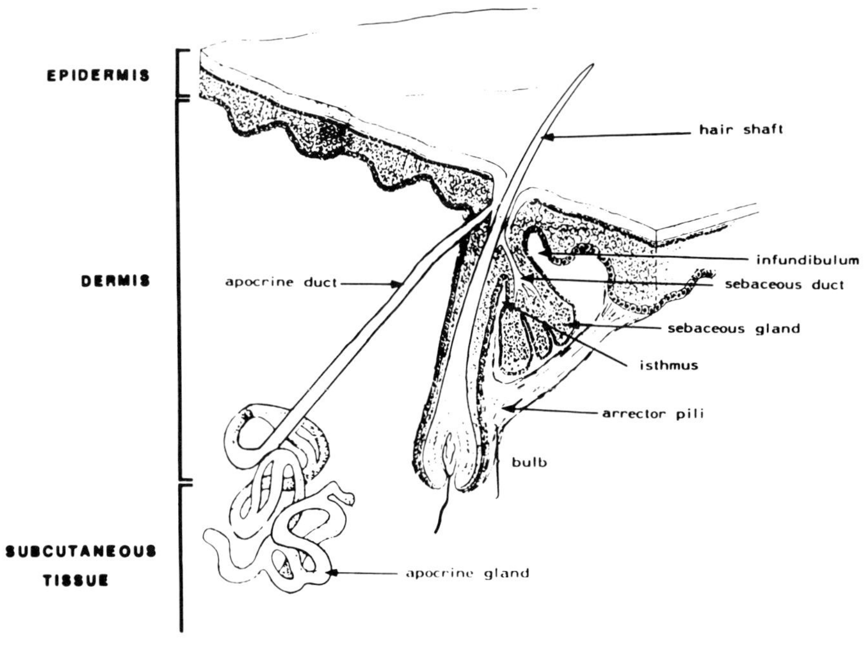


**FIG 5–4.**
Histological structural relationship of the sebaceous gland, hair follicle, and apocrine sweat gland. (From Wright VC, Riopelle MA: *Gynecologic Laser Surgery: A Practical Handbook.* Houston, Texas, Biomedical Communications, Inc, 1982. Used by permission.)

maximal extension was 2.7 mm down a hair shaft located in perianal VIN. The majority of hair shafts with VIN extension do not demonstrate disease beyond 1 mm.

## The Structure of Skin

To develop operative techniques for vulvar intraepithelial neoplasia, it is necessary to understand the structure of skin and its underlying appendages, for some of the latter structures are involved by disease extension to varying depths. The structures of concern are the external hair root sheath, the sebaceous gland and its duct, and the apocrine and eccrine glands and ducts (Figs 5–4 and 5–5). The external hair root sheath is a downward continuation of the epidermis. The squamous epithelium is stratified to the isthmus, including the entrance of the sebaceous duct, and produces keratin in the same manner as the vulvar skin surface. Below this level the sheath is not stratified and does not produce keratin. Because the upper parts of the hair root sheath and the lining of the sebaceous gland duct are contiguous with the surface epithelium and are not composed of similar cells, these areas are susceptible to extension of disease (Figs 5–4 and 5–5).[10] Involvement of hair root sheaths to depths up to 2.75 mm has been documented.[9,11] Involvement of the sebaceous duct, which is secondary to that of the sheath, occurs less often. The ducts of the eccrine and apocrine glands are lined by their own independent epithelium, which is not contiguous with the surface epithelium (see Figs 5–4 and 5–5). Because of this, these structures do not appear prone to exhibit VIN extension.

## Colposcopy of the Vulva

The colposcopic techniques and observations that one would employ on the cervix are also applicable to the vulva. Table 5–3 provides an outline for vulvar colposcopic exam-

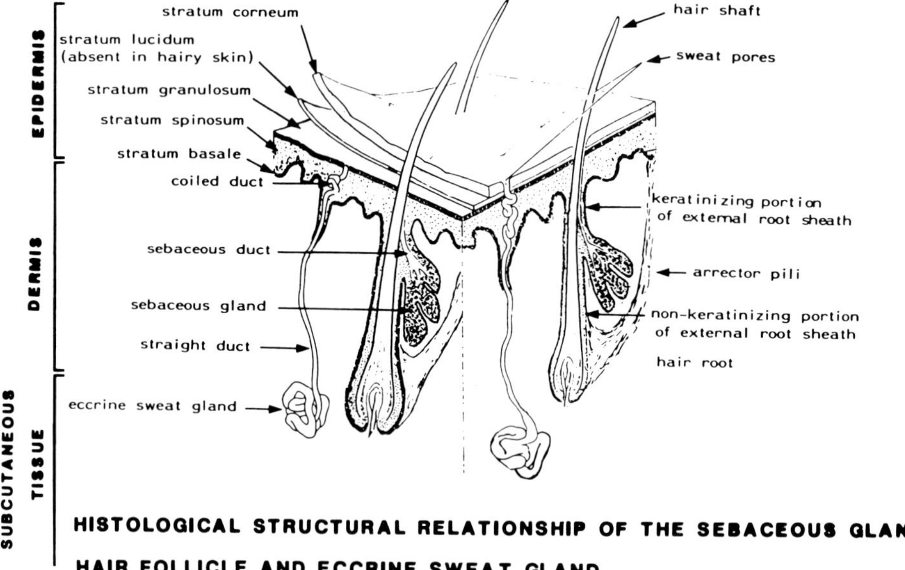


**FIG 5–5.**
Histological structural relationship of the sebaceous gland, hair follicle, and eccrine sweat gland. (From Wright VC, Riopelle MA: *Gynecologic Laser Surgery: A Practical Handbook.* Houston, Texas, Biomedical Communications, Inc, 1982. Used by permission.

**TABLE 5–3.**
VIN Diagnostic Procedures

| |
|---|
| Colposcope plus 2% to 3% acetic acid, or |
| Hand lens plus acetic acid |
| Nuclear staining with 1% Toluidine Blue |
| Careful magnification inspection |
| Entire vulva |
| Perianal skin |
| Anus |
| Anal canal |
| Vagina |
| Cervix |
| Adequate mapping and recording with colpophotograph or sketches |
| Tissue sampling by Keyes Dermatological Punch (4 to 6 mm size) or local scalpel excision |

ination. Observations should include color tone, surface pattern, lesion border, blood vessel patterns and intercapillary distance. However, the latter two points of evaluation are frequently lacking (i.e., blood vessel patterns and intercapillary distance).

The VIN lesions involving the hair portions of the vulva frequently appear well demarcated, elevated, and white even before the application of acetic acid and magnification. The whiteness is enhanced after acetic acid application. The higher-grade lesions usually have an irregular surface contour (Fig 5–6). Hair shafts can frequently be seen coming out of the lesion. Because of hyperkeratosis, colposcopic evaluation can be difficult indeed (Fig 5–7). If the lesions are large with hyperkeratosis, numerous biopsies or a complete excisional biopsy may be required to determine whether invasive disease is present (Figs 5–8 and 5–9).

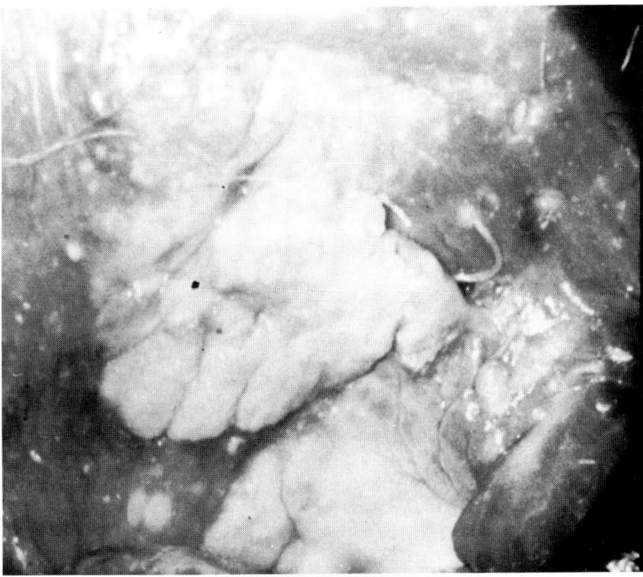

**FIG 5–6.**
VIN III lesions involving the hairy portions of the vulva appear well demarcated, elevated, and white even before acetic acid application. The hair shafts are seen within this lesion. The whiteness is enhanced after acetic acid application. (From Wright VC, Lickrish GM (eds): *Basic and Advanced Colposcopy: A Practical Handbook.* Houston, Biomedical Communications, Inc, in press. Used by permission.)

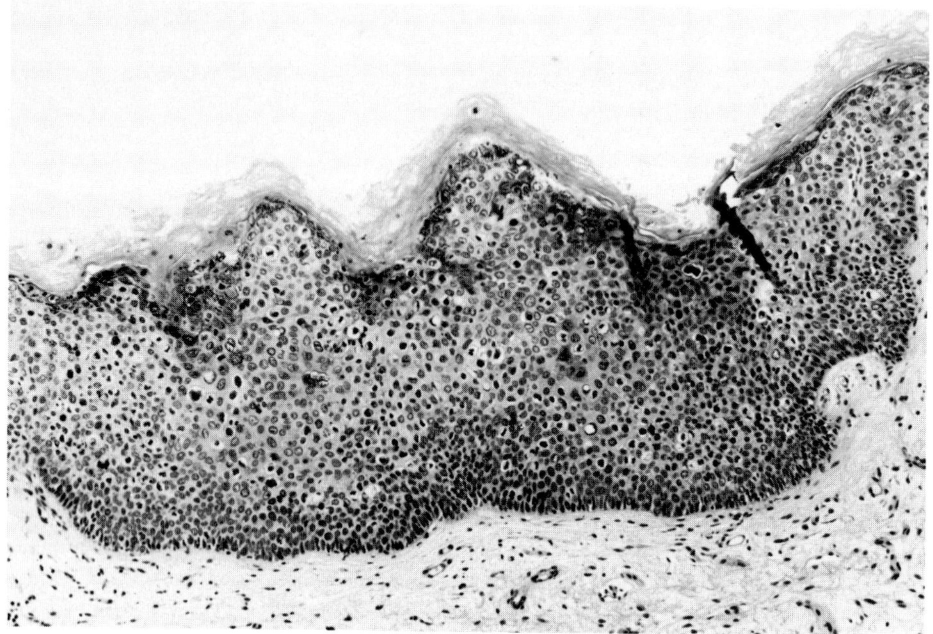

**FIG 5–7.**
Histology of carcinoma in situ of the vulva. Keratin is present on the surface. The average thickness of the epithelium including keratin is 0.46 mm. (From Wright VC, Lickrish GM (eds). *Basic and Advanced Colposcopy: A Practical Handbook.* Houston, Biomedical Communications, Inc, in press. Used by permission.)

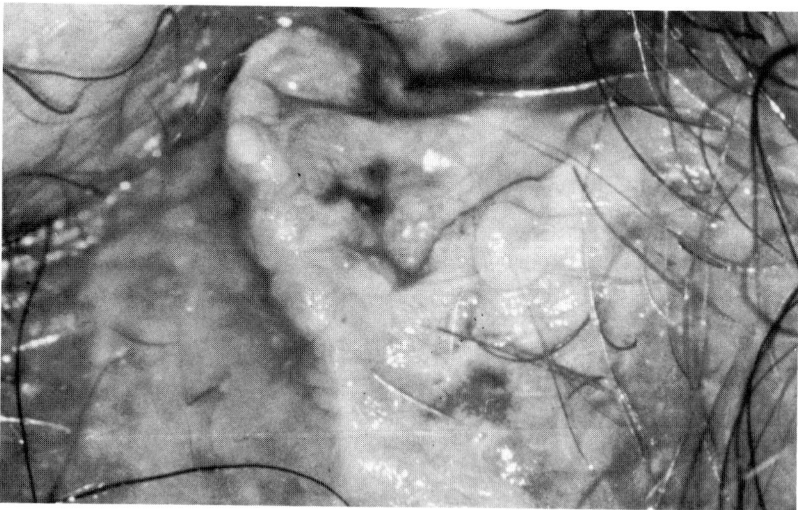

**FIG 5–8.**
A well-demarcated, elevated white lesion occupies the posterior fourchette and extends to the perineum. Colposcopy with biopsies may not rule out invasive cancer; therefore, with such hyperkeratotic surfaces, complete scalpel excision is advised. (From Wright VC, Lickrish GM (eds): *Basic and Advanced Colposcopy: A Practical Handbook.* Houston, Biomedical Communications, Inc, in press. Used by permission.).

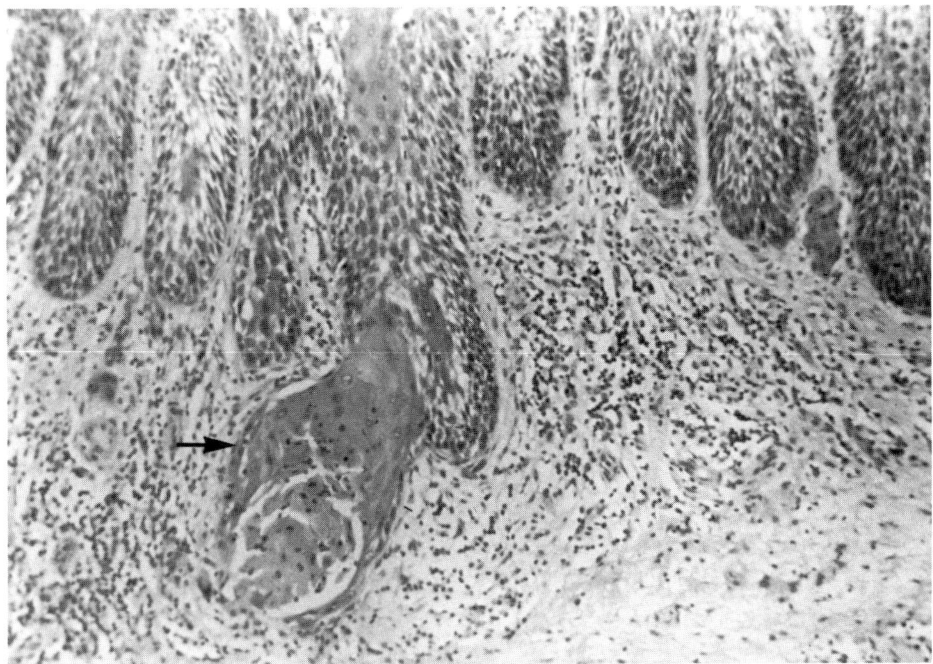

**FIG 5–9.**
This represents the histology of the clinical lesion depicted in Figure 5–8. Microinvasive cancer (indicated by the arrow) was found penetrating to a depth of 0.4 mm from the tip of the rete peg. (From Wright VC, Lickrish GM (eds): *Basic and Advanced Colposcopy: A Practical Handbook.* Houston, Biomedical Communications, Inc, in press. Used by permission.)

In the non-hairy areas, the color tone varies greatly after acetic acid application. The lesions occupying the mucous membrane are frequently macular and pink or red in color. The dense white irregular surface contours are not as prominent as a result of less keratin (see Figs 5–1 and 5–3). The lesions usually have a more poorly defined border than lesions in hairy areas (see Fig 5–6). On occasion, blood vessel patterns are seen.

Multicentric disease can involve any site on the vulva including the clitoral hood and perianal skin (see Figs 5–3 and 5–10). The highest percentage of multifocal disease occupies the non-hairy areas. It is unusual to see disease exclusively confined to hairy sites (see Table 5–2).

## Principles of Laser Surgery for Vulvar Intraepithelial Neoplasia

Because hair roots are absent in the non-hairy areas, it is unlikely that vulvar intraepithelial neoplasia will be deeper than the thickness of the diseased epidermis (less than 500 to 600 microns with keratin) (Fig 5–11). Therefore, laser vaporization for VIN occupying the non-hairy sites should be limited to vaporizing the epithelial thickness only. This results in a histological depth of less than 1 mm and allows preservation of very important anatomical structures such as the labia and the clitoris. Some heat conduction will extend the injury into the underlying superficial dermis; however, underlying tissue necrosis should be less than 100 microns with a limited duration of exposure. This heat conduction turns the papillary dermis a light tan color, which can be recognized by gently washing off any carbon particles. It is not difficult to identify this histological tissue plane with

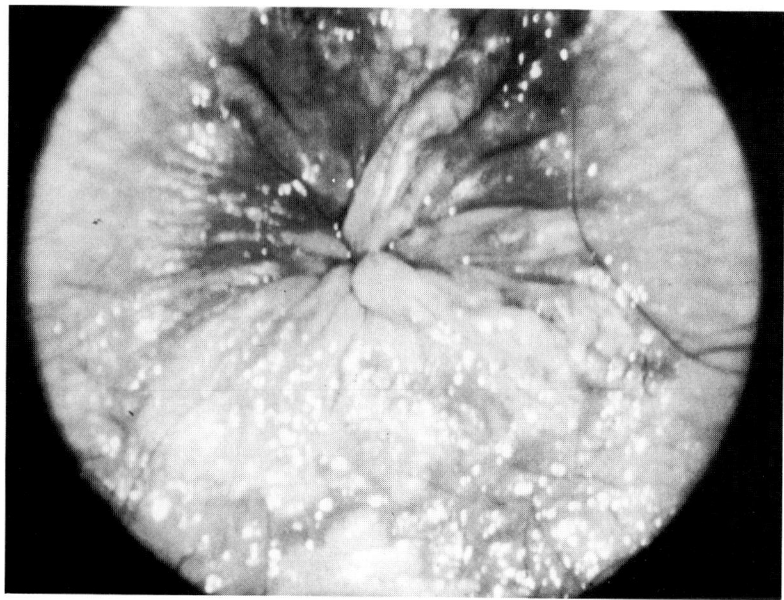

**FIG 5–10.**
Perianal VIN III is illustrated. This primarily occupies the perimucosal tissue. The disease appears white after acetic acid application. Its boundaries are identified with a 3.5× magnification. (From Wright VC, Lickrish GM (eds): *Basic and Advanced Colposcopy: A Practical Handbook.* Houston, Biomedical Communications, Inc, in press. Used by permission.)

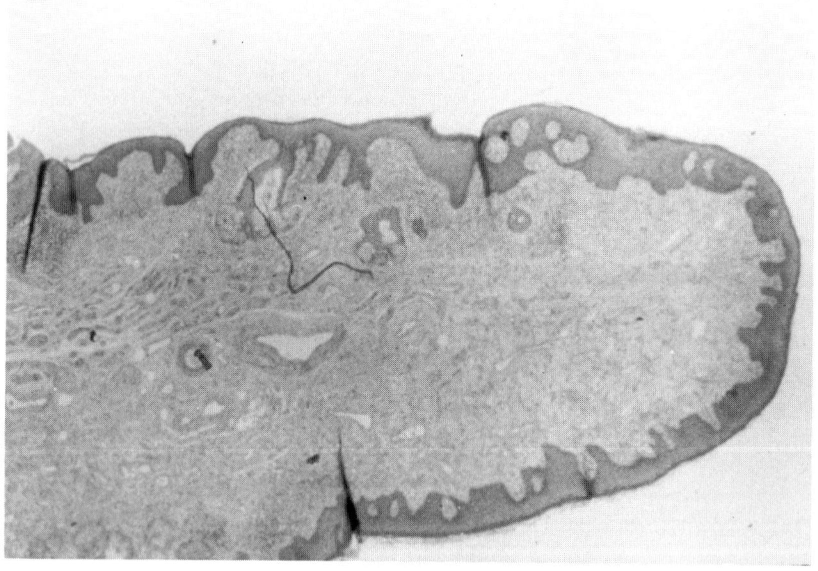

**FIG 5–11.**
Carcinoma in situ involving the tip of a labia minora. The epithelial thickness measures 0.35 mm.

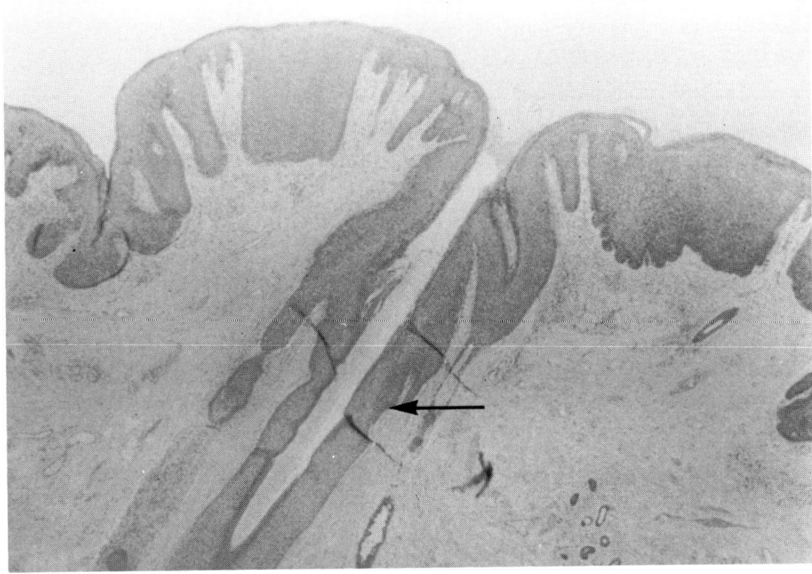

**FIG 5–12.**
Carcinoma in situ extends down the shaft of a hair follicle. The total depth as demarcated by the arrow measures 0.9 mm.

magnification. When this histological layer is identified, no further vaporization depth is required. The suggested safe guidelines for epithelial vaporization are listed in Table 5–4.

Heat conduction may produce edema and later discomfort in the form of a burning pain. This type of injury requires 21 to 28 days to heal, but scarring should not occur with epithelial vaporization only.[9]

## Management of VIN Occupying the Hairy Areas

VIN occupying the hairy areas can extend down hair shafts as much as 2.75 mm (Fig 5–12). In the author's experience, the deepest extension occurred in a perianal hairy area. Usually the extension does not exceed 1 mm. However, the thickness of the dermis on the vulva varies and the level of the hair bulb in the dermis varies. Wright and Davies (unpublished data) found the usual range of the hair bulb depth to be 1.22 to 1.40 mm into the dermis. Eradicating disease in hairy areas, therefore, could require vaporization into the dermis up to 3 mm to be certain that potentially involved appendages (hair root and duct of sebaceous gland) are destroyed. In some areas of the vulva, this would virtually include full thickness vaporization and result in destruction of the epidermis, dermis, and some complete epidermal structures. Such extensive depth of vaporization results in

**TABLE 5–4.**
Laser Vaporization Guidelines for Epithelial VIN

| Laser Vaporization Guidelines for Epithelial VIN |
|---|
| $CO_2$ laser attached to operating microscope |
| Effective laser beam diameter of 2 mm |
| 25 to 40 watts (power density of 625 to 1000 watts/$cm_2$) |
| Working distance of 300 mm (focal length of microscope's main objective lens = 300 mm) |
| Continuous mode |
| Alternately, superpulse mode |

delayed healing, possible scarring, and loss of hair growth (alopecia of the vulva). For these reasons, the author recommends local scalpel excision with approximation of the skin edges in hairy areas. The site of the scalpel excision should be nicely healed within 7 to 14 days. Laser-excised surfaces on the vulva do not heal as well and at times interfere with histological interpretation of the specimen base and margins.

## Combination of Laser Vaporization and Scalpel Excision

In approximately 15% of cases, the VIN occupies both the hairy and non-hairy areas. In this situation, the author recommends scalpel excision of the hairy portion and laser vaporization of the involved epithelium in the non-hairy area. Since these areas frequently are confluent, the surgeon will sometimes approximate the excised dermal edges containing surface epithelium (hairy area) to the dermis edge of the vaporized part (non-hairy area) without epithelium. This produces an excellent cosmetic result (Figs 5–13 to 5–16). In the author's experience, these methods have virtually replaced the skinning vulvectomy procedure. This approach to surgery for VIN on the basis of the histological depth of disease appears to be a reasonable alternative to more radical surgical procedures and seems a logical way of eliminating lesions and minimizing complications.

## Healing and Postoperative Care

Within 12 to 24 hours after laser surgery, induration, exudation, and edema can be noted. The labia minora are prone to swell if lasered, and a Foley catheter may be required. Pain appears to be maximal from 2 to 10 days after the laser surgery. The suggested postoperative care after vulvar laser surgery is outlined in Table 5–5.

Tannic acid was once used in burn units (1928 to 1948), but its use was discontinued because of its severe toxicity resulting from excessive surface absorption.[12] However, the

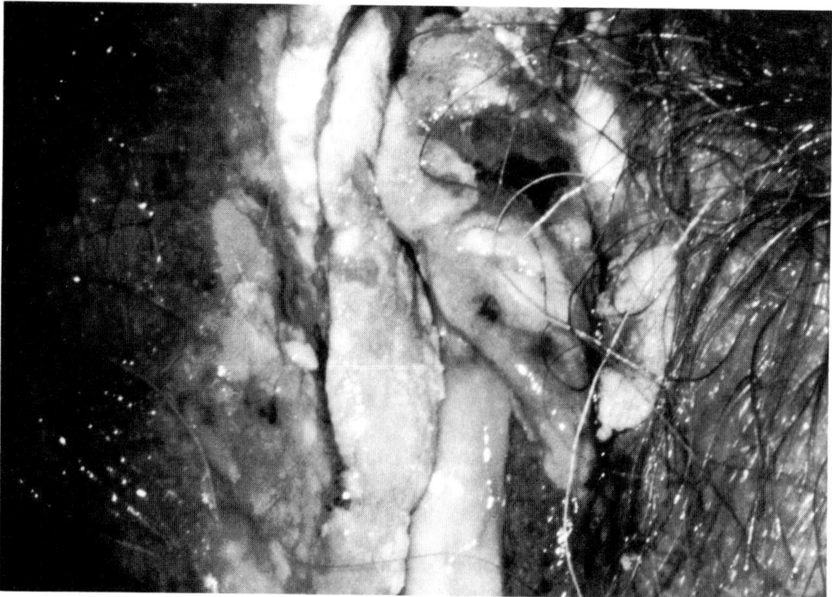

**FIG 5–13.**
Extensive carcinoma in situ of the vulva occupying both hairy and non-hairy areas.

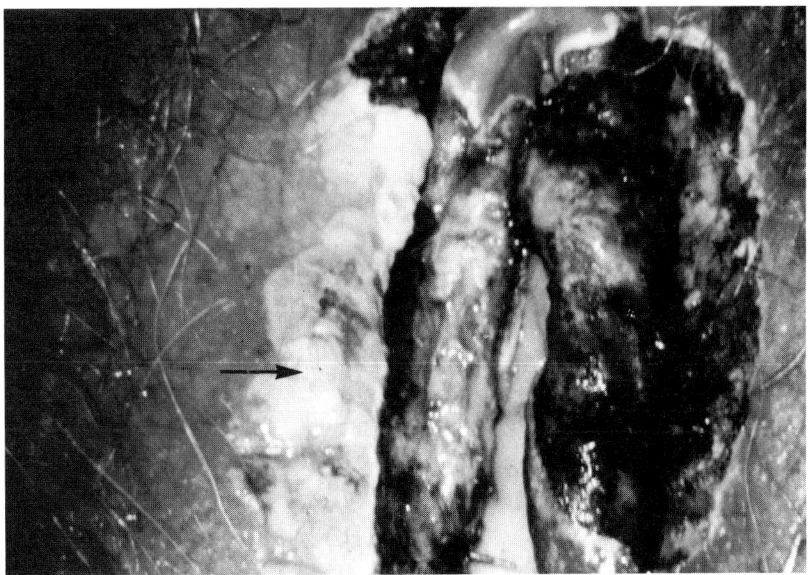

**FIG 5–14.**
Same case as illustrated in Figure 5–13. The disease occupying the non-hairy areas is vaporized down to the level of the papillary dermis. The disease occupying the hairy area, as indicated by *arrows,* will be excised with the scalpel.

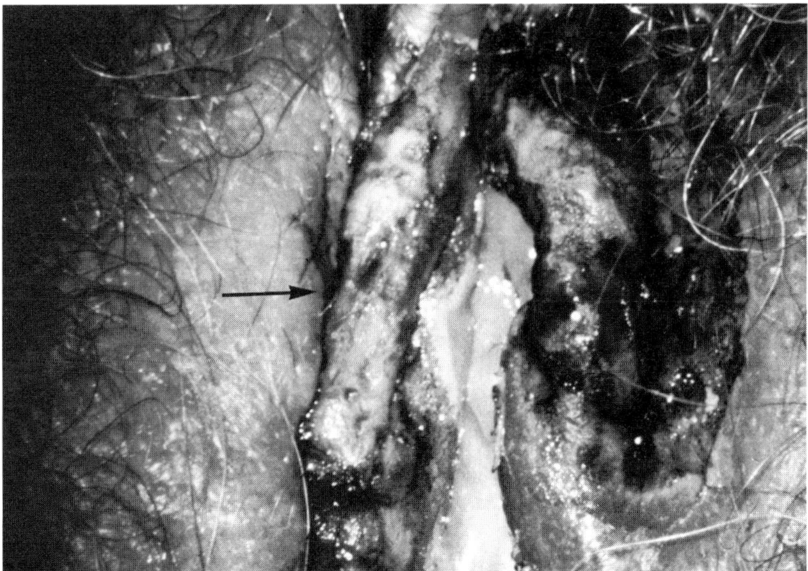

**FIG 5–15.**
After the hairy, diseased portion is excised, the outer margin containing dermis (covered by normal squamous epithelium) is approximated to the vaporized portion by a subcutaneous suture in the dermis *(arrow).*

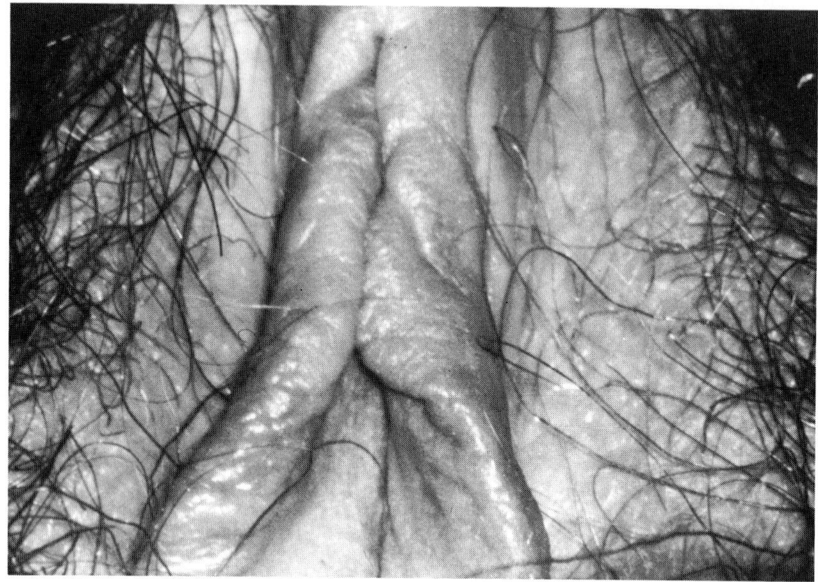

**FIG 5–16.**
The end result of Figures 5–13 to 5–15 results in a normal cosmetic vulva with all anatomical and histological structures preserved.

genital area comprises only 1% of total body area and absorption is nil. In a study by the author (unpublished data), liver enzymes and function tests evaluated after the tannic acid regimen demonstrated no alterations from normal. Genital use is effective and safe. The use of topical Aloe is also extremely effective for instant pain control and also as an antipruritic.[13]

Edema, induration, and discomfort subside towards the end of the second week. Complete re-epithelialization occurs between 3 to 6 weeks. Normal topography is achieved (see Figs 5–13 to 5–16).

Coaptation of the labia is a potential problem in cases requiring extensive lasering of the surface epithelium of opposing surfaces. This complication is prevented by educating patients in postoperative care and particularly in stressing the need to separate the labia at least once a day.

**TABLE 5–5.**
Postoperative Care After Vulvar Laser Surgery

| |
|---|
| Tea sitz baths or warm tea bag compresses four times a day or more. |
| Tannic acid ointment (composed of 5% tannic acid and 95% PCAA concentrate* (supplied in a 50 to 100 g container) applied three times a day. |
| One-quarter strength hydrogen peroxide sitz baths as needed (one part hydrogen peroxide and four parts water) should a cleansing agent be necessary. |
| Use of a hair dryer to dry the skin after bathing and sitz baths. |
| Silver sulfadiazine applied topically as necessary to control superficial bacterial infection. |
| Topical Aloe (99.5% pure Aloe juice stabilized in Vitamin C, 0.5%) sprayed topically for acute severe pain control. |
| Analgesics as necessary. |
| Avoidance of constricting clothing. |
| No intercourse until the area is healed. |
| Careful manual separation of the labia at least once per day to prevent coaptation. |

*Professional Compounding (Canada), Inc, 3 Centre Street, London, Ontario, Canada, N6J 1T4

### Results of Laser Surgery and Scalpel Excision for VIN III

Despite the excellent cosmetic results and therapeutic effectiveness that can be achieved with the three operative methods, the new disease rate exceeds 30% when these patients are monitored continuously. This information is based on the findings of 60 patients with VIN III disease (severe dysplasia, carcinoma in situ, or both) managed as discussed. The preliminary study is published elsewhere.[9]

The persistent and new disease rate within the first 12 months is approximately 30%.[9] It appears that new disease develops early. The highest failure rate occurs in patients diagnosed with multifocal disease. However, after 12 months of disease-free follow-up, the new disease rate is 18% during a seven-year follow-up. More new disease can be expected to occur in patients previously treated for multifocal disease (3 of 12, or 25%) compared to those treated for unifocal disease (7 of 44, or 15.9%)

It is well known that patients diagnosed with VIN are prone to develop new disease during long-term follow-up regardless of the methods of treatment.[8] However, the likelihood of subsequent disease diminishes as time progresses. In the author's experience, the use of the laser vaporization methods described for non-hairy areas and scalpel excision for hairy areas, or a combination of both procedures always provides for excellent cosmetic results. Persistent disease, recurrent disease, or new disease can be managed by these techniques without loss of organ function or disfigurement.

## VULVAR CONDYLOMATA ACUMINATA

The human papillomavirus infection can involve any site on the vulva (Figs 5–17 and 5–18). The most common sites appear to be the non-hairy areas, with the maximal concentration being on the posterior two-thirds of the vulva (Fig 5–19). The most common

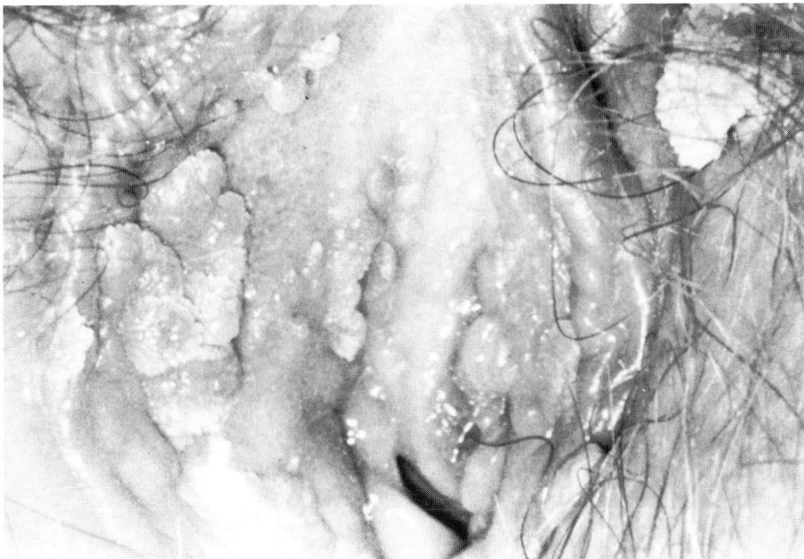

**FIG 5–17.**
Multiple accuminate warts are seen scattered on the vulva. The majority of the wart population occupies the non-hairy areas.

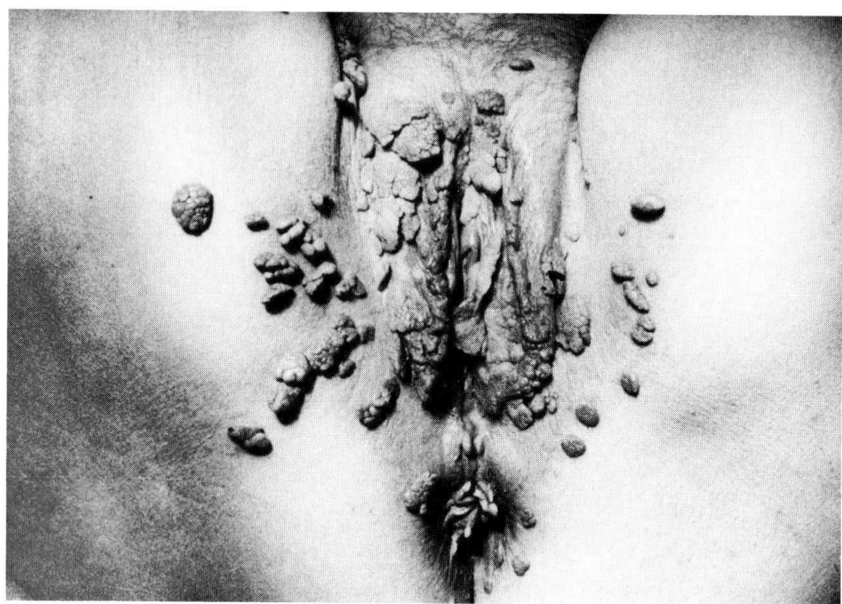

**FIG 5–18.**
Mature-appearing condylomata occupy both the hairy and non-hairy parts of the vulva including the perianal area.

site appears to be the posterior fourchette. The warty areas may assume the form of flat condyloma, florid condyloma, or may appear as micropapillary projections—the latter representing the subclinical HPV infection. The flat-appearing condylomata must be differentiated from vulvar intraepithelial neoplasia, particularly when the disease is located in the non-hairy posterior two-thirds of the vulva. On some occasions the malignant variety

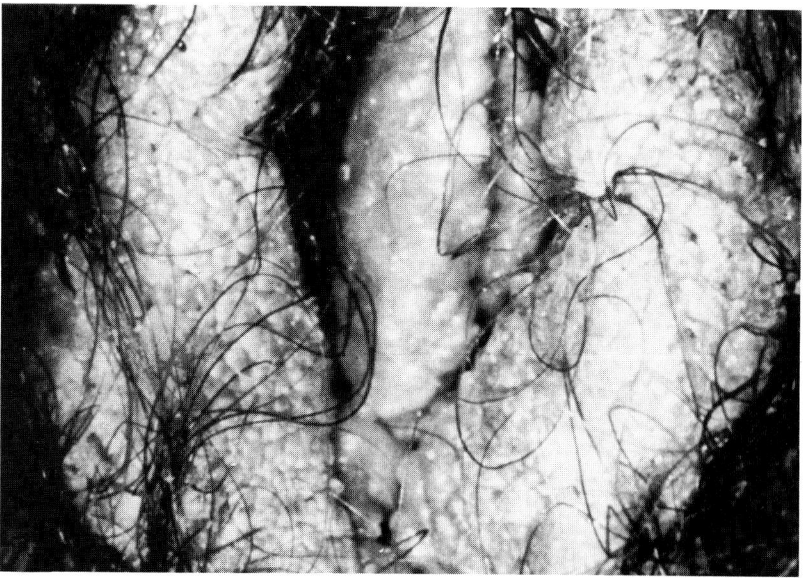

**FIG 5–19.**
Exophytic acuminate warts matted together completely replacing the normal vulvar architecture in an immunosuppressed patient.

is identified (Fig 5–20). It is essential to carry out the standard colposcopic evaluation, as previously described under the section regarding vulvar intraepithelial neoplasia. It may be appropriate to take selected biopsies of questionable areas.

This disease is usually first identified on the vulva, but patients with condylomatous lesions must be carefully and completely evaluated to determine the presence of other lesions. The upper vagina, cervix, anal canal, and perineum must be colposcopically scrutinized. All lesions that are detected must be completely eliminated. Because the virus most likely resides in normal-appearing skin between and surrounding the obvious infected areas, these must be treated as well to prevent the subsequent emergence of lesions in other areas.

## Principles of Laser Surgery for Vulvar Condylomata Acuminata

The type of anesthesia required for employing the carbon dioxide laser for vulvar condylomata depends on the number and extent of the lesions. Small patches of disease can be infiltrated with local anesthesia, but extensive disease will require a general anesthetic. Some patients can be treated on an outpatient basis, but patients with extensive and particularly with refractive condyloma often require hospitalization after the surgery.

Because heat conduction into the surrounding and underlying tissue with resultant

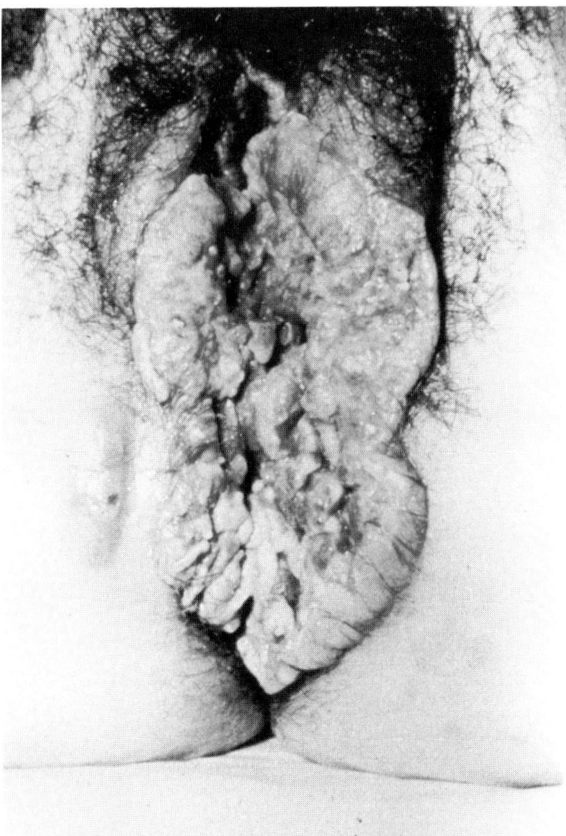

**FIG 5–20.**
This large exophytic growth is completely replacing the vulva and anus. The lesion grossly appears destructive. Biopsies confirmed a verrucous carcinoma of the involved parts.

thermal damage increases the exposure time, exposure of tissue to the beam must be minimized and volumetric destruction maximized. For vulvar laser surgery, this is accomplished by employing a high power density (i.e., ranges of 650 to 1,200 watts/$cm_2$) and by quickly moving the beam across the target surface. It is important to remember to use the highest power density that the laser surgeon can control. Each lesion that is colposcopically identified must be vaporized, but the depth should be carefully controlled. Because the HPV infection is contained within the epithelium only, it is not necessary to vaporize down into the papillary or reticular dermis. Beam penetration into the dermis could result in scarring, and there is no disease in this region.

## Laser Operative Technique for Vulvar Condylomata

For best performance, it is mandatory that the carbon dioxide laser be attached to the operating microscope since microscopic scrutiny is essential. A working distance of 300 mm is required (this equals the focal length of the main objective lens of the microscope). A laser beam diameter of at least 2 mm is advocated. If condylomatous lesions of the vagina or cervix, or both, are noted, these must be managed as well. It has been recommended that even though no obvious condylomata are noted on the cervix, patients with vulvar condyloma have the transformation zone of the cervix vaporized in the fashion traditional for treating cervical intraepithelial neoplasia. This is then followed by "flashing" the laser beam over the remainder of the squamous epithelium of the cervix, still above vaporization threshold power density, to use the brief heat effect to kill superficial latent virus and to prevent new warts.[14]

Each individual condyloma is vaporized down to the papillary dermis. Normal saline or acetic acid can be used to wash off any carbon. The papillary dermis is then recognized as a tan color. This is easily identified using the operating microscope. It is unnecessary to extend into this histological layer. After each individual condyloma is vaporized down to the level of the papillary dermis, the laser beam is then "flashed" over normal-appearing

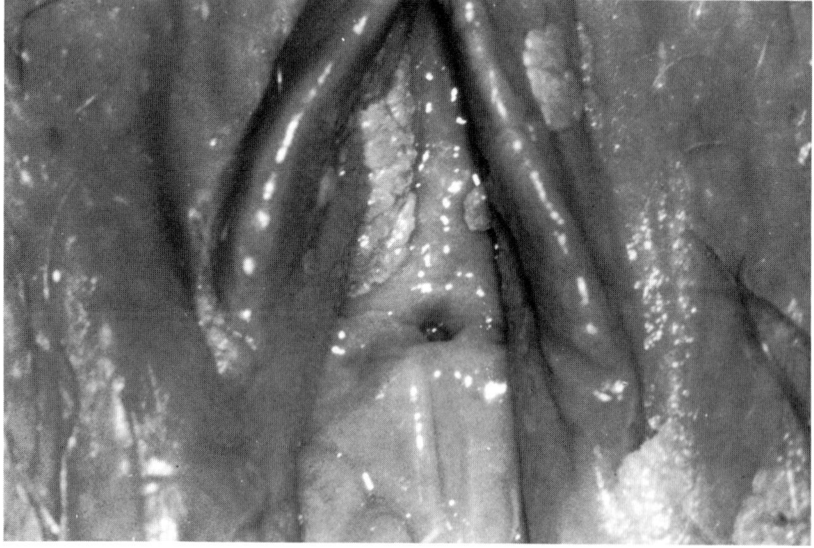

**FIG 5–21.**
Genital condylomata are seen scattered over the vulva.

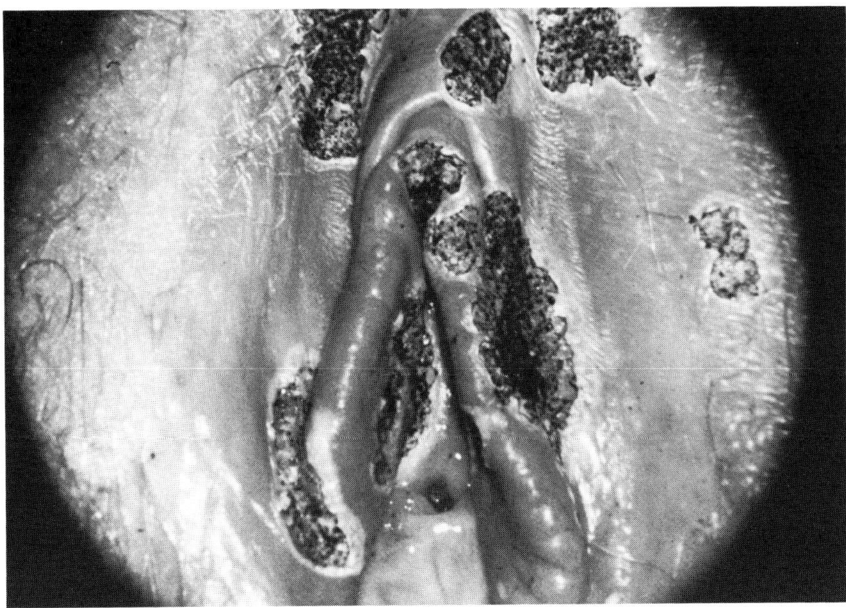

**FIG 5–22.**
The condylomata as shown in Figure 5–21 are laser vaporized down to the level of the papillary dermis. The surrounding normal-appearing tissue is also vaporized to kill latent virus.

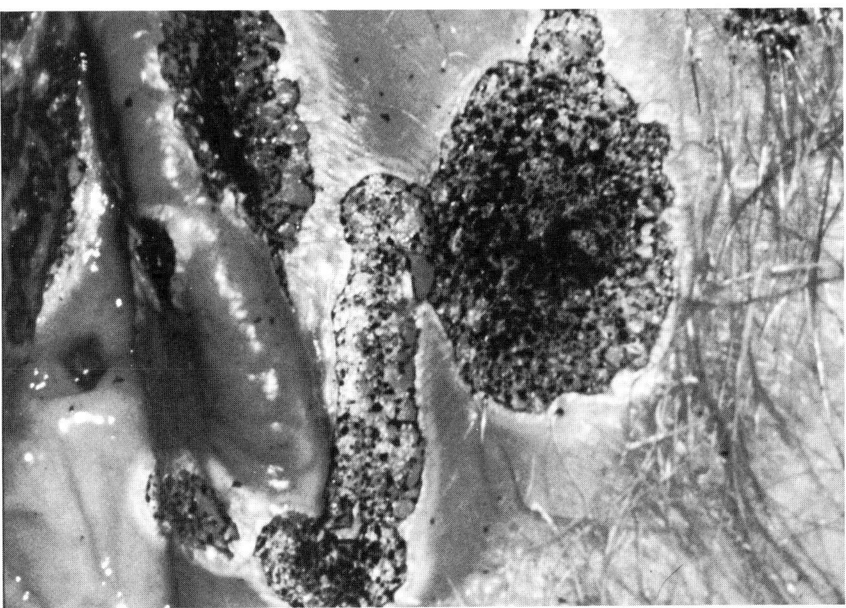

**FIG 5–23.**
A high magnification of Figure 5–22. The small amount of carbonization can be washed away with normal saline. The underlying papillary dermis will appear tan colored.

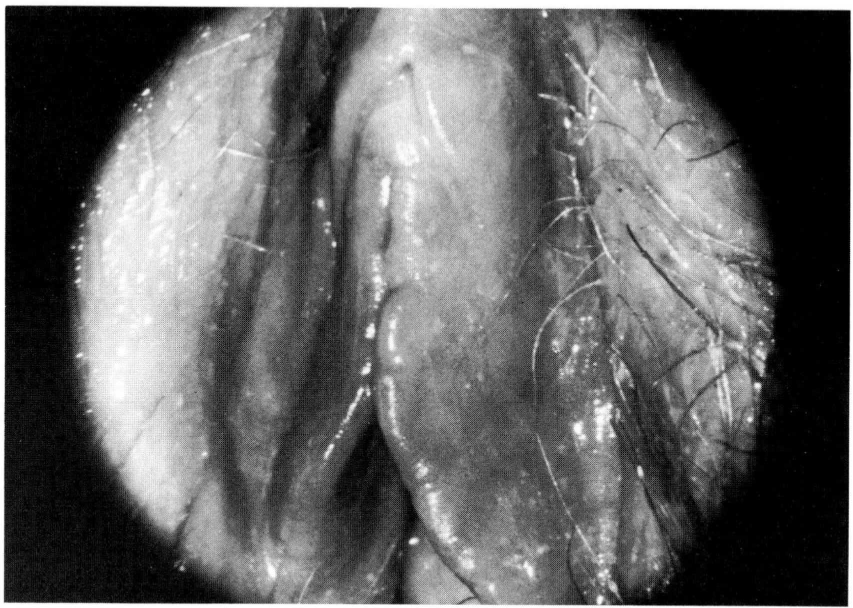

**FIG 5–24.**
The same patient as in Figures 5–21 to 5–23 taken at 6 weeks. Scarring does not occur regardless of disease extent as long as vaporization does not involve the dermis.

adjacent epithelium to kill any latent virus (Figs 5–21 to 5–24). Ferenczy, et al., found that the latent virus can be identified in normal-appearing epithelium up to 2 cm from the individual condyloma.[15]

For patients who have extensive vulvar condyloma, it is necessary to stage the procedure. Figs 5–25 to 5–29 illustrate a large vulvar condyloma completely covering the

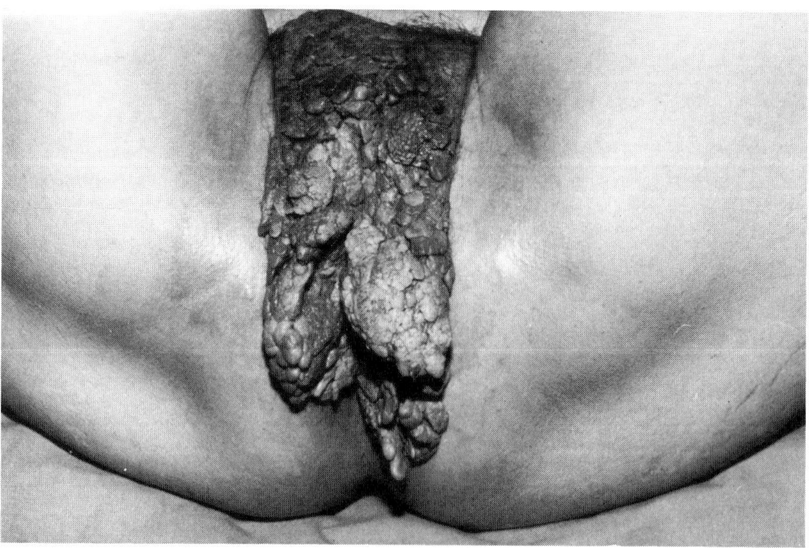

**FIG 5–25.**
A large contiguous mass of condyloma completely covers the mons pubis, vulva, and anus. This problem is best treated in stages.

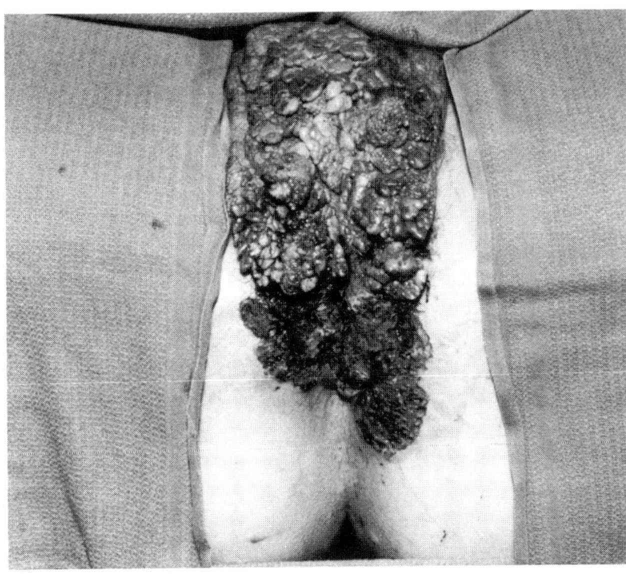

**FIG 5–26.**
Beginning posteriorly, chunks of condyloma can be quickly cut with the monopolar cautery to a level of 8 to 10 mm above the epidermis. The carbon dioxide laser coupled to the operating microscope is then used to vaporize the remaining condyloma to the level of the papillary dermis.

vulva, perineum, and anus. Beginning posteriorly and using the cutting mode of the electrocautery, small chunks of the disease can be removed to a level of approximately 8 to 10 mm above the epithelial surface. Bleeding will be encountered; however, this can be suctioned out of the field. This requires a trap in the suction line that allows blood to go into the trap; the plume will continue on through the filtering mechanism. The laser is then

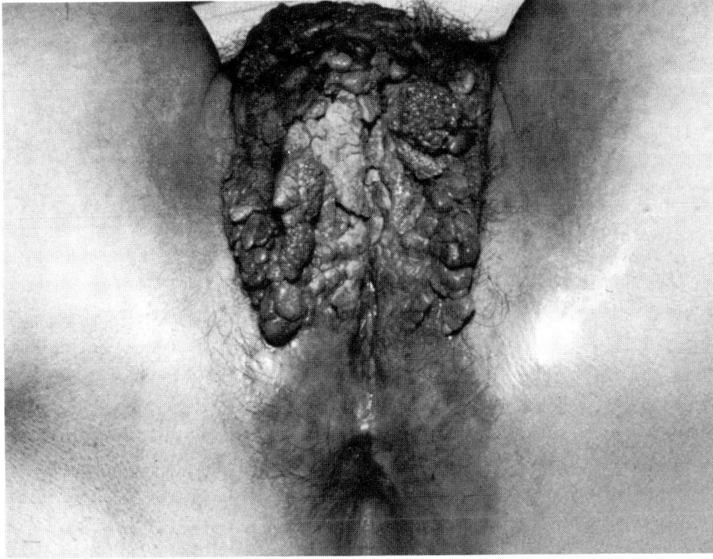

**FIG 5–27.**
This shows the same patient 2 months later prior to the second stage procedure. The area of previous surgery has healed with an excellent cosmetic result.

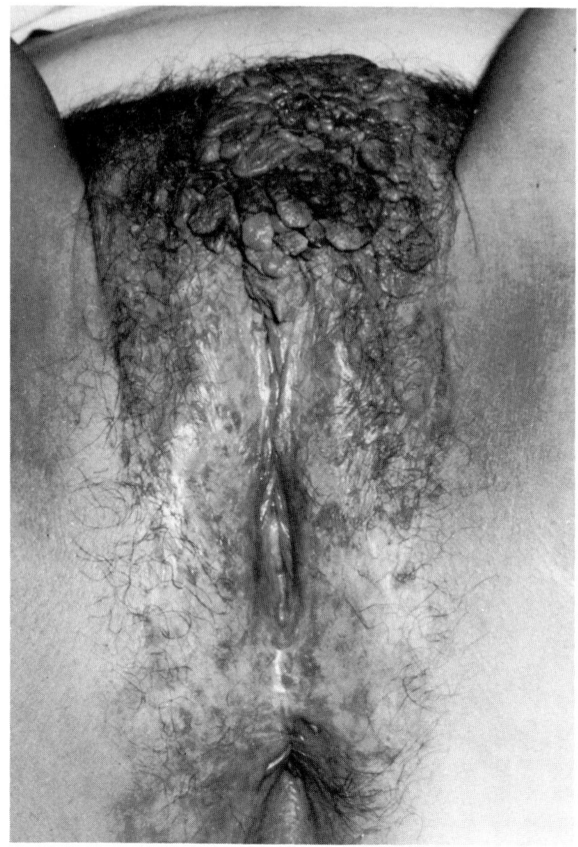

**FIG 5–28.**
Further surgery as described in Figure 5–26 is completed, again with excellent healing. The remaining condyloma on the mons pubis is managed in a similar manner.

used to vaporize the remaining condyloma down to the papillary dermis. After each planned stage of the operation is completed, the areas are allowed to heal before subsequent surgery. Figure 5–29 shows the excellent cosmetic result that can be achieved from such a staged procedure.

## Management of the Postoperative Patient

Management after laser surgery for vulvar condyloma is identical to that described for laser surgery of vulvar intraepithelial neoplasia. In summary, this requires the use of tannic acid (tea) sitz baths, the use of a hair dryer, and application of topical Aloe. Topical silver sulphadiazine can be applied should topical bacterial infection be suspected.

## Anticipated Results

Depending upon the severity of the disease being treated, a 65% to 85% success rate can be anticipated after one laser surgery.[16] Those cases with extensive, and particularly with previous, refractory condyloma can expect an even lower success rate. This must be explained to and understood by the patient. Any persistent or recurrent vulvar condyloma

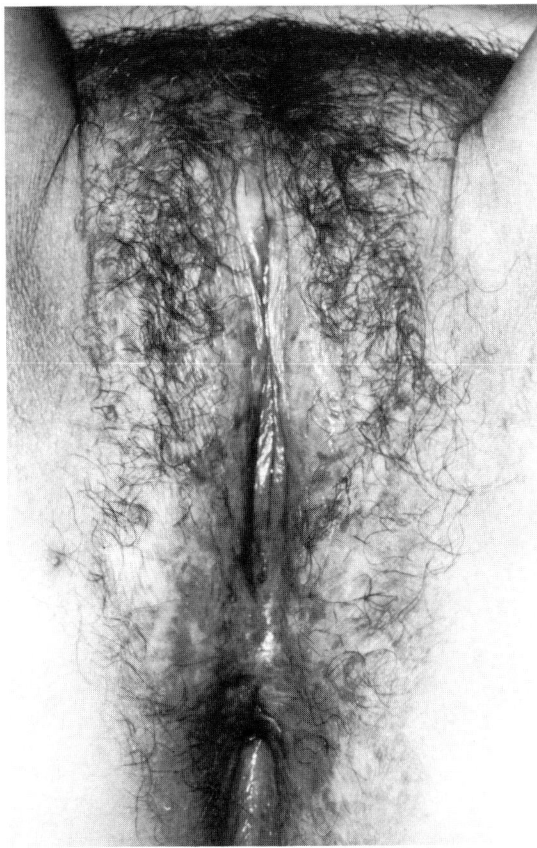

**FIG 5–29.**
This photo demonstrates the final result of the case illustrated in Figures 5–25 to 5–28. An excellent cosmetic result has been achieved with preservation of normal vulvar architecture and hair growth.

can be treated by 50% to 85% trichloral acetic acid or repeat laser surgery with local anesthesia. Although some patients require more than one surgical intervention in the operating room, eventually the condyloma will be eradicated. However, because of the latent virus, there is no guarantee that new areas will not recur during long-term follow-up. In such cases, it is highly recommended that male consort(s) be fully evaluated.

## VAGINAL INTRAEPITHELIAL NEOPLASIA

### Clinical Histology and Anatomy of the Vagina

The vagina is covered by stratified squamous epithelium that also extends onto and covers the vaginal cervix to the squamocolumnar junction. This epithelium is superimposed upon a tunica propria consisting of collagenous and elastic connective tissue that reaches into the epithelial basal layer in the form of papillae similar to the dermal papillae of the normal skin (Fig 5–30). The stratified squamous epithelium is composed of different cell types which are divided into the basal cell, transitional cell, and spindle or prickle cell layers. The superficial cells contain some keratin but normally show no gross cornification in women of reproductive age. The epithelium has a thickness that varies between

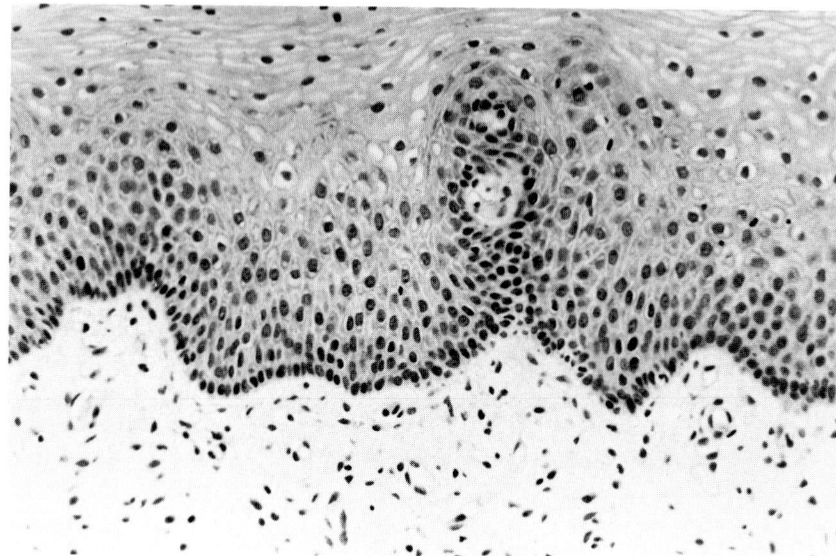

**FIG 5–30.**
The normal histology of the vagina. The epithelial thickness measures 0.27 mm.

100 to 500 microns (0.1 to 0.5 mm) (see Fig 5–30). The epithelium appears to be thickest in the presence of vaginal intraepithelial neoplasia with keratin formation. The smooth muscle beneath the lamina propria is divided into internal circular and external longitudinal muscle groups. Inferiorly, these muscle groups interlace with the stratified fibers of the levator ani muscles. An extensive blood supply nourishes the vagina. The vaginal artery lies external to the muscular coat and supplies smaller branches into the lamina propria.

Under normal conditions there are no glands or crypts in the vagina. Under rare conditions a few glands may be found in the fornix; however, these usually represent aberrant cervical glands or glandlike tubules derived from the vestigial wolffian duct. These findings indicate that vaginal intraepithelial neoplasia (VAIN) and vaginal condyloma are confined to the epithelium.

## Vaginal Intraepithelial Neoplasia

Vaginal intraepithelial neoplasia is uncommon. It can occur in patients with or without a cervix. Frequently, if the cervix is present, VAIN appears as an extension of cervical intraepithelial neoplasia. It is reported to occur in 0.9% to 6.8% of patients who have had a hysterectomy for benign disease.[17–19] Also, 28% of VAIN cases have been reported to occur after hysterectomy for preinvasive or invasive disease.[18] All cases of VAIN do not progress to cervical cancer.[20] The histological grading system for the vagina is similar to that of the cervix: VAIN I, mild dysplasia; VAIN II, moderate dysplasia; VAIN III, severe dysplasia or carcinoma in situ.[21]

The time interval between previous treatment of genital tract neoplasia and the diagnosis of VAIN varies with the type of initial treatment.[18] Patients with preinvasive and invasive cervical disease treated surgically have a decreasing incidence of VAIN as time progresses. Most cases of VAIN occur within ten years after surgical procedures. In contrast, those patients treated with radiation for other genital tract malignancies demonstrate an increasing incidence of disease as times passes.[18]

Because vaginal intraepithelial neoplasia is an epithelial disease, it is confined to that histological level; that is, the vagina does not have underlying adnexal structures like the vulva. Under normal situations it also does not have glandular structures when compared to the cervix.

Patients most often present with abnormal Papanicolaou smears and usually without symptoms. Careful colposcopic examination of the cervix (if present), vagina, vulva, and perianal area is necessary and should be part of the initial examination. It is necessary to inspect the entire vagina before and after the application of any solutions (e.g., acetic acid or Schiller's solution). It may be necessary to apply the acetic acid every 2 to 3 minutes to enhance the pattern. After the application of Schiller's solution (1 part iodine, 2 parts potassium iodide, 300 parts water), the normal vaginal epithelium immediately stains a deep brown. The color fades within a few minutes, but the epithelium can be restained as many times as necessary. If glycogen is absent, the epithelium will not stain. Thus, in preparation for a colposcopic evaluation of the vagina in a non-estrogenic woman, it will be necessary to give the patient either oral or vaginal estrogen so that a proper staining with Schiller's solution can be accomplished. A positive Schiller's test occurs when any of the normal-appearing squamous epithelium fails to stain brown. In the author's experience, Schiller's solution is frequently more useful in identifying the suspect areas than is acetic acid.

Higher-grade lesions are frequently hyperkeratotic and are not difficult to identify. On occasion, an accompanying mosaic pattern is seen. The disease can be multifocal; however, most lesions are found in the upper one-third of the vagina.[22]

Various treatment modalities have been used for VAIN including radiation, local resection, total or partial vaginectomy with or without skin graft, electrocautery, and topical 5-fluorouracil.[22, 23] It has been demonstrated that 5-fluorouracil can achieve high cure rates.[22–24] Because of the nonaggressive nature of VAIN and the difficulty of conventional surgical therapy, carbon dioxide laser vaporization has become another excellent method of treating VAIN.[24] Lesions demonstrating hyperkeratosis appear to respond well to vaporization by the $CO_2$ laser. Lesions located within the upper lateral vaginal folds, particularly post-hysterectomy "dog ears," are sometimes inaccessible to both 5-fluorouracil and the laser beam. Because of mechanical problems, these areas are best surgically excised. It is not possible to know the amount of vaginal epithelium buried during the closure or healing of the vaginal vault after hysterectomy or whether buried epithelium is diseased. Should there be any doubt, such areas must be surgically excised.

## Laser Surgery for VAIN

The carbon dioxide laser provides excellent hemostasis and the procedure is usually easily performed once excellent exposure is achieved. The laser sites heal without scarring. Because the vaginal wall is thin and in close proximity to the underlying vascular plexus, careful beam control is essential.

The normal vaginal epithelium is less than 300 microns in thickness (see Fig 5–30). The epithelium containing disease, even with a keratinized surface, is usually less than 500 microns (0.5 mm). Because VAIN is an epithelial disease, laser vaporization should be confined to this depth.

### Laser Operative Procedure

Many patients will require a general anesthetic to permit adequate exposure and operative manipulation. A small isolated area of VAIN, however, can be treated by laser vaporization under local anesthesia in an office or clinic setting.

Regardless of the type of anesthesia, excellent exposure is mandatory. All lesions should be re-identified by using both acetic acid and Schiller's solution. Control of power density is necessary. It is always important for the laser surgeon to work at the highest power density that is controllable and to move the laser beam as quickly as possible. In the author's experience, power densities ranging between 650 to 1,200 watts/$cm_2$ are controllable in the vagina. An effective laser beam of 2 mm and a working distance of 300 mm (this equals the focal length of the main objective lens of the microscope) are recommended, and a smoke evacuation system is required. Each lesion, including 3 mm of normal-appearing tissue beyond its periphery, is encircled with the beam. The lesions are ablated by cautiously moving the controlled laser beam in multiple directions over the diseased area(s). Vaporizing to a depth not exceeding 1.5 mm should account for any disease distribution and uneven rugae.

The author has also used topical 5-fluorouracil in the vagina immediately after laser surgery and for two subsequent applications to reduce any activation of the disease in what appears to be normal vaginal epithelium.

### Postoperative Care

The vagina heals more slowly than the cervix and vulva. Patients should be instructed not to put anything into the vagina until it is completely healed, which usually takes 4 to 6 weeks. This means no douching, no tampons, and no intercourse. The first follow-up visit is usually at approximately four weeks, at which time the physician can advise the patient on healing progress and usually identify any persistent disease.

### Results of Carbon Dioxide Laser Surgery

Cure rates with the laser are acceptable, although there is no evidence to suggest that laser vaporization is superior to topical 5-fluorouracil.[24] The cure rate after laser surgery varies between 50% to 85%.[18, 24, 25] Using a combination of vaporization and 5-Fluorouracil increases cure rates (unpublished data).

## VAGINAL CONDYLOMATA

The human papillomavirus (HPV) causing condyloma in the genital area appears to be sexually transmitted. In patients presenting with vulvar condylomata, approximately one-third will also have vaginal condylomata and half will have the human papillomavirus present on the cervix. The DNA-containing human papillomavirus types responsible for genital condylomata are thought to be types 6 and 11, a subgroup of the Papovaviridae family. Types 16 and 18 are found exclusively in high-grade cervical intraepithelial neoplastic lesions.[26] The human papillomavirus invades the tissue and must be considered to potentially involve all cellular layers with involvement depending upon the stage of cellular replication. Vaginal condylomata can be of the florid or flat type and can be of clinical or subclinical states. Warts can occupy any part of the vagina, although the most common sites include the upper one-third and posterior one-third, which can also include the area surrounding the introitus (Fig 5–31).

It is necessary to colposcopically inspect the entire vagina. Acetic acid as well as Lugol's iodine solution can be very effective in coating the areas of involvement. The HPV infections are associated with abnormal Papanicolaou smears. Because the HPV is associated with genital neoplasia, selected biopsies may be necessary when an abnormal colposcopic pattern or an abnormal Papanicolaou smear is identified.

Many different therapies have been advocated for the treatment of vaginal condylomata including topical 5-Fluorouracil, laser vaporization, and topical interferon. The response to topical 5-Fluorouracil varies, depending upon the type of condyloma present and the dose of the agent used. Ferenczy found the $CO_2$ laser more effective than 5-Fluorouracil in eradicating flat condylomata.[16] Both methods appeared equally effective for the florid type. Using a once-weekly regimen of topical 5-Fluorouracil for a period of 10 consecutive weeks, Krebs has successfully treated vaginal condylomata.[27] He further found that the once-weekly regimen controlled 85% of the flat condylomata, which appeared to be as effective a therapy as the carbon dioxide laser. The superficial nature of the disease makes it amenable to limited-depth laser vaporization, particularly when the chemical methods fail.

## Technique of Laser Surgery for Vaginal Condylomata Acuminata

The patient is placed in the lithotomy position and the legs are placed comfortably in stirrups. A non-reflecting, bivalved vaginal speculum is placed into the vagina. Attached to the speculum is a smoke-evacuating system. The laser must be attached to an operating microscope or colposcope with a working distance of 300 mm. The effective laser beam diameter should be at least 2 mm. It must be remembered that the vaginal wall is very thin and that the thickness of the epithelium is less than 500 microns. Because of the known

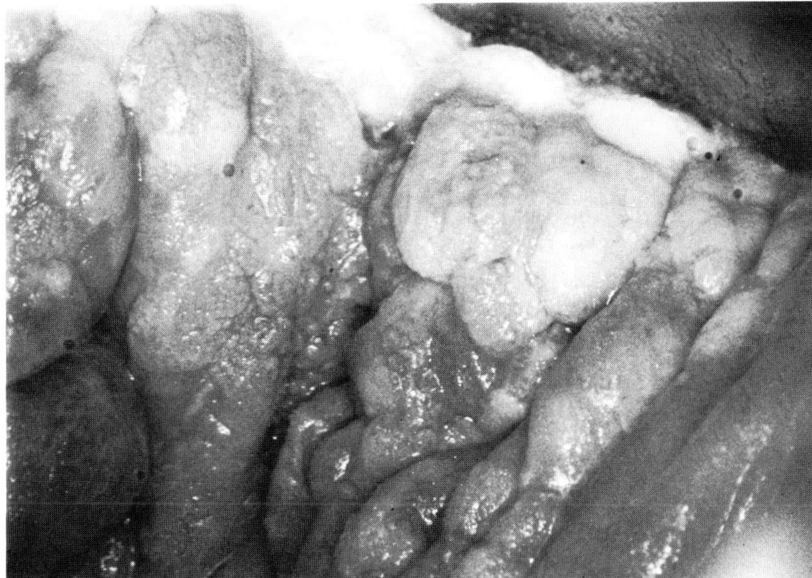

**FIG 5–31.**
Contiguous masses of condylomata occupy most of the vaginal wall.

histological and anatomical situation, it is important to control the power density and resulting vaporization depth. A power density range between 650 and 1,200 watts/cm$^2$ is satisfactory. The surgeon should keep in mind the great vascularity surrounding the vagina. Penetration into this plexus of vessels could present very troublesome bleeding.

Each individual vaginal condyloma is vaporized along with a 3-mm border of normal-appearing epithelium without penetrating into the underlying subcutaneous tissue. Total laser vaporization depth should not exceed 1 mm, which should account for the extension of any dermal papillae. The laser beam should be quickly "flashed" over all the remaining vaginal epithelium to create a brief thermal effect that will destroy any latent virus contained within the epithelial cells in what appears through the microscope to be normal vaginal epithelium.

Resistant vaginal condyloma can be re-treated with the carbon dioxide laser plus the insertion of topical 5-Fluorouacil into the vagina immediately after the surgery and for 2 successive nights. In the author's experience this is extremely effective in achieving high cure rates. For those patients who are prone to develop new disease, the prolonged (i.e., 6 to 8 weeks) use of topical 5-Fluorouracil has been proposed.[27]

## Condylomata of the Cervix

Approximately 50% of patients who have vulvar condylomata will have evidence of HPV infection on the cervix. These can be found in different forms and include flat condylomata, florid condylomata, or the presence of micropapillary projections occurring in acetowhite areas both within the transformation zone and elsewhere (Figs 5–32 to 5–34). The laser is attached to an operating microscope with a working distance of 300 mm. A speculum is placed into the vagina, and a smoke-evacuating system is attached to the speculum. The depth of destruction of the condyloma on the cervix is similar to the depth of vaporization of cervical intraepithelial neoplasia (6 to 8 mm at least), as previously

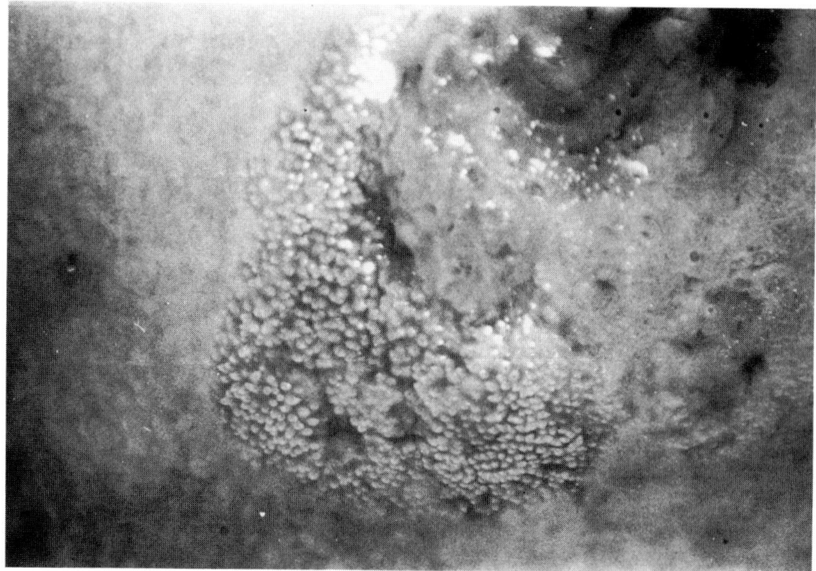

**FIG 5–32.**
Subclinical papillomavirus involving the transformation zone of the cervix. The micropapilliferous appearance is easily seen after acetic acid application.

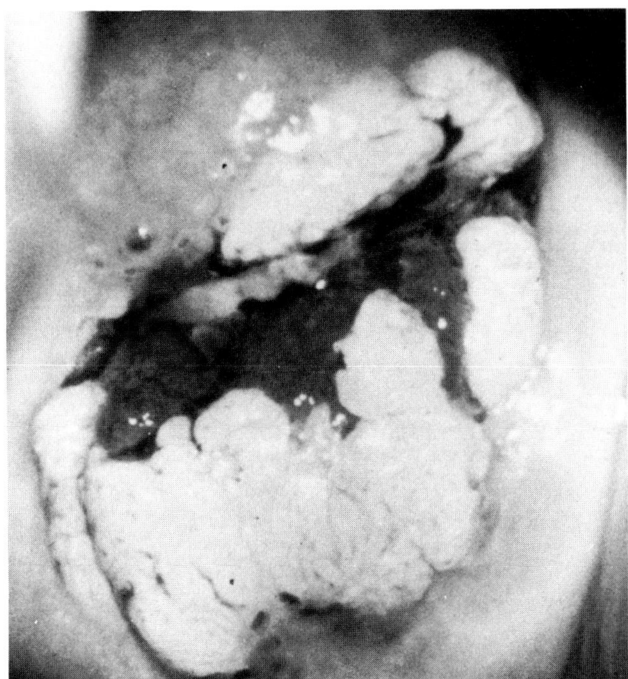

**FIG 5–33.**
Florid condylomata of the cervix.

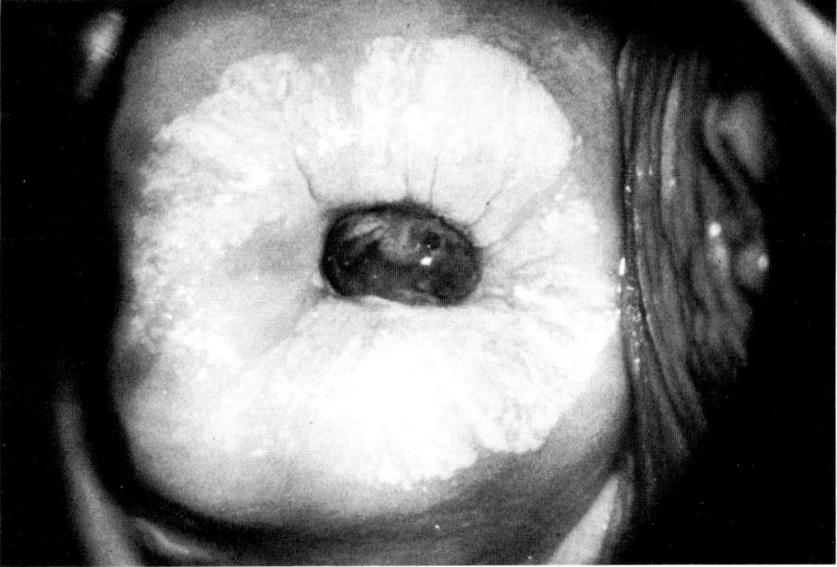

**FIG 5–34.**
Flat cervical condylomata are frequently seen with magnification before the application of acetic acid. The lesions appear to glisten after acetic acid application. In this case the condylomata are found covering cervical squamous epithelium.

described.[14] Since the virus may be harbored in the normal-appearing epithelium, the entire surface of the cervix should be routinely "flashed." For persistent or recurrent condylomata of the cervix, retreatment with the laser plus 5-Fluorouracil appears to be effective in the author's experience.

### Postoperative Care

Postoperative care of patients having laser surgery for vaginal condylomata is identical to the care after laser vaporization of VAIN. Persistent lesions are re-treated in various ways, depending on their extensiveness.

### Results

Condylomata can be stubborn and require multiple treatments and combined modalities, especially laser plus 5-Fluorouracil. However, most patients can be eventually returned to normal. Small persistent or recurrent lesions can be treated in the clinic with topical trichloral acetic acid as they are identified during follow-up.

## REFERENCES

1. Woodruff JD, Julian C, Purvy T, et al: The contemporary challenge of carcinoma in situ of the vulva. *Am J Obstet Gynecol* 1973; 115:667–670.
2. Lupulescu A, Mehregan AH, Rahbari H, et al: Venereal warts versus Bowen's disease. *JAMA* 1977; 237:2520–2524.
3. Kovi J, Tillman RL, Lee SM: Malignant transformation of condyloma acuminatum. *Am J Clin Pathol* 1974; 61:702–705.
4. Jagella J, Stegner HE: Histopathologic and cytophotometric study of dysplastic and precancerous condylomata acuminata. *Arch Gynecol Obstet* 1974; 216:119–123.
5. Forney JP, Morros CP, Townsend DE, et al: Management of carcinoma in situ of the vulva. *Am J Obstet Gynecol* 1977; 127:801–806.
6. Kaufman RH, Gardner HL: Intraepithelial neoplasia of the vulva. *Clin Obstet Gynecol* 1965; 8:1035–1040.
7. Buscema BA, Woodruff DJ, Parmley TH, et al: Carcinoma in situ of the vulva. *Obstet Gynecol* 1980; 55:225–230.
8. DiSaia PJ, Rich WM: Surgical approach to multifocal carcinoma in situ of the vulva. *Am J Obstet Gynecol* 1981; 140:136–145.
9. Wright VC, Davies E: Laser surgery for vulvar intraepithelial neoplasia. *Am J Obstet Gynecol* 1987; 156:374–378.
10. Moschelle SL, Hurley HJ: *Dermatology*, 2nd ed. Toronto, Ontario, Canada, WB Saunders, 1985.
11. Mene A, Buckley CH: Involvement of vulvar skin appendages by intraepithelial neoplasia. *Br J Obstet Gynaecol* 1985; 92:634–638.
12. McClure RD, Lam CR, Romence H: Tannic acid and the treatment of burns. *Ann Surg* 1944; 120:387–405.
13. Anton R, Haag-Berrurier M: Therapeutic use of natural anthraquinone for other than laxative actions. *Pharmacology* 1980; 20:104–112.
14. Wright VC, Riopelle MA: *Gynecologic Laser Surgery: A Practical Handbook.* Houston, Texas, Biomedical Communications, Inc, 1982.
15. Ferenczy A, Mitao M, Nagai N, et al: Latent papillomavirus and recurring genital warts. *N Engl J Med* 1985; 313:784–787.

16. Ferenczy A: Comparison of 5-fluorouracil and $CO_2$ laser for treatment of vaginal condylomata. *Obstet Gynecol* 1984; 64:773–778.
17. Benedet JL, Sanders HB: Carcinoma in situ of the vagina. *Am J Obstet Gynecol* 1984; 148:695–698.
18. Lenehan PM, Meffe F, Lichrich GM: Vaginal intraepithelial neoplasia: Biologic aspects and management. *Obstet Gynecol* 1986; 68:333–337.
19. Gallup DG, Morley GW: Carcinoma in situ of the vagina—a study and review. *Obstet Gynecol* 1975; 46:334–340.
20. Guthrie D, Way S: Immunotherapy of non-clinical vaginal cancer. *Lancet* 1975; 2:1242–1243.
21. Richard RM: Natural history of cervical intraepithelial neoplasia. *Clin Obstet Gynecol* 1967; 10:723–730.
22. Woodruff JD, Parmley TH, Julian CG: Topical 5-FU in the treatment of vaginal CIS. *Gynecol Oncol* 1975; 3:124–127.
23. Bolten KA: Practical colposcopy in cervical and vaginal cancer. *Clin Obstet Gynecol* 1967; 10:808–810.
24. Petrilli ES, Townsend DE, Morrow CP, et al: Vaginal intraepithelial neoplasia: Biologic aspects and treatment with topical 5-fluorouracil and the carbon dioxide laser. *Am J Obstet Gynecol* 1980; 138:321–328.
25. Wright VC: Laser surgery for carcinoma in situ of the vagina, in Shapshay SM (ed): *Endoscopic Laser Surgery Handbook*. New York, Marcel Dekker, Inc, 1987.
26. Crum CP, Mitao M, Levine RU, et al: Cervical papilloma viruses segregate within morphologically distinct precancerous lesions. *J Virol* 1985; 54:675–679.
27. Krebs HB: Prophylactic topical 5-fluorouracil following treatment of human papillomavirus-associated lesions of vulva and vagina. *Obstet Gynecol* 1986; 68:837–840.

Chapter 6

# Laser Therapy of the Cervix

Roger B. Yandell, M.D.

Tung Van Dinh, M.D.

Edward V. Hannigan, M.D.

Laser treatment of gynecologic lesions was first done a little more than a decade ago, but it is already widely used for preinvasive lesions of the cervix and is gradually becoming the standard of care. In this chapter we will briefly present a historical perspective and the natural history and histology of preinvasive and invasive carcinoma of the cervix, including an overview of nonlaser therapeutic modalities. We will then describe the history of and the rationale for the use of lasers in treating cervical disease, and will discuss the advantages and disadvantages of the different wavelengths currently available, as well as the techniques for both ablative and excisional procedures using the laser. We then will compare the results of laser therapy with those more conventional methods of treatment.

## HISTORICAL PERSPECTIVE

Gynecology was first recognized as a discipline in the Kahun Papyrus in 2000 B.C., but it was not until 450 B.C. that Hippocrates' writings first mentioned cancer of the uterus.[1] Other writings on the subject continued to appear throughout the periods of the Greek and Roman empires, including the works of Galen and Celsus during the first century A.D.[2] In the late 1500s, Ambroise Paré spoke on the use of the vaginal speculum and was probably the first to perform excisions of the cervix. His writings were soon followed by those of Tulipus of Amsterdam in 1652.[3] It is believed that these procedures were high amputations of the uterine cervix performed for what the surgeons believed to be cancer.

The first procedure that resembled the cone biopsy of today was performed by Lisfranc in 1815.[4] It was similar to an open conization wherein a wedge-shaped portion of the cervix was removed and left to heal without suturing the wound closed. In 1851, Sims devised a modification of this procedure in which he freed a section of vaginal mucosa and stretched it to serve as a flap to cover the defect, using silver wire to close the margins.[5] A number of modifications to the Sims technique were reported, but only the Sturmdorf modification continues to be used today.

The next 3 decades saw the introduction of 3 important areas in the study of the cervix. In 1925, Von Hinselmann developed the colposcope, which became very popular throughout Europe. He was followed in 1938 by Martzloff, who promoted the diagnosis of premalignant lesions using cervical biopsy, and finally by Papanicolaou and Traut in 1943, who described the diagnosis of uterine cancer using exfoliative cytology from the vaginal fornix.[6]

Surgical treatment of the cervix has focused mainly on excising the lesions–both the chronic inflammatory processes and cervical cancer—but more recently has evolved into a concentration on early diagnosis of the preinvasive lesions.[7] Laser therapy has developed as an important part of this task.

## THE EPIDEMIOLOGY OF CERVICAL INTRAEPITHELIAL NEOPLASIA

In the early 20th century, the number one cause of cancer deaths among women in the United States was carcinoma of the cervix. With the wide use of the colposcopically directed cervical biopsy and mass screening with the Pap smear, the death rate from cervical cancer declined steeply and is now surpassed by that from lung, breast, colon, and ovarian cancer, as well as that from the leukemias and lymphomas. Even during the last decade, the incidence of new cases has decreased by approximately 20%. The prediction from the American Cancer Society of 12,900 new cases and 7,000 deaths from cervical cancer during 1988[8] represents a promising trend, but it must be taken in light of the other shifts in the epidemiology of cervical disease: a notable increase in the number of preinvasive lesions of the cervix along with a drop in the average age of the patients.

The first studies on the epidemiology of cervical cancer were reported by Rigoni-Stern in 1842. By studying mortality records in Verona, Italy, he found that the patients were more often married and that the disease virtually never occurred in nuns. He also observed that it first occurred in the 30- to 40-year-old age groups and that the incidence increased to age 60, after which it dropped rapidly. After his study, little was written on the subject until the 1940s, when a great deal of demographic information was gathered as cervical screening programs were undertaken.

To the epidemiologic characteristics reported by Rigoni-Stern and others, these have been added: marrying at an early age, being of low socioeconomic status, being nonwhite, experiencing early pregnancy, and being a prostitute. Also implicated were human semen, the absence of circumcision in the sexual partner, and the presence of syphilis or Trichomonas, although subsequent studies have not supported these as risk factors. Also at higher risk are immunocompromised patients. It seems reasonable to assume that the immune system plays an important role in the development of cervical neoplasia. Cigarette smoking and deficiencies in vitamin A, vitamin C, and folic acid have also been associated with an increased risk of cervical neoplasia.

Our understanding of the risk factors for cervical neoplasia is now more refined, even though the exact etiologic agent—or agents—are still disputed. Because of the conspicuous absence of cervical neoplasia in virginal women, it appears obvious that the carcinogen is sexually transmitted. The two most important risk factors appear to be onset of intercourse before the completion of cervical metaplasia (approximately age 20), and exposure to multiple sexual partners. Other proven epidemiologic risk factors (low socioeconomic status, use of oral contraceptive agents or intrauterine devices, and failure to participate in screening programs) may correlate so highly with the above as to be relatively insignificant if examined alone.

Women at strikingly high risk are those whose current sexual partner had a previous consort who developed cervical neoplasia, strongly supporting a venereal etiology. The fact that the increased incidence of cervical intraepithelial neoplasia (CIN) has closely paralleled increases in herpes, chlamydia, and human papillomavirus (HPV) has motivated extensive study of these entities to search for an association with CIN. The evidence supporting an association with herpes and chlamydia, however, remains suspect, and they are believed to be, at most, cofactors in the disease process. On the other hand, the evidence for an association with HPV has grown rapidly over the last decade. DNA hybridization studies and epidemiologic studies have yielded enough evidence of an association that many physicians now believe subclinical papilloma infections of the cervix and the lower genital tract are synonymous with grade I intraepithelial neoplastic lesions (see Chapter 4).[9]

## THE BIOLOGY AND NATURAL HISTORY OF CERVICAL INTRAEPITHELIAL NEOPLASIA

Cervical dysplasia begins at the squamocolumnar junction of the transformation zone as a unicellular abnormality. It appears to be derived from either the underlying reserve cells or the basal cells. In the presence of a neoplastic stimulus during metaplasia, a period of neoplastic potential can occur. It has been observed that normal metaplasia resulting in normal squamous epithelium does not give rise to a field of neoplastic potential.[10] Cervical intraepithelial neoplasia represents a continuum of a disease process in that the neoplastic potential begins with mild dysplasia (CIN I) and, in many cases, ends in invasive cancer if not treated. The median transit time for progression of CIN I to severe dysplasia or carcinoma in situ (CIN III) is approximately 58 months. The median transit time for CIN III to invasive carcinoma is approximately 10 years.[11] Currently, it is not possible to determine by any method which lesions will ultimately stabilize, regress, or progress. However, numerous investigators have shown evidence that HPVs are etiologically related to the development of anogenital squamous cell carcinoma.[12–15] For example, lesions containing HPV types 6 and 11 often regress and only in rare instances progress to invasion. However, patients with lesions containing HPV types 16 or 18 carry a significantly greater risk for developing cancer than those without such lesions.[16]

Extrapolation from previous prospective studies on patients with CIN suggests that the relative risk (RR) of patients developing invasive cancer can be correlated with the grade of CIN and the ratio of HPV 6/11 to 16/18. For example, the RR of CIN I is 1,200 and the proportion of HPV 6/11 to 16/8 is in favor of 6/11. CIN II lesions have mainly HPV 16/18 types and the RR is 1,500, whereas essentially all CIN III lesions are 16 or 18 type lesions and have a 2,000 greater RR than that of the general population.[16]

Cervical intraepithelial neoplasia can extend into the underlying cervical crypts. Anderson and Hartley measured the maximum glandular depth and maximum depth of neoplastic involvement in 343 cone specimens done for CIN III.[17] They found that the deepest uninvolved gland measured 7.83 mm from the surface, while the deepest involved gland was 5.22 mm and the mean depth was 1.24 mm. They concluded that destruction to a depth of 3.8 mm would eradicate disease extension in 99.7% of the cases.

In 1982, Abdul-Karim et al. published similar data in which the depths of all grades of neoplasia were measured with the respective linear length of disease.[18] They found the mean depths of CIN I, II, and III to be 0.42, 0.93, and 1.35 mm, respectively, and estimated that a depth of 4.80 mm was required to achieve the same 99.7% confidence level in treatment. They also noted a very strong positive correlation between linear length and both the severity of the CIN and the depth of glandular involvement. These studies conclude that destruction to a depth of at least 5 mm is required to achieve high cure rates when treating cervical intraepithelial neoplasia.

The linear length of CIN varies between 2 and 22 mm.[19, 20] The average lesion length varies between 6 and 10 mm. It is further observed that CIN lesions do not extend more than 22 mm up the endocervical canal when measured from the outermost border of the lesion.[19]

The transformation zone recedes into and up the endocervical canal with age.[20] It is well known that colposcopic examination is more often unsatisfactory in older patients. In contrast, Shingleton et al. found that only 2.5% of patients under the age of 30 required conization for adequate assessment of abnormal Papanicolaou smears.[21] Invasive cancer occurs on the canal side, that is, the worst disease is located centrally.[22, 23]

## NON-LASER THERAPY OF CIN

### Cryotherapy

Although the freezing of tissues to treat gynecologic disease dates back to the nineteenth century, modern cryotherapy began in 1967 when Crisp[24] reported using cryosurgery instruments in the treatment of cervical intraepithelial neoplasia. Since that time, this has been the most commonly used conservative method for the treatment of CIN, largely because of the simplicity of the procedure.[25]

The uncertainty of the depth of destruction is a large problem with cryocautery. This uncertainty is due to the variability in blood flow through the vessels beneath the cervical surface: an area with a large flow is a heat sink around which tissues do not freeze. This phenomenon may be responsible for the varying success rates cited for cryocautery. In 1980 in an extensive review of the literature, Charles and Savage found success rates varying from 27% to 96%.[26] Arof subsequently reported an overall cure rate of 84% for 393 patients treated for CIN I, II, and III.[27] They found that lesion size alone was the major determinant of the success rate, showing a 99% and 93% cure in patients with one- and two-quadrant lesions, respectively. However, the success rate dropped to 61% with three- and four-quadrant lesions. They also observed that extension of the lesion into the endocervical canal (even though the extent was seen) reduced the success rate to 64%. In 1985, Berget and Lenstrup summarized published data on approximately 3,000 cases and showed overall treatment successes in 94% of CIN I, 91% of CIN II, and 85% of CIN III lesions.[28] Although other authors have been more successful, the general tendency holds that as the severity of the CIN increases, the lesions are generally larger and extend deeper into the cervical glands, which decreases the cure rate with cryocautery.

The procedure itself is virtually painless and, other than the heavy watery discharge encountered as the necrotic tissue sloughs over the two weeks following the procedure, patients seldom have clinically significant side effects. The cervical defect is filled with granulation tissue and is subsequently covered with a mature squamous epithelium. This epithelium extends up into the canal to the extent that subsequent colposcopic examination is inadequate in 40% to 70% of these patients. Patients with persistently abnormal cytologic findings or recurrence of disease after cryocautery may have a fibrotic and stenotic external os, constricted to the point that subsequent endocervical curettage may not be possible. This patient will ultimately require an excisional cone biopsy for evaluation of abnormal cytologic findings, thus negating the ultimate goal of conservative management.

In spite of these problems, cryotherapy remains extremely popular. The procedure is very simple, is essentially painless, and can be performed very easily in the clinic setting. The equipment is inexpensive and can be easily transported from one facility to another.

### Electrocoagulation Diathermy

This procedure has maintained great popularity in Australia since first being reported in 1971 by Chanen and Hollyock.[29] It entails the destruction of the cervical tissue by using heat delivered through needle-and-ball electrodes placed in the substance of the cervix. As the heating occurs, mucus boils from the cervical glands. The procedure is continued to a depth of 10 mm or until the mucus production ceases.

The success rate of this procedure in the eradication of CIN is outstanding, with Chanen and Rome reporting a 97.3% success rate in 1,864 patients after a single diathermy treatment.[30] Problems with infection, cervical stenosis, or subsequent fertility are minimal. The major drawback encountered is the need for general or regional anesthesia, thus making the procedure more expensive and dangerous than cryocautery.

### "Cold" Coagulation

The term "cold" coagulation is somewhat of a misnomer. In 1966, Semm treated chronic cervicitis by means of an instrument that would allow tissue destruction by thermal heating to the range of 50°C to 120°C.[31] Energy is delivered to the tissue via a Teflon probe called a cold coagulator to distinguish it from instruments used for electrocoagulation diathermy, which reach much higher temperatures.

As with cryocautery, the use of the "cold" coagulator in the treatment of CIN is simple and virtually pain-free. Duncan has reported a success rate of 95% in the treatment of CIN.[31] Most failures reported by Duncan were present in patients with CIN III. Haddad et al. reported limited depth of destruction.[32] Their data showed tissue destruction of 2.6 to 3.5 mm, which corresponds to that believed to occur with cryocautery. The device has been used very little in North America. Although this method is promising, further evaluation is necessary before it can attain widespread use.

## LASER TREATMENT OF CIN

### $CO_2$ Laser Vaporization

The $CO_2$ laser permits surgeons either to vaporize or excise CIN of the cervix. Its advantage is that the surgeon can create surgical craters or defects of virtually any size or shape. In other words, surgeons can limit excision to only diseased tissue, sparing surrounding normal tissue. In the cervix, three basic surgical patterns account for the distribution of CIN. These three surgical procedures include a shallow, domed cylinder for ectocervical CIN, a tall cylinder for canal disease, and a moderately tall cylinder surrounded by a doughnut or inner tube configuration for disease occupying the endocervical canal and extending beyond a radius of 8 mm onto the ectocervix (Fig 6–1).[33] Depending on the geometry of the lesion, the laser surgeon will choose whether to ablate or excise the CIN.

The criteria to be fulfilled prior to laser vaporization or ablation include (1) the CIN must occupy the ectocervix with no extension into the endocervical canal; (2) correlation must exist between cytology, colposcopy, and histology; and (3) the diagnosis of microinvasive and invasive cancer must have been eliminated. The geometry of ectocervical intraepithelial neoplasia is illustrated in Figure 6–2. The end result is a central cylindrical

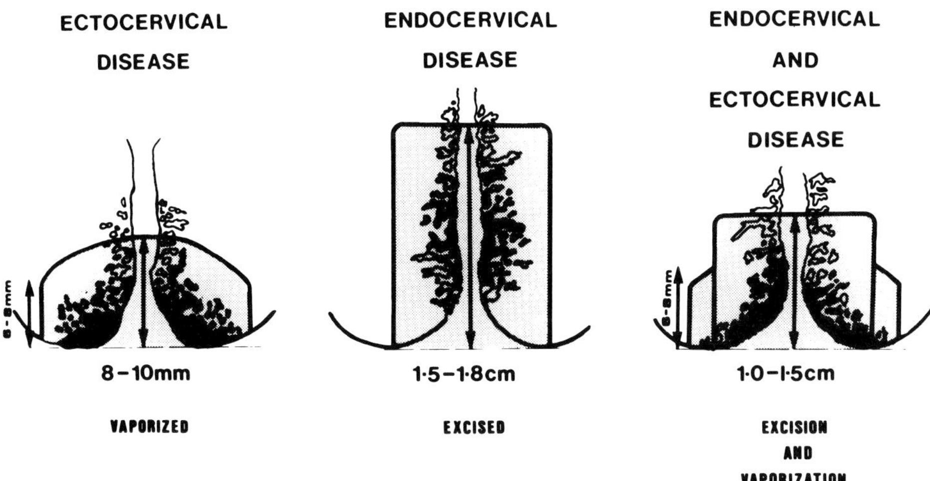


**FIG 6–1.**
Diagrammatic representation of the tissue defects appropriate for the three characteristic configurations of CIN. These defects are vaporized, excised, or both by the $CO_2$ laser as indicated; but it should be noted that excision of the vaporized portions of exocervical lesions can also be accomplished using the argon and KTP-532 lasers. An example of a specimen submitted to pathology is seen in Figure 6–14. (From Wright VC, Riopelle MA: *Gynecologic Laser Surgery: A Practical Handbook*, 2nd ed. Houston, Texas, Biomedical Communications, Inc, 1982. Used by permission.)

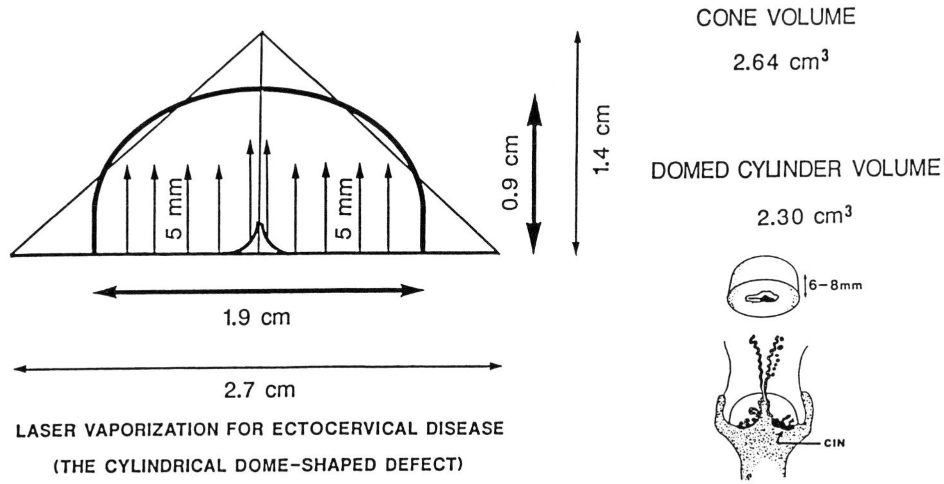


**FIG 6–2.**
Diagrammatic representation showing the volume and configuration of the tissue destroyed by laser vaporization compared to a cone-shaped excision of suitable size to remove the same disease. (From Wright VC, Riopelle MA: *Gynecologic Laser Surgery: A Practical Handbook*, 2nd ed. Houston, Texas, Biomedical Communications, Inc, 1982. Used by permission.)

dome-shaped defect, which incorporates both the ectocervical linear length (radius 9.5 mm in the example in the figure) and the underlying crypt involvement (height at least 5 mm along the entire lesion and transformation zone).

This procedure is easily done in the office or clinic setting. The procedure is usually well tolerated with approximately half of the patients having no appreciable discomfort. Approximately 10% will require local anesthetic infiltration into the cervical stroma or a paracervical block to complete the procedure. Alternately, the laser surgeon can locally anesthetize all patients if desired and give a preoperative nonsteroidal anti-inflammatory drug. Should discomfort occur, it is most likely a result of heat transfer. Prior to the procedure, it must be determined that all equipment is in functioning order and that the helium:neon and the $CO_2$ beams are aligned.

The procedure is done by inserting a dulled, nonreflective speculum to adequately expose the cervix. (Although the color of the speculum is irrelevant for use with the $CO_2$ laser, blackened instruments do absorb the argon, KTP-532, and Nd:YAG wavelength more readily.) The cervix is washed with 3% acetic acid and colposcopy is repeated to re-identify the disease and the transformation zone. A smoke evacuation system is at-

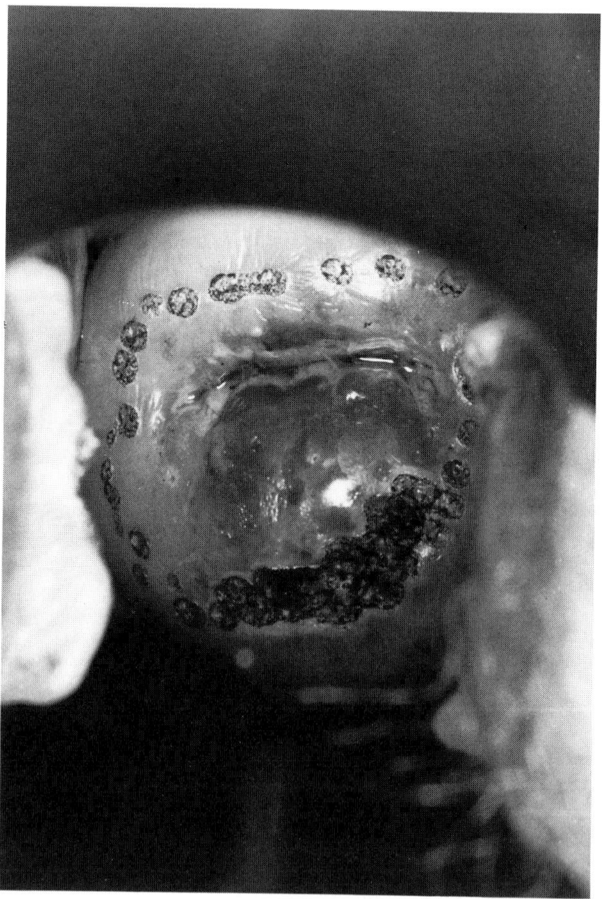

**FIG 6–3.**
Carbon dioxide laser vaporization of the cervix is begun by first outlining the original squamocolumnar junction, taking care to include 2 to 3 mm of normal-appearing tissue around any colposcopically visible lesion.

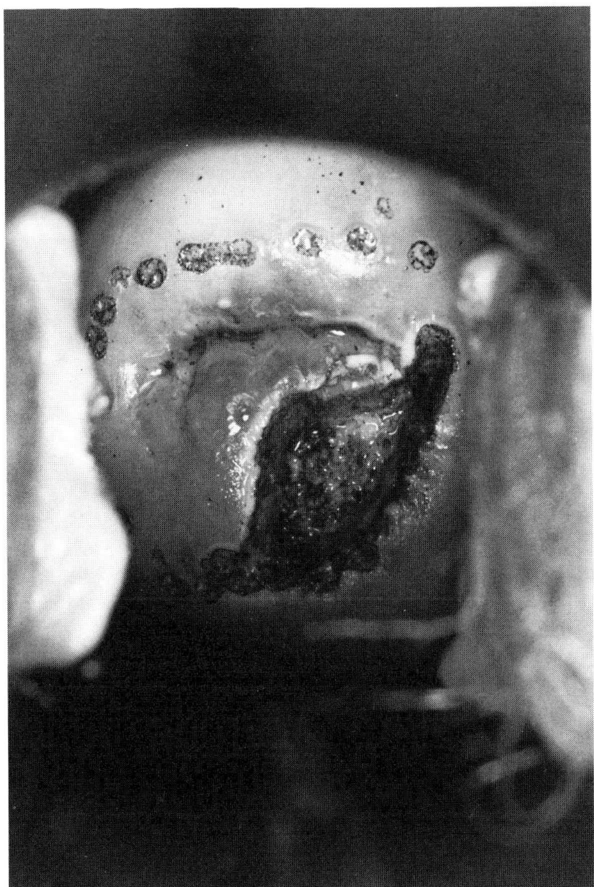

**FIG 6–4.**
As a second step in carbon dioxide laser vaporization of the cervix, the cervix is divided into four quadrants and each quadrant is vaporized to the appropriate depth prior to moving to the next area.

tached to the speculum. A power density in the range of 750 to 2,000 W/cm$^2$ is recommended. An effective laser beam diameter of 1.5 to 2 mm is appropriate for vaporization; it is achieved when the laser is attached to the colposcope (or operating microscope). The recommended magnification is 3.0 to 3.5 times, for a diameter of view of approximately 67 to 37 mm. Higher magnifications provide a greatly decreased diameter of view and make the procedure technically difficult. The recommended working distance is 300 mm, which equals the focal length of the main objective lens(es) of the colposcope.

The original squamocolumnar junction is identified and the intended defect is marked with the beam. Care should be taken to ensure that the cervical lesion is surrounded by a margin of approximately 3 mm of colposcopically normal tissue in all directions (Fig 6–3). This outline of the tissue to be ablated is advantageous because once vaporization is begun, dehydration of the tissue causes the outer edges to shrink and fall in on themselves, which can distort the normal cervical anatomy.

The cervix is then mentally divided into four quadrants, and vaporization is begun in one of the lower quadrants. Because of tissue shrinkage and control of bleeding (should it occur), it is advantageous to complete the intended depth in a single quadrant before moving to the next (Fig 6–4). Vaporization is done by moving the micromanipulator joystick in such a manner as to draw vertical, horizontal, and diagonal lines within the designated circumference over the area to be vaporized. Care should be taken not to cause furrowing or to extend the vaporization deeper than 7 mm (Fig 6–5). A flat, uniform defect base is desirable at least 6 mm along the entire transformation zone.

As a surgeon becomes more skilled in the manipulation of the laser beam, both the power density and speed of manipulation should be increased. The higher power density will allow less heat transfer into the tissues below and will result in significantly less uterine cramping as well as reduced operative time. If cramping begins, the surgeon may move to another quadrant of the cervix or pause for dissipation of heat.

While vaporization is taking place in the depth of tissue where the cervical glands are, the surgeon may notice mucus bubbling up from the base of the lesion. Once bubbling has ceased, it can be assumed that the deepest glands have been destroyed. This will occur somewhere between 5.5 and 8 mm in depth in a plane perpendicular to the

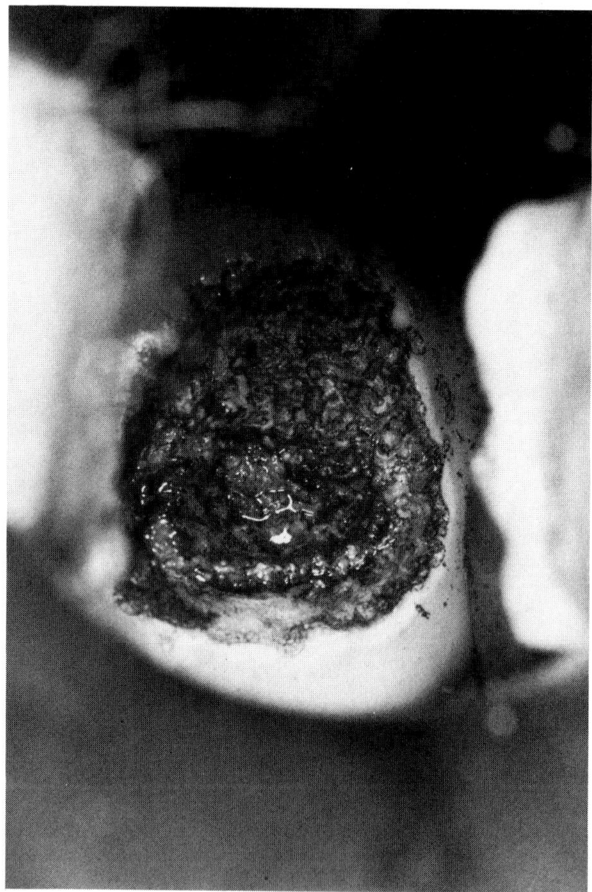

**FIG 6–5.**
Carbon dioxide laser vaporization of the cervix is completed when mucus ceases to bubble in the base of the crater, indicating that the cervical glands have been destroyed. Any irregularities in the base should then be flattened by the beam. The depth at the edges of the defect should measure 6 to 8 mm, as measured by a microruler. The depth at the center or around the os should be 8 to 12 mm measured from the most external plane of the ectocervix. The carbon particles along the defect's surface can be wiped away with a wet cotton swab.

surface of the cervix. As vaporization moves toward the endocervical canal, it may appear that the area being vaporized is greater than 8 mm. In fact, this is true if it is measured from the most distal aspect of the exocervix, but not if the lesion is measured from the original curved cervical surface.

The most commonly encountered problems associated with conservative methods of management are the lack of inclusion of both the entire linear extent of the lesion and the inadequate depth of destruction. The beginning laser surgeon may inadequately treat these patients by removing too little tissue. Because of this, a microruler should be used to ensure a depth of 6 to 8 mm along the lateral walls and 8 to 12 mm in the region of the cervical canal. Although the defect may appear extremely large when visualized through the colposcope, the tissues immediately adjacent to this are healthy and the defect will disappear completely in 3 to 4 weeks after the surgery. Following this type of ablative procedure, the new squamocolumnar junction will be visible in 90% to 95% of patients and the incidence of cervical stenosis is low. The latter, if it occurs, is related to an inadequate power density and an increased exposure time, which allows the heat to destroy adjacent tissue and cause scarring. The end result of optimal laser vaporization for ectocervical intraepithelial neoplasia is a cylindrical dome-shaped defect. This procedure usually takes between one and six minutes to perform, depending mostly upon the linear length of the disease and the volume to be removed.

The most significant complication encountered during laser vaporization is intraoperative bleeding. The $CO_2$ laser beam is not in itself a hemostatic instrument, nor is the 10,600-nm wavelength preferentially absorbed by hemoglobin to cause coagulation of blood. The hemostasis that does occur with the $CO_2$ laser beam is a product of thermal transfer through tissues as a result of energy absorption and subsequent boiling of water within the surface cells.

As the power density of the beam is increased, the beam should be moved faster over the tissue to control depth. This causes less and less thermal transfer around the zone of vaporization. As long as there is enough heat absorbed by the smaller vessels (up to 0.5 mm in diameter), coagulation of the blood will occur as the vessel is transected and the field will remain hemostatic. But, with structures as vascular as the uterine cervix, one must expect at some point to transect a larger vessel or to move the beam too quickly for the heat effect and be forced to deal with bleeding. The power density can be kept at a very low level, causing large amounts of heating and coagulating all of the vessels prior to ablation. However, under these circumstances, the patient will encounter a great deal more uterine irritability and pain. Also, the procedure will take substantially longer to perform if the power density drops significantly below 200 watts/cm$^2$, and a large zone of thermal necrosis will result with the possibility of stenosis and cervical incompetence.

Assuming that normal vaporization power densities are being used, several steps can be taken upon encountering bleeding. The first observation in the face of active bleeding is that, once blood has completely covered the operative surface, any attempt to use the laser to stop the bleeding simply coagulates this surface blood so that the energy never reaches the target. In many cases, if the beam is immediately turned back toward the spot at the instant where bleeding is first noted, there will be enough energy absorbed in the vessel to facilitate coagulation at the vessel opening. If this effort is not successful, the first thing that must be done is to remove the blood from the surface of the cervix by the use of suction or by cotton-tip applicators. Once the surface is dry, the laser may be used to coagulate the vessel in one of two methods. The power density may be decreased by either decreasing the power of the instrument or by defocusing and enlarging the spot size. This will increase the thermal effect and coagulate the vessel. Another method is to direct the laser beam to the areas immediately adjacent to the bleeding point, causing heating around the vessel wall with subsequent coagulation. If this is not immediately successful, the tamponade and cautery should be performed, using either silver nitrate sticks or Monsel's solution. Following 2 to 3 minutes of continuous tamponade, if the vessel continues to bleed, it may become necessary to place hemostatic sutures.

## $CO_2$ Laser Excisional "Cone" Biopsy

The laser "conization" (which is, in fact, a cylindrical removal of tissue) is recommended as a substitute to scalpel conization and is appropriate when (1) the disease occupies the endocervical canal; (2) discrepancies exist between cytology, colposcopy, and histology and invasive cancer cannot be ruled out; (3) colposcopy is unsatisfactory; or (4) colposcopically directed biopsy reveals microinvasive cancer or adenocarcinoma in situ.

Figure 6–6 illustrates the geometry of endocervical intraepithelial neoplasia and the configuration of an excisional laser cone. The cylindrical removal of tissue accounts for the linear length of the CIN (1.5 cm in the hypothetical case in the figure) and potential underlying cervical crypt extension (indicated by horizontal arrows). This cylindrical ap-

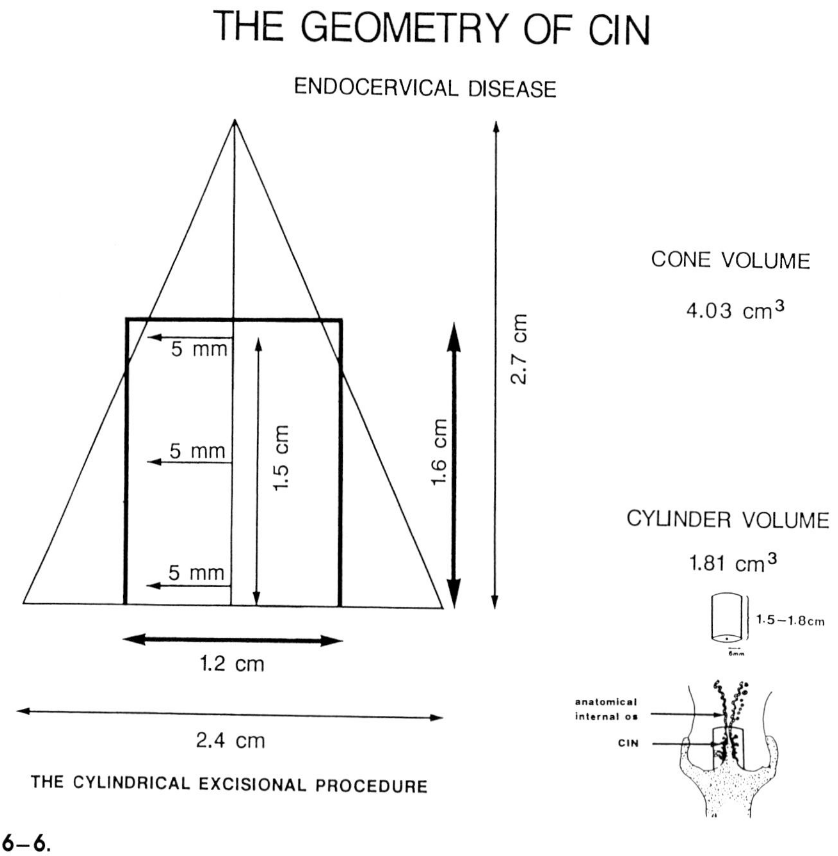

**FIG 6–6.**
Diagrammatic presentation of the configuration and volume removed during the cylindrical excision procedure compared to the volume of a geometric cone required to encompass the same diseased tissue. It is important to note that the cone volume is substantially more than twice that of the cylinder. (From Wright VC, Riopelle MA: *Gynecologic Laser Surgery: A Practical Handbook,* 2nd ed. Houston, Texas, Biomedical Communications, Inc, 1982. Used by permission.)

proach removes less than half the volume of tissue required by a traditional cone-shaped specimen to remove all disease (indicated by triangle).

This procedure can be accomplished either in a clinic setting with local anesthesia or as ambulatory day-care surgery with general anesthesia. The latter approach is preferred because of discomfort to patients necessitated by cervical and vaginal retraction to achieve adequate exposure. The cervix is exposed by placing a weighted speculum in the vagina. A tenaculum is placed at the 12 o'clock position, and the cervix is positioned so that the incision will be made parallel to the endocervical canal (Fig 6–7, A). A Pitressin (vasopressin) solution not exceeding one pressor unit is injected into the cervical stroma circumferentially. The vasopressin solution decreases the lumen size of the blood vessels so that the brief thermal effect of the beam will seal them. Further, to decrease the inflow of blood into the cervix, hemostatic sutures may be placed at the 9 and 12 o'clock positions.

The procedure is best performed with the laser attached to the operating microscope, although the handheld component has been used. With the laser attached to the operating microscope and the use of the micromanipulator, greater precision is achieved. The other problem encountered with handheld laser delivery is the relatively short focal length of handpiece lenses which causes difficulty in keeping the laser beam in focus.

With the laser attached to the operating microscope, a matching lens system of 300 mm is recommended (that is, the laser light-capturing lens of 300 mm equals the 300 mm focal length of the main objective lens of the operating microscope). The smallest effective laser beam diameter is usually about 0.5 mm in this situation. It is adequate in diameter for rapid incision without destroying too much extra tissue yet has a sufficient beam area to seal blood vessels during the procedure. Larger beam diameters can be selected by adjusting the variable spot size mechanism in the articulated arm.

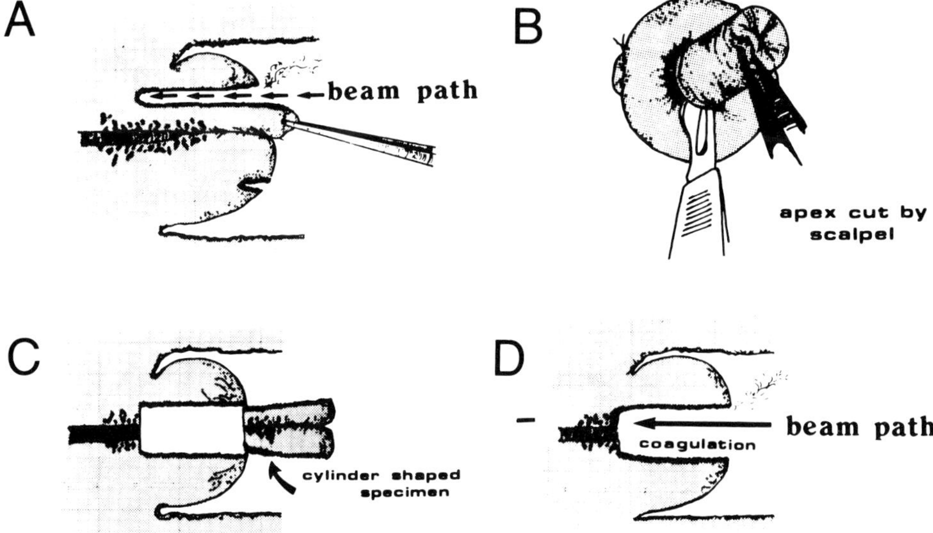


**FIG 6–7.**
The laser cylindrical excision is performed by directing the laser beam straight into the substance of the cervix to a depth of 1.5 to 1.8 cm. The incision should circumscribe the cervical canal at a radius of 6 to 8 mm. Once this is completed, the cylindrical specimen is lifted away from the cervix and severed using a scalpel or tonsil snare. The procedure is completed by coagulation of the base using a lower power density. (From Wright VC, Riopelle MA: *Gynecologic Laser Surgery: A Practical Handbook*, 2nd ed. Houston, Texas, Biomedical Communications, Inc, 1982. Used by permission.)

The laser procedure is begun by encircling the external os with a radius of 6 to 8 mm. A power density of 12,000 to 20,000 W/cm$^2$ permits rapid cutting. The specimen is developed with its sides parallel to the endocervical canal (Fig 6–7, A). It is important to obtain the desired height at each arc of the circle before moving onward; that is, it is advisable not to keep encircling the cervix. This leads to excessive thermal damage of the specimen. Forceps or an iris hook provide traction of the specimen away from the plane of the laser beam. The traction is applied at the 3, 6, 9, and 12 o'clock positions, respectively. The incision is continued to a depth of 1.5 to 1.8 cm in the reproductive-aged patients. This radius of 6 to 8 mm and height of 1.5 to 1.8 cm usually incorporates the underlying crypt involvement and linear extent of disease. Also, the specimen is adequate to diagnose microinvasive and invasive cancer. The recommended height should be below the anatomical internal os and thus avoid creating an incompetent cervix. Once this depth is achieved, the specimen is severed at the apex transversely with scissors, a scalpel, or a tonsil snare and removed (Fig 6–7, B and C). The apex of the defect usually appears white because of the effects of the Pitressin solution. A laser beam diameter of 2 mm is now substituted, yielding a power density in the range of 650 to 1,200 W/cm$^2$ to quickly "flash" the surface of the apex to seal the blood vessels, thus taking advantage of beam heat (Fig 6–7, D).

Should any bleeding be present, this can be suctioned out of the field and followed by the application of the laser beam as described under laser vaporization. Should this fail, then an appropriate suture(s) is required. It is important never to chase a bleeder with the $CO_2$ laser because further vaporization will continue and the beam may enter an undesirable area. The entire excisional procedure usually requires 6 to 8 minutes to complete. The amount of blood loss varies between 2 and 8 cc under normal circumstances.

## $CO_2$ Laser Excision Plus Laser Ablation (The Combination Procedure) for Endocervical and Ectocervical CIN

In approximately 18% of CIN cases, extensive disease occupies the transformation zone on the ectocervix but also extends beyond colposcopic vision into the endocervical canal.[33] Although cytology and colposcopy indicate only CIN, histologic examination of the endocervical tissue is necessary to completely evaluate this area. Figure 6–8 illustrates a suitable defect incorporating the ectocervix and lower endocervical canal to eliminate the disease. As previously stated, the worst histology is present centrally. The combination procedure is employed when the ectocervical component of disease has a radius greater than 8 mm. The advantage of this approach is that the total volume of tissue removed is much less than that of a traditional cold-knife cone.

With the patient usually under general anesthesia (or, alternately, paracervical block), the central cylinder is removed first for histologic evaluation. Specimen heights usually range from 1.0 to 1.8 cm. This part of the operation is surgically similar to the laser cylindrical excision just described. In many cases the approximate depth of the central excision can be identified by examination of the endocervical canal using a contact hysteroscope. Then, employing a 2-mm $CO_2$ laser beam, the remaining peripheral disease and transformation zone are vaporized to a uniform depth of 6 to 7 mm. This results in a "cowboy hat" configuration (Fig 6–8). If the lesion extends onto the vagina, vaporization to a depth of 1.0 to 1.5 mm can be carried out and is sufficient to eradicate vaginal intraepithelial neoplasia.

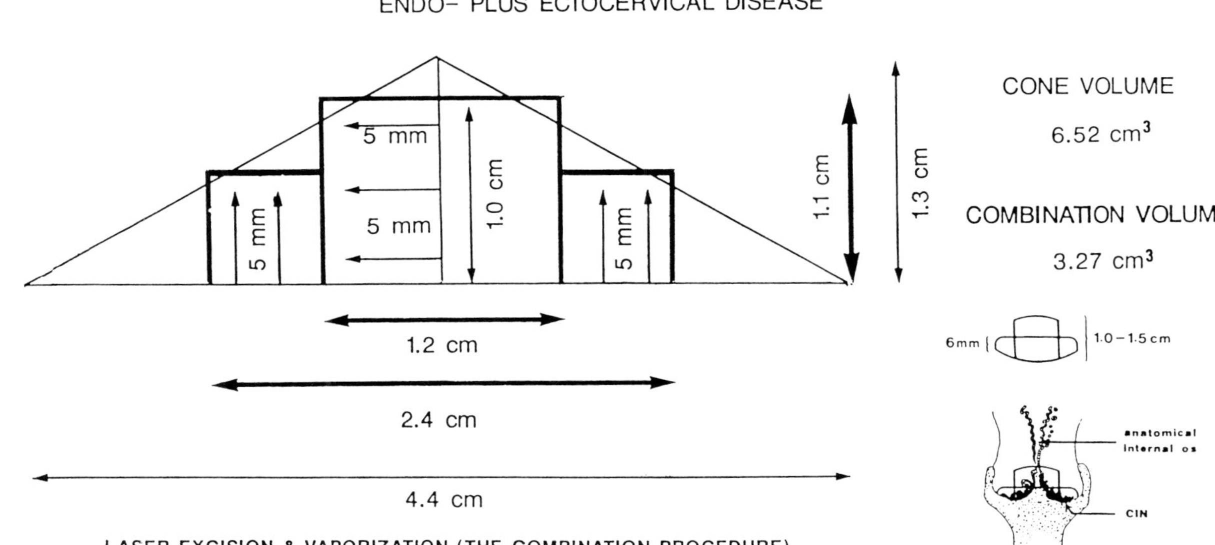


**FIG 6–8.**
The volumes of tissue required to eliminate disease by a cylindrical and by a conical approach are compared. Endocervical disease is excised for examination and disease on the portio is vaporized. To incorporate disease by a conical specimen, twice as much tissue must be excised. The same anatomically correct removal of tissue can be performed using the argon or KTP lasers in a pure excisional fashion. (From Wright VC, Riopelle MA: *Gynecologic Laser Surgery: A Practical Handbook,* 2nd ed. Houston, Texas, Biomedical Communications, Inc, 1982. Used by permission.)

## Follow-up After $CO_2$ Laser Surgery

Postoperative care after these procedures is minimal. Patients are instructed to refrain from placing anything in the vagina for 2 or 3 weeks. Minor bleeding or spotting occurs in approximately 10% of patients; major bleeding, requiring some type of clinical intervention, occurs in less than 1% of patients. Postoperative pain is usually minimal. The patients will experience some discharge, although this is substantially less than that encountered following cryosurgery. After healing, the new squamocolumnar junction forms at the level of the external os in 90% of patients.[33]

The patients should have follow-up cytologic sampling 4 months after the procedure. Some authors also recommend at least one colposcopic examination after healing. Cytology is repeated every 4 months for the first year and then every 6 months for the next year before returning the patient to an annual examination schedule.

Depending upon the grade of disease, these three procedures have shown a cure rate between 92% to 95%. Usually any persistent disease can be retreated with the $CO_2$ laser so that the eventual hysterectomy rate for CIN is approximately 1/200 cases originally treated.[33]

These three procedures, $CO_2$ laser vaporization of a dome-shaped cylinder, $CO_2$ excision of a cylindrical specimen of endocervix, or a combination of both, appear to be quite effective for eliminating CIN regardless of histological grade, lesion size, or disease location. This is probably because the surgical approaches are designed to remove appropriate tissue volumes based on the solid (i.e., three dimensional) geometry of CIN. The defects created always have a base and sides to promote healing. This planned volume of tissue removed does not appear to increase the premature delivery rate or produce an incompetent cervix.[33] This is likely related to the fact that these three $CO_2$ laser procedures are designed to remove disease but not to encroach upon the anatomical internal os in the reproductive female.

## Conization With Argon, KTP-532, and Nd:YAG Lasers

Recent advances in technology have made the argon, KTP-532, and Nd:YAG lasers practical for the excision of cervical lesions. Although the number of cases reported to have been performed with these instruments is indeed small, the fiberoptic delivery system coupled with the greatly superior hemostatic characteristics of their wavelengths ultimately may confirm their speculative value as superior to the $CO_2$ laser for performing cervical procedures, particularly in terms of bleeding incidence. With these lasers, the added tactile sensation and the ability to curve the fiber inside the limited confines of the vaginal space allow the surgeon to hemostatically excise an anatomically correct exocervical or endocervical specimen without the use of vaginal retractors or stay sutures.

The argon and KTP-532 lasers are very similar in their clinical applications. There are several characteristics of the "green" lasers that make their use in cervical procedures advantageous when compared to the $CO_2$ laser. First and most important is the extremely high absorption coefficient of the blue-green wavelength in hemoglobin, coupled with the virtual absence of absorption in water. This allows the laser energy to travel a short distance through the cervical tissue before absorption, allowing coagulation of vessels of substantial size before the vessel wall is destroyed. This has allowed for the virtual elimination of what is probably the largest single complication of cervical excisional cone biopsies—excessive blood loss.

The other significant difference is the ability of the laser beam to travel through a highly flexible quartz fiber. Because of this, the energy may be applied to the cervix at virtually any angle, using a long tubular hand piece with a 30- to 45-degree curve at the tip. This allows sculpting of excisional cones without significant cervical or vaginal retraction (Figs 6–9 to 6–14). The large excisional cone specimen in Fig 6–14 was obtained using only a Graves laser speculum and two skin hooks. Paracervical block was used, and the estimated blood loss was approximately 25 cc.

The argon and KTP-532 wavelengths do result in a larger coagulation defect on the surgical specimen than does the $CO_2$ laser. We have measured these depths and found them to be still significantly less than 1 mm and to allow pathologic evaluation of the affected tissue.[34] Although the $CO_2$ laser is a much more powerful incisional tool, the KTP-532 uses 15 to 20 W through a 400- or 600-micron fiber, allowing a power density approaching 20,000 W/cm$^2$. Using the methods previously described, the experienced surgeon can complete an excisional cone procedure in approximately 15 to 20 minutes. It should also be noted that these power densities are satisfactory for ablation procedures, again without the worry of excessive blood loss during the procedure.

Postoperative care is essentially the same as with other cervical laser surgery. Although the number of cases reported is still relatively small, there have been no reports of major postoperative bleeding. Because they allow all ablative and excisional cones to be performed in the outpatient clinic, these instruments deserve a very serious evaluation by the medical community.

Yandell et al. reported data on a series of ten consecutive excisional "cones" performed using the KTP-532 laser in 1988.[34] Each procedure was performed using only a Graves laser speculum for exposure and smoke evacuation and without the use of stay sutures or vasopressin. The endocervical margin was excised sharply with a knife. The average blood loss was 25 ml; in five patients, blood loss was limited to 0 to 1 ml. The last procedure was performed under paracervical block. A specimen, as submitted to the pa-

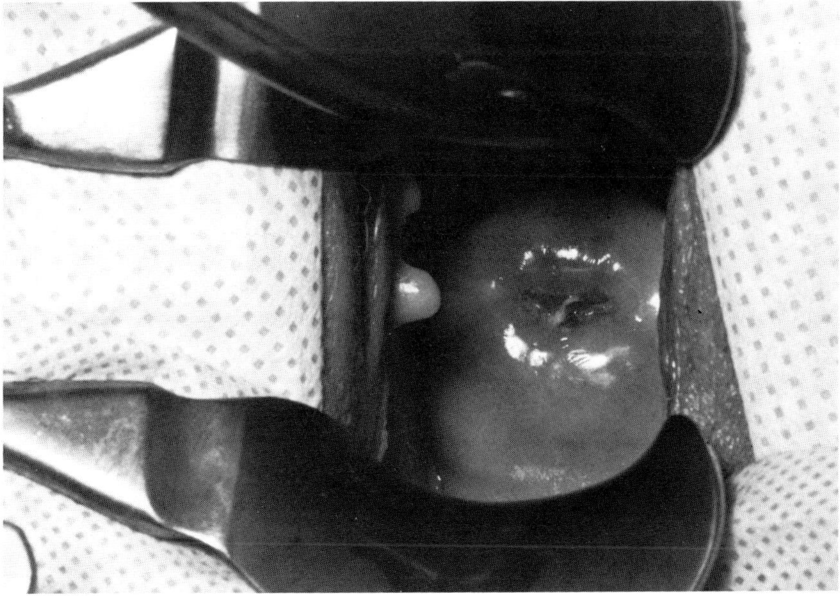

**FIG 6–9.**
Excisional cone biopsy performed using the KTP laser. The only retraction required is a Graves laser speculum.

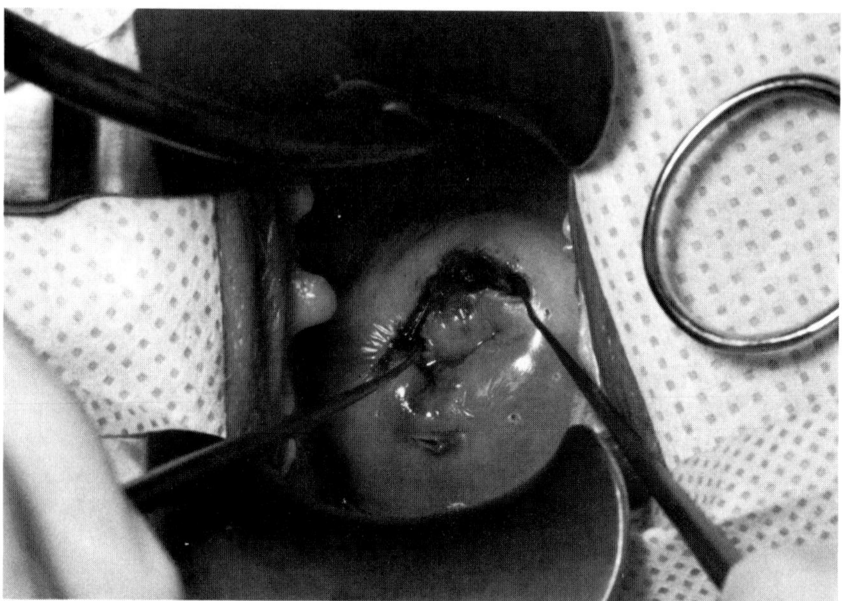

**FIG 6–10.**
Excisional cone biopsy using the KTP laser. The procedure is begun by outlining the original squamocolumnar junction and creating an initial incision of sufficient depth to allow attachment of skin hooks (2 to 3 mm depth).

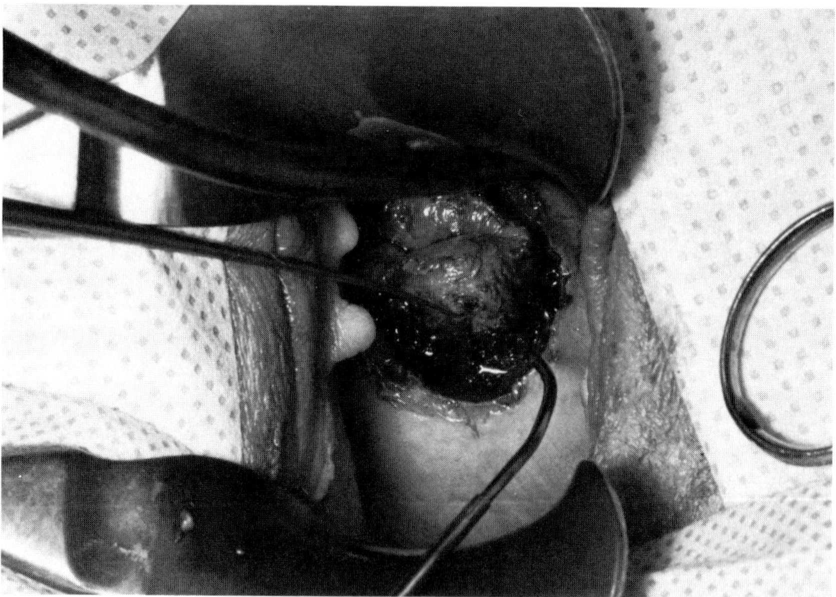

**FIG 6–11.**
Excisional cone biopsy of the cervix using the KTP laser. The narrow, curved hand piece, which contains the quartz fiber, is seen entering the field at a sharp angle from the 5-o'clock position on the cervix.

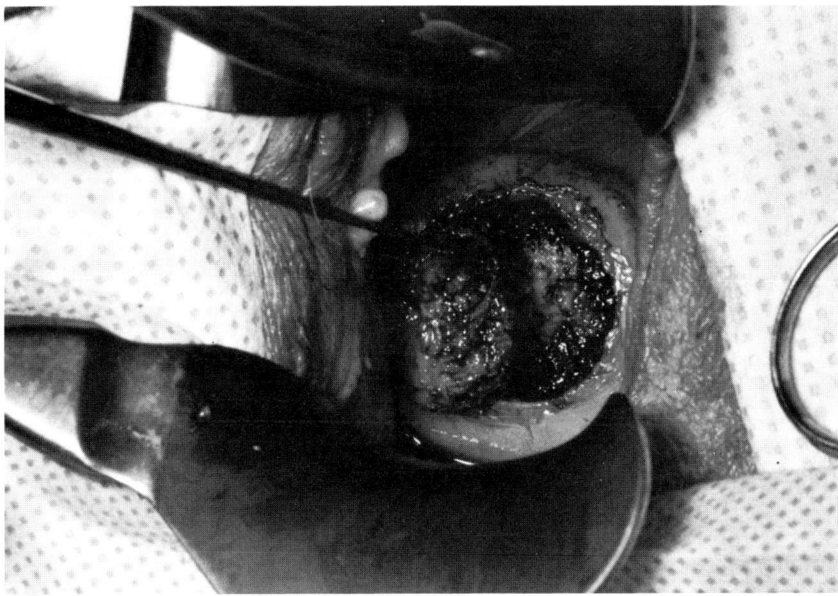

**FIG 6–12.**
Excisional cone biopsy of the cervix using the KTP laser. Most of the excision has been completed. Because of the coagulation defect, the laser is not used to incise the tissue immediately adjacent to the endocervical canal. Note the complete lack of blood in or around the surgical field.

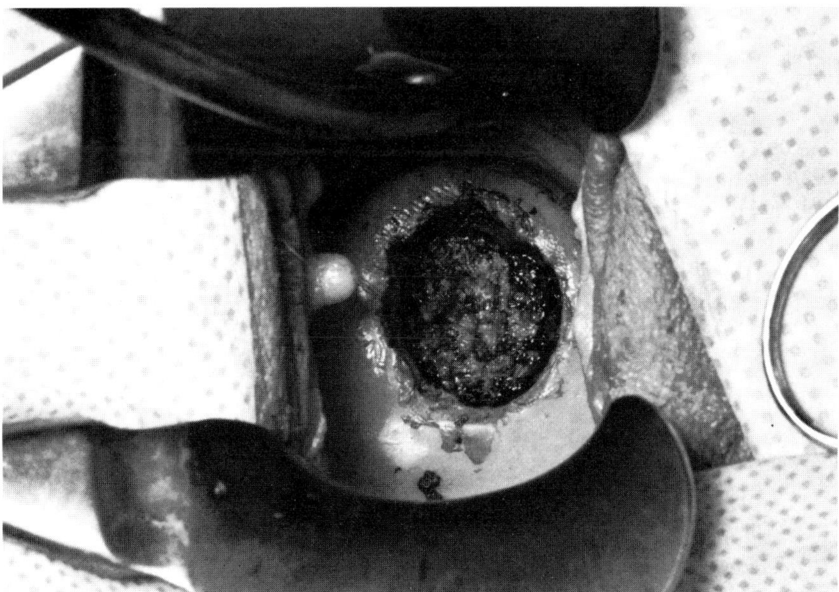

**FIG 6–13.**
Excisional cone biopsy of the cervix using the KTP laser. The specimen has been sharply excised using a scalpel and the base of the lesion photocoagulated using the laser. The carbon may be removed from the tissue with a wet sponge. In an effort to decrease the possibility of postoperative hemorrhage, the laser may be defocused by backing the fiber 5 to 10 mm from the surface and brushing the entire excised surface area.

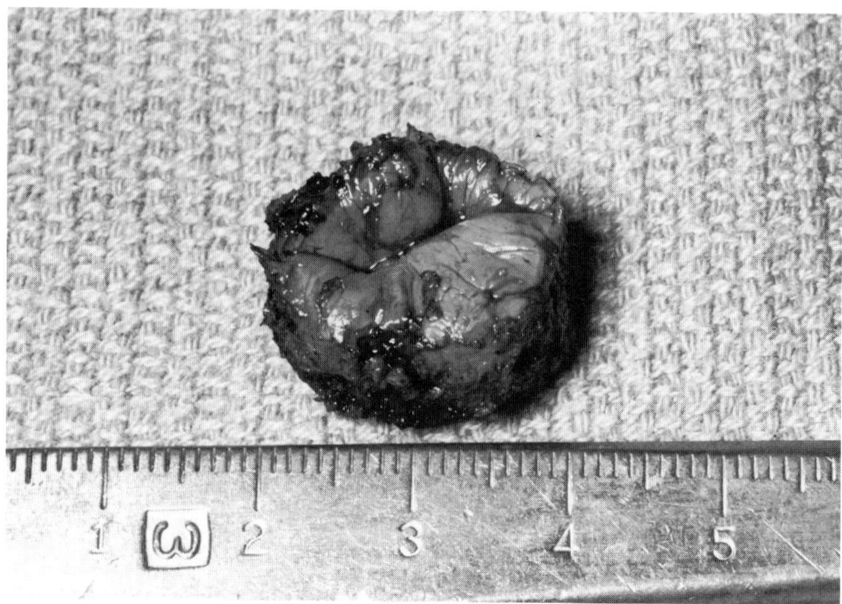


**FIG 6–14.**
Excisional cone biopsy of the cervix using the KTP laser. This is the final excised specimen as it appears immediately after surgery. Coagulation necrosis may vary from 0.4 to 1.0 mm. This may be kept to a minimum by angling the fiber away from the surgical specimen during the excisional process.

thologist, is seen in Fig 6–14. The coagulated defects on the ten specimens ranged from 480 to 1,360 microns in extent (10 to 14 times those of the $CO_2$ thermal injury).

The authors have also performed the same procedure using the argon laser and the Nd:YAG laser with contact surgical sapphire tips attached to the fiber's end.

In the past, the Nd:YAG laser had been of relatively little value in cervical surgery because of its enormous scattering effects within tissue and its significant penetration. Its use had been restricted to coagulation procedures. However, with the development of artificial sapphire tips for contact laser surgery, the characteristics of the instrument's tissue effects have changed substantially. Although the Nd:YAG laser is still of little use in cervical ablation procedures, the use of the sapphire tip as a cutting instrument has resulted in very rapid and almost completely hemostatic excisional procedures.

This procedure is performed using 20 to 30 W of power with the beam delivered via the air-cooled coaxial fiber. With this range of settings, the average excision can be completed in 2 to 5 minutes, with a resulting coagulation defect of less than 0.5 mm. The respective coagulation defects observed histologically in specimens created with the $CO_2$, KTP-532, Nd:YAG, and argon lasers are shown in Plates 5 to 8, respectively. In each case the specimen is adequate for pathologic evaluation. A drawback to the use of the Nd:YAG laser in contact mode is the inflexibility of the sapphire tip because it is attached to the handpiece, thus allowing slightly less maneuverability and fewer cutting angles than are possible using the KTP-532 and argon lasers.

## CONCLUSION

Throughout this chapter, we have examined the different methods currently available for the treatment of cervical intraepithelial neoplasia and found drawbacks or problems associated with each. Initial studies showing the use of lasers to be inferior to traditional methods were largely the result of failures in technique. With current ablative and excisional methods, the treatment of CIN has been very satisfactory. Laser procedures are even beginning to show a superior success rate with regards to the more advanced lesions.

In 1985, in an in-depth review of the literature, Berget and Lenstrup[28] compared almost 3,000 cryosurgery procedures to the same number of laser vaporization cases. The cumulative success rate after one treatment was identical in CIN I at 94%; however, the success rate after one treatment of CIN III lesions was 91% for laser procedures versus 85% for the cryocautery. In the same series, the patients who were treated more than once using the laser had a success rate approaching 98%. Perhaps this is the most significant aspect of these findings. The cervix may actually be treated more than once with laser ablation because of the rapid return to relatively normal cervical architecture, thus allowing subsequent colposcopy to visualize the transformation zone of these cases.

One of the most commonly cited negative aspects regarding the use of lasers for CIN is the initially high expense involved with the purchase of the instrument. True cost savings to the patient are a result of the reductions in hospitalization and anesthesia expenses. Certainly, if one reviews the preliminary data currently being collected on the use of the argon, KTP-532, and Nd:YAG lasers for these procedures, it becomes apparent that the need for hospitalization for the treatment of intraepithelial neoplasia will soon be a thing of the past.

## REFERENCES


1. Shingleton HM, Orr JW: *Cancer of the Cervix: Diagnosis and Treatment*. New York, Churchill Livingstone Publishers, 1987.
2. Mann M: *A System of Gynecology*. Pennsylvania, Lea & Febiger, 1887.
3. Leonard VN: Post-operative results of amputation of the cervix. *Surg Gynecol Obstet* 1913; 16:390.
4. Lisfranc MJ: Memoire sur l'amputation du col de l'uterus. *Gaz Med de Par* 1834; ii:385.
5. Sims M: Amputation of cervix. *Tr Med Soc New York*, 1861.
6. Papanicolaou GN, Traut HF: Diagnosis of uterine cancer by the vaginal smear. *Commonwealth Fund* New York, 1943.
7. Larsson G: Conization for preclinical cervical carcinoma. *Acta Obstet Gynecol Scand Suppl* 1983; 114:7–40.
8. American Cancer Society: Ca-A cancer journal for clinicians. *Cancer Statistics* 1988; 38:1.
9. Kaufman R, Koss LG, Kurman RJ, et al: Statement of caution in the interpretation of papillomavirus-associated lesions of the epithelium of uterine cervix. *Am J Obstet Gynecol* 1983; 146:125.
10. Coppleson M: The origin and nature of premalignant lesions of the cervix uteri. *Int J Gynecol Obstet* 1970; 8:539-547.
11. Peterson E, Hoeg K, Kolstad P: Mass screening for cancer of the uterine cervix in Ostfold County, Norway: An experiment. *Act Obstet Gyn Scand Suppl* 1971; 11:1–18.
12. zur Hausen H, Scheider A: The role of papillomaviruses in human genital cancer, in Hawley P, Jabzmann NP (eds): *The Papilloma-virus*. New York, Plenum Press, 1985, pp 245–259.
13. Richard RM: Causes and management of cervical intraepithelial neoplasia. *Cancer* 1987; 60:1951–1956.
14. Shah KH, Lewis MC, Jensen AB, Kurman RJ: Papillomavirus and cervical dysplasia. *Lancet* 1980; 2:1190–1193.
15. Gissman L: Papillomaviruses and their association with cancer in animals and man. *Cancer Surv* 1984; 3:163–167.
16. Ferenczy A: HPV infection and genital neoplasia. *ACOG Syllabus on Lasers in Gynecology*; 1988, p 169.

17. Anderson MC, Hartley RB: Cervical crypt involvement by intraepithelial neoplasia. *Obstet Gynecol* 1980; 55(5):546–550.
18. Abdul-Karim FW, Fu YS, Reagan JW, et al: Morphometric study of intraepithelial neoplasia of the uterine cervix. *Obstet Gynecol* 1982; 60(2):210–214.
19. Przybora LA, Plutowa A: Histological topography of carcinoma in situ of the uterine cervix. *Cancer* 1959; 12:268–273.
20. Hamperl H, Kaufmann C: The cervix uteri at various ages. *Obstet Gynecol* 1959; 14:621–625.
21. Shingleton H, et al: Outpatient evaluation of patients with atypical Papanicolaou smears: Contributions of endocervical curettage. *Am J Obstet Gynecol* 1976; 121:122.
22. Gusberg SB, Moore DB: The clinical pattern of intraepithelial carcinoma of the cervix and its pathologic background. *Obstet Gynecol* 1954; 2:1–14.
23. Carson RP, Gall EA: Preinvasive carcinoma and precancer metaplasia of the cervix. *Am J Pathol* 1954; 30:15–19.
24. Crisp WE, Asadourian L, Romberger W: Application of cryosurgery to gynecologic malignancy. *Obstet Gynecol* 1967; 30:668.
25. Townsend DE, Ostergard DR: Cryocauterization for preinvasive cervical neoplasia. *J Reprod Med* 1971; 6:55–60.
26. Charles EH, Savage EW: Cryosurgical treatment of cervical intraepithelial neoplasia. *Obstet Gynecol Surv* 1980; 35(9):539–548.
27. Arof HM, Gerbie MV, Smeltzer J: Cryosurgical treatment of cervical intraepithelial neoplasia: Four year experience. *Am J Obstet Gynecol* 1984; 150(7):867–869.
28. Berget A, Lenstrup C: Cervical intraepithelial neoplasia. Examination, treatment and follow-up, REVIEW. *Obstet Gynecol Survey* 1985; 40(9):545–552.
29. Chanen W, Hollyock VE: Colposcopy and electrocoagulation diathermy for cervical dysplasia and carcinoma in situ. *Obstet Gynecol* 1971; 37:623.
30. Chanen W, Rome RM: Electrocoagulation diathermy for cervical dysplasia and carcinoma in situ. A 15 year survey. Obstet Gynecol 1983; 61:673–679.
31. Duncan ID: The Semm cold coagulator in the management of cervical intraepithelial neoplasia. *Clin Obstet Gynecol* 1983; 26(4):996–1006.
32. Haddad N, Hussein I, Blessing K, et al: Tissue destruction following cold coagulation of the cervix. *Colposcopy and Gynecologic Laser Surgery* 1988; 4(1):23–27.
33. Wright VC: Carbon dioxide laser surgery for the cervix and vagina: Indications, complications and results. *Compr Ther* 1988; 14:54–64.
34. Yandell RB, Dinh TV, Dillard EA, et al: Evaluation of the KTP-532 nm laser for excisional cone biopsy of the cervix. Abstract presented at the Proceedings of the Combined Clinical Meeting of the American Society for Culposcopy and Cervical Pathology, and Gynecologic Laser Society, April 1988.

# Chapter 7

# Intrauterine Laser Surgery

Milton H. Goldrath, M.D.

Gynecologists have long recognized the need for intrauterine surgery. Until recent times, major uterine surgery has required a laparotomy and uterine incision. Examples include the Strassman procedure for treatment of bicornuate uterus[1] and the variety of techniques described by Jones and Roch[2] for the treatment of uterine duplication anomalies. Recently, however, Chervenak and Newirth,[3] DeCherney and Polan,[4] and March, Israel, and March[5] have all described intrauterine surgery for the removal of uterine septa and synechiae using sharp scissors dissection or electrosurgery. Unfortunately, procedures utilizing the scissors have been described as occasionally being quite bloody. In addition, the use of a high-frequency cutting current, while hemostatic, does have some disadvantage, in that it is impossible to determine the extent of electrical spread and tissue damage. Newirth[6] has reported on the hysteroscopic resection of submucous fibroids.

The first reported use of transcervical intrauterine laser surgery was in 1979, by the author, Fuller, and Segal.[7] We used the Neodymium:yttrium-aluminum-garnet (Nd:YAG) laser to photocoagulate and photovaporize the endometrium for the treatment of menorrhagia. Subsequently, we have used the Nd:YAG laser to divide intrauterine septa. Marlowe has also used the carbon dioxide ($CO_2$) laser at laparotomy to remove uterine septa in patients with duplication anomalies of the uterus (Marlowe, personal communication). He found this technique a very useful adjunct in providing hemostasis in this usually bloody operation. The transcervical use of the $CO_2$ laser has been hampered by the inability, up to now, to transmit the $CO_2$ laser energy via a fiberoptic tube. In the near future, this technique may prove to be a clinical reality and would be quite useful in the correction of uterine anomalies and synechiae.

## THE TREATMENT OF MENORRHAGIA BY ENDOMETRIAL PHOTOVAPORIZATION AND COAGULATION

Over the past 35 years, the indications for hysterectomy have been greatly liberalized, and this procedure has been advocated for relief of symptoms in the absence of organic disease. There has been considerable debate in the medical literature, as well as the lay press, concerning the soundness of this liberalization.[8–13] Hysterectomy is the most common major operation performed in the United States.[9] The most common presenting symptom in cases in which a normal uterus has been removed is dysfunctional uterine bleeding.[9–12, 14]

Obviously, large numbers of patients are greatly distressed by excessive menstrual bleeding, whether ovulatory or anovulatory, and are consulting their physicians for relief. Current methods of management consist of curettage, hormones, ergot derivatives, and antifibrinolytic agents.[15] When these methods fail, cause undesirable side effects, or are contraindicated, the gynecologist is currently faced with either performing a hysterectomy or allowing the patient to endure her symptoms and prescribing iron supplements to prevent or treat anemia.

It is not the purpose of this chapter to enter the debate concerning which patients should be subjected to hysterectomy and which should be allowed to live with their symptoms. There are many patients who will not endure even moderately heavy menses, and others who will tolerate profuse menorrhagia and profound anemia rather than undergo a major surgical procedure. In addition, there are patients with blood dyscrasias and other physical disorders that contraindicate or markedly complicate hysterectomy. It is with these thoughts in mind that we explored the treatment of abnormal uterine bleeding with the laser.

Posttraumatic intrauterine synechiae were first described by Fritsch in 1894.[16] More than half a century later, Asherman[17] reported a series of patients and described a syndrome that now bears his name. The major clinical symptoms of intrauterine synechiae are amenorrhea or hypomenorrhea and infertility. The prominent symptoms of amenorrhea or hypomenorrhea and infertility have led to attempts to reproduce the syndrome for control of uterine hemorrhage or for sterilization. A variety of physical and chemical agents have been used for this purpose, including quinacrine hydrochloride, methyl 2-cyanoacrylate, oxalic acid, paraformaldehyde, silicone rubber,[18] intracavitary radium,[19, 20] direct application of super-heated steam,[21] and cryocaogulation.[18, 22–26] All of these substances and agents except for cryocoagulation have been abandoned, however, because they were unsuccessful or otherwise unacceptable. Cryocoagulation holds some promise, and the ingenious applications devised by Droegemueller have been successful in a few patients.[23, 24] Cryocoagulation is basically a blind procedure, however, and areas of endometrium are often spared. Thus, in only a few instances was there complete destruction of the entire endometrium. Frequently, the fundal and cornual endometrium was viable and functioning, often producing hematometra if previous ligation had been performed or if the isthmus was oblierated by cryocoagulation. In addition, Burke, Rubin and Kim[27] reported a case of uterine abscess formation following cryosurgery of the endometrium. This outcome was probably due to excessive necrosis of the uterine wall. The reader is referred to Droegemueller's excellent papers, for he has extensively studied and beautifully described the use of cryocoagulation in both humans and baboons in order to accomplish sterilization and amenorrhea.[18, 23–25]

The endometrium has an amazing capacity to regenerate, and attempts to remove or destroy the tissue in animal models have been largely unsuccessful. Hartman[28] excised the entire endometrial lining at the time of hysterotomy in order to recover early monkey embryos. He attempted to remove the entire endometrium, including the stratum basale. In many of the 103 monkeys studied, the myometrium was wiped as clean as possible with a cotton sponge, so that no vestige of endometrium was visible to the naked eye; yet perfect regeneration occurred.

Shenker and Polishuk[29] studied the effects of local applications of various agents to the rabbit endometrium. The following chemical agents were instilled: 10% formalin, 2% formalin in ethanol, cupric sulfate pellets, talc suspension, sodium lauryl sulfate, and quinacrine hydrochloride. The 10% formalin was the only agent that prevented endometrial regeneration and caused complete occlusion of the uterine cavity by fibrous tissue.

The same authors were able to produce intrauterine adhesions in the rabbit with autologous fibroblast implants.[30, 31] In 1975, Polishuk described the use of homologous fibroblasts in the rat.[32] In the same publication, he described the successful use of autologous fibroblast implantation in a few patients. This procedure is quite an intriguing possibility, but we know of no further animal or human studies.

## PRELIMINARY STUDIES

We proposed to ablate the endometrium by means of Nd:YAG photovaporization under direct vision through a hysteroscope. The human uterus appeared to be an ideal organ for this modality, since it has a relatively thick myometrium (usually greater than 1.5 cm in thickness) and a thin endometrium (usually less than 1 mm in thickness). This relationship provides a great safety factor.

Initially, we attempted to approach the hormonal state occurring in the postabortal or puerperal uterus by placing each patient on a regimen of danazol, 800 mg/day for 3 weeks prior to the procedure. We continued the danazol for approximately 2 weeks after the procedure, with the objective of allowing healing and scar formation to occur prior to a return to ovarian cyclic activity and estrogenic stimulation of the endometrium. As we followed these patients, we learned that healing did not occur for as long as 4 to 5 months. Therefore, we did not continue the danazol after the surgical procedure was performed. The danazol produced a very atrophic endometrium, which greatly facilitated the procedure, and therefore we have continued to use it preoperatively with very satisfactory results.

From those lasers whose energy can be transmitted via fiberoptics we selected the Nd:YAG laser because of its greater energy output and greater degree of tissue penetration.

In addition, we used dextran to distend the uterine cavity during hysteroscopy, but we found that large bubbles were produced in this viscous medium. Therefore, we substituted 5% dextrose in physiologic saline for the dextran, with satisfactory results.

Among our initial studies was an investigation of the possible thermal damage to adjacent organs. We first used the laser on the endometrium of hysterectomy specimens, which when hand-held did not produce any sensation of heat through the thick myometrial wall. This finding was reassuring, for there is even greater heat dissipation in the intact uterus, because of circulating blood and the large amount of irrigating solution that flows continuously through the uterine cavity.

In an effort to predict the potential for transmural necrosis created by Nd:YAG laser photocoagulation of the endometrium, the following study was performed. The Nd:YAG laser, delivering 55 W of 1.06-μm laser energy via a 0.6 mm fiberoptic tube, was used. Two copper-constantan thermocouples, each placed inside a 25-gauge needle, were imbedded in freshly excised hysterectomy specimens 1 cm from the endometrial surface. These thermocouples had a system response time of less than 100 ms. The tissue specimens with the imbedded thermocouples were then placed inside a saline bath and both the tissue and the bath were permitted to equilibrate thermally at 37° C. The laser fiber was placed in contact with the tissue specimen perpendicular to the tip of the thermocouple probe. The laser was then fired onto the tissue for 5 seconds. The termperature rise, as measured by the thermocouples, was recorded on a graphic recorder with a linearizing thermocouple amplifier. Mean and peak values of temperature were recorded and averaged. The mean temperature at the serosal surface was 46.0 ± 1.0° C, with a peak temperature of 48.6 ± 1.3° C, far below that required for tissue necrosis and coagulation.

These results are even more reassuring, for two reasons. First, this study represents a worst-case analysis of tissue temperature rise during laser photovaporization, because the tissue was deprived of its circulation, which has a cooling effect. Second, the experiment was performed in a static bath of saline that was held constant at 37° C. In the application of the laser to the intact uterus at surgery, the saline is at room temperature and is rapidly flowing across the photovaporized site. Both of these factors have a cooling effect on the tissue. In addition, in the clinical application of this technique, the fiber is moved across the tissue at a velocity of approximately 0.25 cm/sec, as estimated by analysis of motion pictures of the procedure and confirmed by our surgeon's observations. As a result, the fiber is in contact with each area of the tissue for less than 0.5 second. In the in vitro study, the laser was in contact with the tissue for 5 seconds, 10 times longer than in the clinical case. Even with these conditions, the maximum temperature was well below the threshold for enzyme and protein denaturation. Henriques and Moritz[33] stated that "temperatures in excess of 52° C will result in danaturation within a relatively short exposure time." For an exposure time of 5 seconds, temperatures in excess of 55° C will cause irreversible damage.[34]

## CLINICAL STUDIES

### Patient Selection

From 1979 to 1988, 335 of our patients were carefully selected for this procedure. All had excessive and disabling uterine bleeding and were unable or unwilling to use other methods for control, although all could have been considered candidates for hysterectomy. All of the patients, of course, stated that future childbearing was not desired. In addition, many of the patients had had prior tubal sterilization.

In order to prevent the irrigation solution from entering the peritoneal cavity during hysteroscopy, Yoon rings were initially applied laparoscopically to the fallopian tubes of patients who had not had prior sterilization.[35] Although destruction of the endometrium would most likely produce sterility, additional protection against the serious sequelae of pregnancy in these patients was thought to be afforded by the Yoon ring application. In the subsequent follow-up of patients who had ablation of the endometrium with the Nd:YAG laser, we found that there was no communication of the fallopian tubes to the endometrial cavity (or what remained of it) after a period of several months, and we therefore discontinued the application of Yoon rings on those patients who had not been sterilized. To date (over 5 years), there have been no pregnancies in these patients.

Curettage had been performed in all patients and was unsuccessful in controlling the symptoms. Many of the patients had had multiple curettages, and in these patients endometrial biopsy was performed within 6 months of the procedure. All of these patients had a normal proliferative or secretory endometrium. One patient with a blood dyscrasia refused to stop oral contraceptives to allow the curettage, because when she had done so previously, serious bleeding had ensued. It is most important in these patients to rule out any malignant or premalignant change in the endometrium.

The age range of the patients was from 12 to 53 years. Ninety-two of the patients had leiomyomata, of which 57 were submucous in their location. Twenty-two patients were thought to have adenomyosis, either by history or by hysteroscopic findings. Sixteen patients had diagnosed clotting disorders, from conditions that included warfarin sodium (Coumadin) therapy, von Willebrand disease, idiopathic thrombocytopenic purpura, Bernard-Soulier syndrome, and storage pool disease. The one 12-year-old in this series had

Bernard-Soulier syndrome, a severe platelet disorder. The patient apparently had suffered a cerebral hemorrhage at birth, as a result of the condition, and since then has been markedly mentally retarded. During her first menstrual period, she became severely anemic. Attempts to control her menorrhagia with hormones led to severe exacerbation of her convulsive disorder, and it was decided to treat her endometrium with the laser.

Loffer has performed endometrial ablation in 100 women with menorrhagia or menometrorrhagia.[36] Like those patients of ours, his patients underwent endometrial ablation because they were poor medical risks for hysterectomy, were reluctant to have a hysterectomy, or could not afford the recovery time that follows a hysterectomy. All of his patients had undergone preoperative hysteroscopy or endometrial sampling or both. Patients with polyps, submucous myomata, endometrial hyperplasia, a uterus greater than 10 cm in depth, or a structural abnormality of the uterus were usually not considered candidates for endometrial ablation.

Following endometrial sampling, Loffer administered 400 mg danazol twice a day for 3 to 4 weeks before the procedure. Finally, all of the patients were informed that, while the chance of becoming pregnant after the procedure was small, if pregnancy were to occur it might be associated with a problem of implantation or it might be ectopic.

## Surgical Technique

The operation is performed with the patient under general or spinal anesthesia. The cervix is grasped with a tenaculum and dilated to allow insertion of a continuous-flow hysteroscope.

The hysteroscope is advanced through the cervical canal into the endometrial cavity, with continuous flushing of the irrigating solution, using 5% dextrose in 0.9% sodium chloride. Continuous irrigation is maintained by gravity. Adequate outflow from the hysteroscope is achieved by suction.

Following inspection of the endometrial cavity, the 0.6-mm fiber is inserted through the operating channel of the hysteroscope. A transparent protective filter is placed over the eyepiece of the hysteroscope to prevent injury to the operator's eye.

The endometrial photovaporization is performed under direct vision. With the use of a power output of 55 W, the endometrial surface is destroyed by systematically and continuously moving the hysteroscope from one point to another, with the fiberoptic tip in close approximation to the surface. It is convenient to start at the cornual and fundal areas, moving in a transverse direction, and then proceed down the anterior and posterior surfaces of the corpus, up to and including the isthmus. It is difficult to distinguish the isthmic surface from the endocervical surface hysteroscopically. To avoid treating the endocervix, the cervical length is marked on the hysteroscope sheath. Repeated inspection of the endometrial surface will frequently reveal areas that were skipped, since treated areas change color from pinkish-white to brownish-black because of carbonization of the underlying myometrium. The topography of the treated areas appears as rough channels and holes, in contrast to the smooth, velvety untreated endometrial surface. Care is taken to avoid perforation in the regions of the tubal ostia, which are the thinnest portions of the myometrium. The procedure takes 30 to 40 minutes. One hundred fifty milligrams depomedroxy progesterone acetate is administered intramuscularly at the time of the procedure.

Loffer performs endometrial ablation with a power setting between 55 and 70 W and a bare 600-micron fiber passed through the operating channel of a standard 25° or 30° fore-oblique hysteroscope.[36] A 0° hysteroscope does not allow the surgeon to view the lateral walls adequately, and a 70° hysteroscope may not allow the surgeon to view the end of the fiber when it is advanced into the endometrial cavity. In addition, he introduces a 7 French outflow catheter through a second operative channel of the hysteroscope to aid in the removal of blood, debris, and bubbles from the intrauterine cavity. The use of the catheter eliminates the need to over-dilate the cervix and, therefore, aids in maintaining sufficient intrauterine pressure to distend the uterus.

While viewing the procedure on a video monitor, Loffer begins by clearing any blood or debris from the cavity and coagulating a band of endometrium from one ostium to the other. This separates the endometrial cavity into an anterior half and a posterior half and gives the surgeon a point of reference during the procedure. He then uses a no-touch technique to coagulate the cornual regions (using at least 65 W) and completes the ablation by dragging the fiber (by the touch technique) along the anterior, lateral, and posterior walls. This dragging technique creates furrows in the endometrium and makes it easier to determine what surfaces have been treated. If heavy bleeding occurs, he injects diluted vasopressin (Pitressin) into the cervix and paracervical tissues or places the bulb of a Foley catheter in the endometrial cavity.

## Results and Complications

Most patients were discharged on the day after surgery. Several patients went home the day of surgery, and a few stayed for a second postoperative day. A few patients complained of uterine cramps, which were relieved by salicylates. Patients likened the postoperative course to that following a dilatation and curettage. All patients experience various amounts of serosanguinous discharge, which in some instances continued up to 4 to 5 weeks.

The results were tabulated for 335 patients who were followed for more than 2 months postoperatively. Of these patients, 292 were considered to have excellent results. Our definition of an excellent result was amenorrhea (about 50% of patients) or only 2 to 3 days of staining per month. A good result was defined as improvement sufficient to produce what the patient considered to be normal menstrual periods. Seven patients fell into this category. Twenty-two patients had poor results (little or no improvement) and were retreated. Following retreatment, of 11 of these 22 patients, 10 became amenorrheic, and 1 had a hysterectomy, owing to large submucous leiomyomata.

Ten patients had a subsequent hysterectomy. Five of these patients had severe adenomyosis, which caused both recurrent bleeding and considerable pain. Two patients had hysterectomies for ovarian cysts, although they had been amenorrheic following laser therapy. Two patients had subsequent hysterectomies because of large submucous leiomyomata. In retrospect, patients with large submucous leiomyomata are probably poor candidates for this procedure, unless preoperative hysteroscopy reveals that all of the endometrial surfaces are accessible. One patient had a hysterectomy for severe bleeding from the endocervix, which occurred 3 weeks postoperatively. She had an artificial mitral valve and was on warfarin sodium (Coumadin) therapy. Examination of the hysterectomy specimen revealed that the bleeding source was high in the endocervix. Apparently, we had coagulated the endocervix, which sloughed. We now mark the level of the internal os on the hysteroscope, to avoid treating the endocervix.

It can be seen that excellent results were obtained in 87.2% of the patients with one treatment. If we include in this count patients with good results and those who had excellent results with the second treatment, there is an 89.3% success rate.

Hysterograms were obtained 3 to 6 months following the procedure in 18 patients. All showed evidence of marked scarring and deformity of the cavity, which was often extremely contracted. The uterotubal junction was sometimes patent in the first hysterogram; on follow-up hysterograms one and one and a half years later, however, the tubes were closed on all patients. An example is shown in Figures 7–1 and 7–2. Figures 7–3 and 7–4 also show the continued scarring after one year.

Biopsies of the endometrial surface were performed on all patients from 1 to 20 months following laser photovaporization of the endometrium. A Novak suction curet was used for this procedure. In patients with biphasic basal body temperature curves, the biopsies were done after ovulation. Somewhat necrotic myometrium is easily obtained for up to 4 months. This tissue is histologically remarkable by the almost complete absence of inflammatory reaction other than the foreign body giant cells surrounding carbon particles. Polymorphonuclear leukocytes are rare, and there are few areas of sparse round cell infiltration. Only rare endometrial glands are obtained at up to 4 months. After 5 months, no muscle or scar tissue is removed, and only a minute amount of normal-appearing endometrial fragments can be obtained, in spite of vigorous curettage. Semiannual biopsies are planned for the long-term follow-up of these patients.

Twelve patients had a small hematometra found during a postoperative endometrial biopsy. These hematometras responded to dilation of the cervix with a 6 mm suction curet and did not recur. Because of this complication, we feel that the uterus should be sounded in the postoperative healing period at 1 and 3 months.

One patient experienced a uterine perforation during the procedure, when the endometrium was about one-half treated. The perforation occurred during manipulation of the hysteroscope when the fiber was not in use. Antibiotics were started, and the patient was discharged on the third postoperative day. Two months later, bleeding recurred, and it was decided to retreat the patient. At this time, Yoon rings were laparoscopically applied prior to hysteroscopy.[35] The site of perforation was not visible. The hysteroscopic laser ablation was performed again, although the endometrial surface in the previously treated areas showed marked scarring, carbonization, and dense ridges, with the appearance of a healed

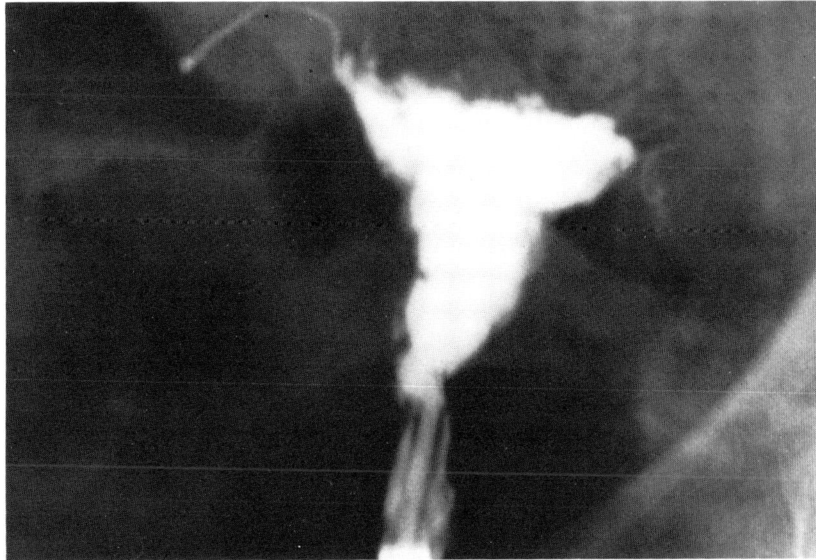

**FIG 7–1.**
HSG 3 months post laser ablation. Beginning synechiae are seen. Note patent uteral tubal junction.

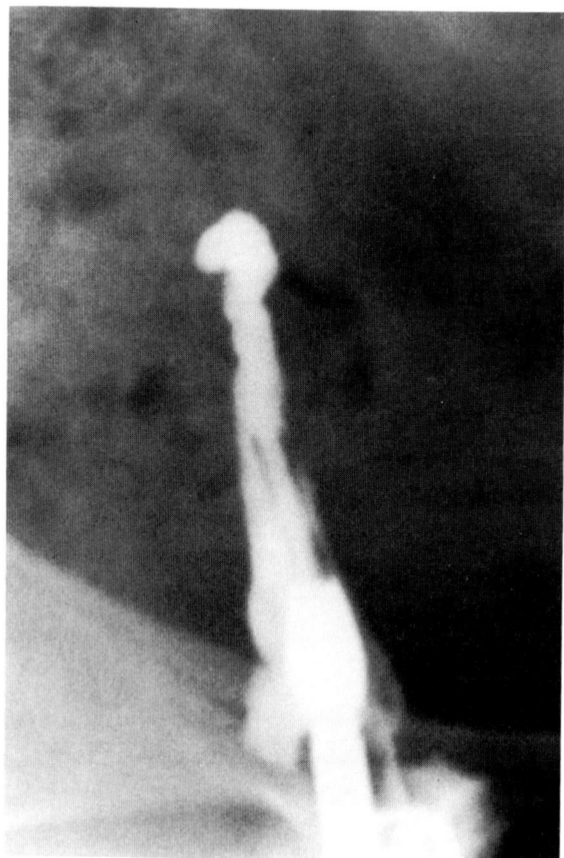

**FIG 7–2.**
Same patient as Figure 7–1. 1½ years post laser ablation with only minimal cavity present. Note no tubal filling.

third-degree burn of the skin. The normal endometrial surfaces were photovaporized. When the procedure was almost completed, the uterus was again perforated, probably in the same location, and the operation was terminated. The patient had an uneventful recovery. The end result was excellent, with the patient having only occasional staining.

Three patients had postoperative urinary tract infections. All responded to outpatient antibiotic therapy. The remainder of the patients had no temperature elevation. One patient had heavy uterine bleeding 4 weeks postoperatively, presumably because of sloughing of the treated areas. This bleeding was controlled by curettage.

The first few patients treated had evidence of fluid overload. There was some facial edema, and the patients complained of marked diuresis during the first 24 hours postoperatively. In one of these patients, in whom we had used 5% dextrose as an irrigating solution, serum electrolytes in the immediate postoperative period were measured as sodium, 124 mEq/L and chloride, 89 mEq/L, indicating a dilutional hyponatremia. The following morning, the electrolytes had returned to normal without treatment. This phenomenon is presumably similar to the dilutional hyponatremia and hypervolemia that complicate transurethral resection of the prostate,[37, 38] in which there is excessive infusion of the irrigating fluid into the open venous sinuses of the prostate. This condition is especially

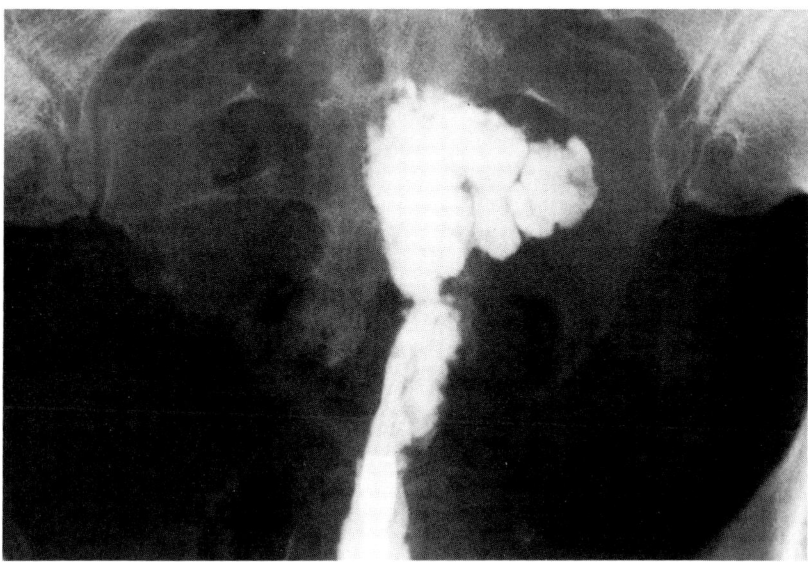

**FIG 7–3.**
HSG 3 months post laser ablation. Note beginning synechiae.

marked if the procedure is prolonged. In laser photovaporization of the endometrium, the venous channels are open, but blood loss is controlled by the pressure of the irrigating fluid. Since this one case of demonstrated dilutional hyponatremia, we are using a solution containing electrolytes: 5% dextrose in 0.9 saline. In addition, we have found that decreasing the operating time and using a continuous flow system has greatly reduced the total amount of solution absorbed. The use of an electrolyte solution is, of course, possible

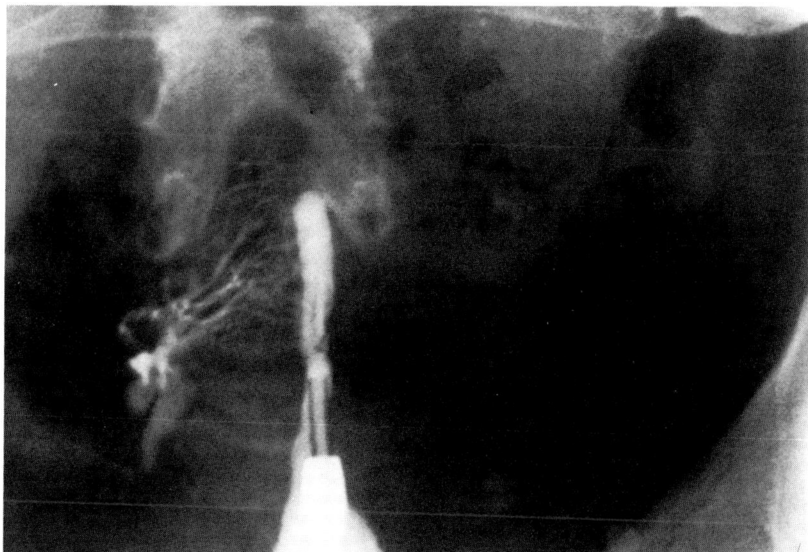

**FIG 7–4.**
Same patient as Figure 7–3. One year post laser ablation with almost complete obliteration of cavity. Note intravasation of dye characteristic of Asherman's syndrome.

**TABLE 7–1.**
Nd:YAG Ablation of the Endometrium*

| Author | Number of Cases | Percent Amenorrhea | Percent Hypomenorrhea | Percent Failed |
|---|---|---|---|---|
| Loffer[36] | 100 | 19 | 76 | 5 |
| Lamano[39] | 62 | 50 | 50 | 0 |
| Daniell[40] | 18 | 39 | 39 | 22 |
| Baggish[41] | 14 | 71 | 21 | 7 |
| Gimpleson[42] | 20 | 40 | 55 | 5 |
| Totals† | 214 | 35 | 57 | 5 |

*Data from references 36, 39–42.
†Note: Totals do not equal 100% because patients with postoperative follow-up of less than 6 months were not included.

with the laser but not with an electrosurgical procedure such as transurethral resection of the prostate. While hyponatremia and hypervolemia produced no ill effects in our patients, they are potentially serious problems and should be avoided by using an electrolyte solution in moderate amounts. Hypervolemia can be treated with diuretics. In general, we are dealing with healthy patients who can handle a fluid overload; but patients with cardiovascular disease or renal disease might have more difficulty.

Others have reported similar results.[39–43] Table 7–1 describes their results.

## Histologic Follow-up

Small amounts of endometrium do survive, as demonstrated by vigorous endometrial biopsy. This phenomenon is similar to the syndrome of recurrent intrauterine adhesions described by Polishuk and Sadovsky.[44] These investigators postulated that in their patients, the scanty endometrium was due to wide areas of fibrosis involving the endometrial surface.

The six hysterectomy specimens obtained after sufficient time for healing to have oc-

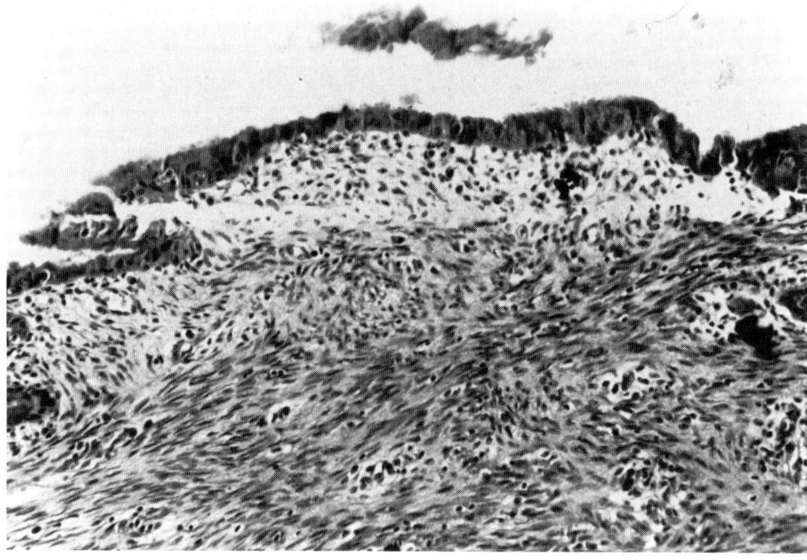

**FIG 7–5.**
Photomicrograph of endometrial surface in hysterectomy specimen. Note absence of glands and very sparse endometrial stroma.

curred show a single layer of simple cuboidal epithelium of an atypical müllerian type, with ciliated and brush borders (Fig 7–5). Cytogenic stroma was sparse, and only rare endometrial glands were present. The epithelium rested directly on the underlying myometrium, with only minimal hemosiderin accumulation. Hardly any carbon particles remained, and there was no inflammation. Healing appeared complete, with virtually no evidence of functioning endometrium. In three patients, marked adenomyosis was present. In reviewing the histories of these patients, it seems evident that they had adenomyosis prior to the laser ablation of the endometrium, although this possibility cannot be proved, of course.

## Laser Metroplasty

Early in this series of patients, several patients were found to have uterus subseptus. It was noted that when the laser fiber was carried across the septum, it opened very widely, thereby creating a single cavity. As a result of this experience, we decided to attempt laser metroplasty to treat septate uterus.

Twenty patients were treated clinically. One had had a midtrimester pregnancy loss and had a very wide septum. This condition was treated very simply by taking the laser fiber, beginning at a safe distance from the tubal ostia, and bringing it down one side of the septum and up the other side. The septum opened widely, much wider than the width of the laser fiber, and one or two sweeps of the laser were enough to take the septum out completely. This patient subsequently had a normal vaginal delivery (Figs 7–6 and 7–7).

Two other patients had a complete uterine septum down to the cervix. The septum was discovered at the time of a hysterosalpingography, during the course of an infertility workup. It was decided to remove the septum prior to a tuboplasty procedure. This removal was done without event. The results are shown in Figures 7–8 and 7–9. Unfortunately, this patient has not as yet conceived.

The third patient was a patient with in utero exposure to diethylstilbestrol. Hysteros-

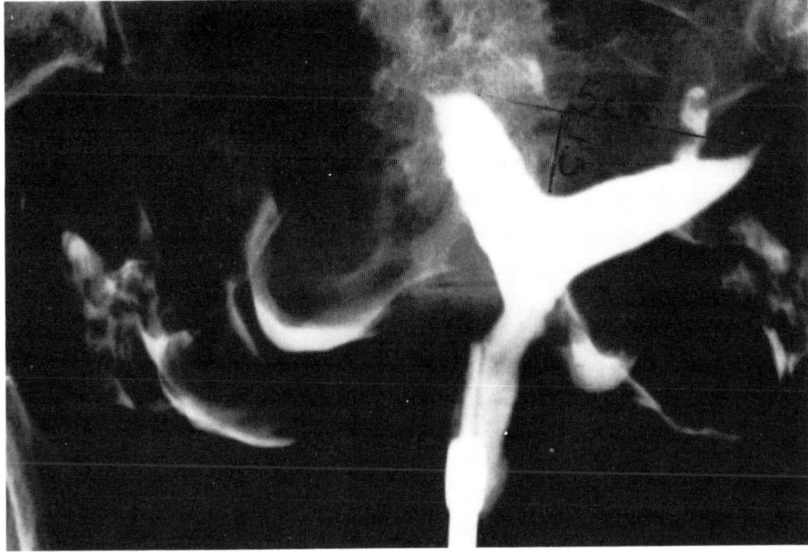

**FIG 7–6.**
HSG of patient with large uterine septum.

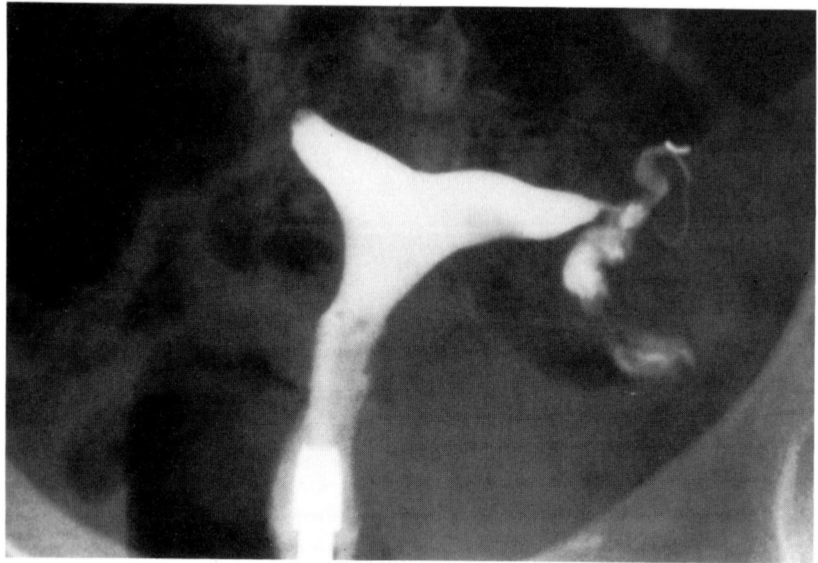

**FIG 7–7.**
Same patient as Fig 7-6 postoperatively. Note large capacity of cavity.

copy revealed a marked uterine septum. The patient had had a prior myomectomy. She was considering pregnancy in the near future. It was thought advisable in view of the diethylstilbestrol-affected uterus, with its decreased capacity, that the septum be removed prior to the pregnancy. This removal was performed without incident. Follow-up results are not as yet available.

Patients undergoing metroplasty can easily be discharged the day after surgery. We will consider doing the metroplasty as an outpatient procedure on our next patients. Postoperatively, there is no pain. As noted previously, the one patient who conceived had a

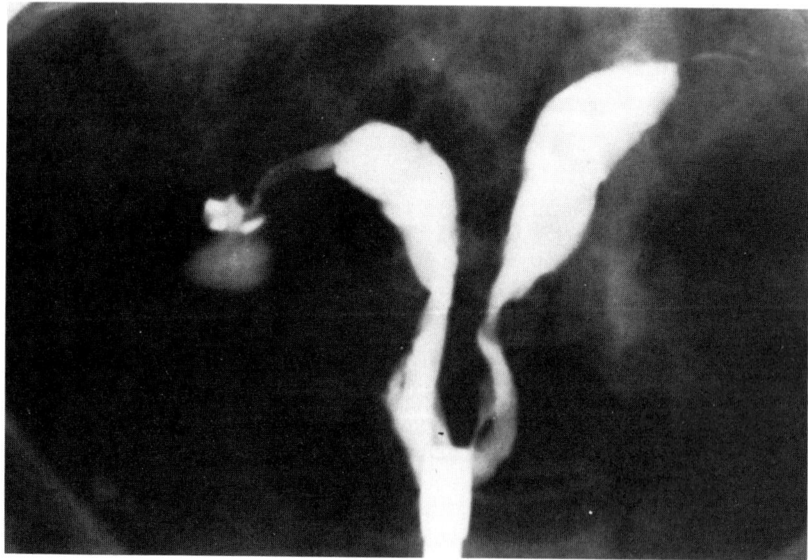

**FIG 7–8.**
HSG of patient with complete uterine septum into the cervix. Note tubal occlusion.

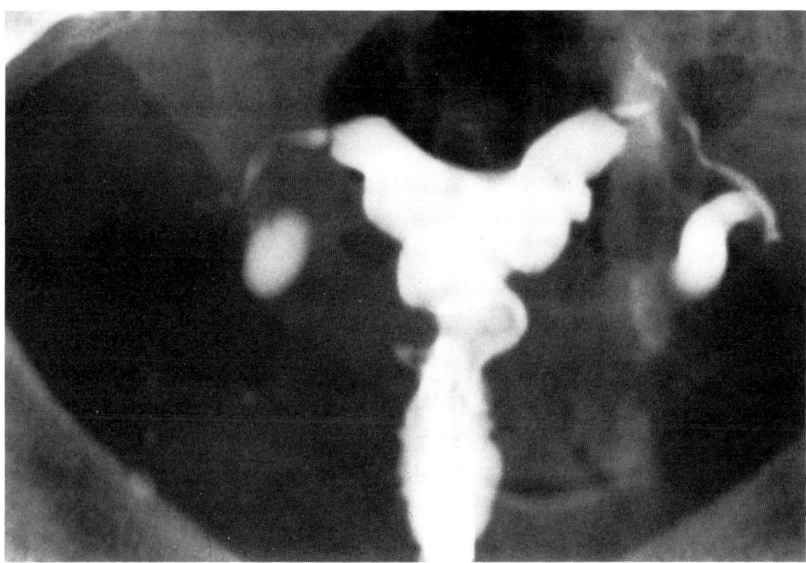

**FIG 7–9.**
Same patient as Fig 7-8 postoperatively. Septum almost completely gone. Note variegated margins of cavity. Patient was still on large dose of estrogen which probably caused very thick endometrium.

normal vaginal delivery. This possibility is in contradistinction to most metroplastic procedures done by the Strassman or Jones method, after which cesarean section is mandatory.

As with most previously described metroplasties, the patients were placed postoperatively on large doses of estrogen, which was withdrawn after 2 months by administration of progestogens. A Lippes loop intrauterine device was inserted in the latter two patients.

It is important that laparoscopy be performed before or during this procedure, to make sure that a bicornuate uterus does not exist. Division of the septum with the laser in a patient with a bicornuate uterus would most likely result in perforation and could be catastrophic.

We believe that laser metroplasty is a useful procedure that is very simple and bloodless and should yield excellent results. The results are preliminary, but we foresee no disadvantage with this technique, compared to division of the septum with a scissors or high-frequency current. The advantage of the laser over the scissors dissection, of course, is that it is virtually bloodless. When compared to an electrosurgical procedure, there is no danger from spread of electrical current to adjacent organs. It is important that the procedure be done immediately following menstruation or after pretreatment with danazol, in order to work in a field with an atrophic endometrium, which gives far better visualization for intrauterine hysteroscopic surgery.

## THE FUTURE OF INTRAUTERINE LASER SURGERY

This chapter summarizes our experience to date with intrauterine laser surgery. It should be remembered that laser surgery, by its nature, is destructive. Tissue diagnosis cannot be obtained unless the laser is used to excise tissue. It is for this reason that we have not chosen to destroy malignant or premalignant lesions of the endometrium with the laser.

It may be possible in the future to treat premalignant lesions with the laser; at this time, however, their response to endocrine therapy precludes the increased risk of progression to malignancy if remnants of premalignant tissue were left.

Until now, we have not used the laser as a method of sterilization by destruction of the uterotubal junction. While sterilization by this method is possible, we do not believe it offers enough of an advantage over laparoscopic tubal sterilization to warrant its use or testing.

Other applications of intrauterine laser surgery will most assuredly come to mind as more gynecologists undertake this approach in the treatment of their patients. We eagerly await the future development of intrauterine laser surgery.

## REFERENCES

1. Strassman EO: Fertility and unification of double uterus. *Fertil Steril* 1966, 17:165.
2. Jones HW Jr, Rock JA: *Reparative and Constructive Surgery of the Female Generative Tract.* Baltimore, Williams & Wilkins, 1983.
3. Chervenak FA, Newirth RS: Hysteroscopic resection of the uterine septum. *Am J Obstet Gynecol* 1981, 141:351.
4. DeCherney A, Polan ML: Hysteroscopic management of intrauterine lesions and intractable uterine bleeding. *Obstet Gynecol* 1983, 61:392.
5. March CM, Israel R, March AD: Hysteroscopic management of intrauterine adhesions. *Am J Obstet Gynecol* 1978, 130:653.
6. Newirth RS: Hysteroscopic management of symptomatic submucous fibroids. *Obstet Gynecol* 1983, 62:509.
7. Goldrath MH, Fuller TA, Segal S: Laser photovaporization of endometrium for the treatment of menorrhagia. *Am J Obstet Gynecol* 1981, 104:14.
8. Burchell RC: Hysterectomy: Functional versus anatomic indications. *CA* 1977; 27:241–242.
9. Cole P, Berlin J: Elective hysterectomy. *Am J Obstet Gynecol* 1977, 129:117–123.
10. D'Esopo DA: Hysterectomy when the uterus is grossly normal. *Am J Obstet Gynecol* 1962, 83:113–122.
11. Dyck FJ, et al: Effect of surveillance in the number of hysterectomies in the Province of Saskatchewan. *N Engl J Med* 1977, 296:1326–1328.
12. Miller NF: Hysterectomy—therapeutic necessity or surgical racket? *Am J Obstet Gynecol* 1946, 51:804–810.
13. Wright RC: Hysterectomy: Past, present, and future. *Obstet Gynecol* 1969, 33:560–563.
14. Parrott M: Elective hysterectomy. *Am J Obstet Gynecol* 1971, 113:531–537.
15. Nilsson L, Göran R: Treatment of menorrhagia. *Am J Obstet Gynecol* 1971, 110:713–720.
16. Oelsner G et al: Outcome of pregnancy after treatment of intrauterine adhesions. *Obstet Gynecol* 1974, 44:341–344.
17. Asherman JG: Amenorrhoea traumatica (atretica). *J Obstet Gynaecol Br Emp* 1948; 55:23–30.
18. Droegemueller W, et al: Cryocoagulation of the endometrium at the uterine cornua. *Am J Obstet Gynecol* 1978, 131:1–9.
19. Crossen RJ, Crossen HS: Radiation therapy of uterine myoma. *JAMA* 1947, 133:593–599.
20. Rongy AJ: Radium therapy in benign uterine bleeding. *J Mt Sinai Hosp* 1947, 14:569–575.
21. Falconer B: The treatment of metropathia haemorrhagica: Suggestions for a therapeutic programme. *Acta Obstet Gynecol Scand* 1947, 27:288–296.
22. Cahan WG, Brockunier A: Cryosurgery of the uterine cavity. *Am J Obstet Gynecol* 1967, 99:138–153.
23. Droegemueller W, Greer B, Makowski E: Cryosurgery in patients with dysfunctional uterine bleeding. *Obstet Gynecol* 1971, 38:256–258.
24. Droegemueller W, Makowski E, Macsalka R: Destruction of the endometrium by cryosurgery. *Am J Obstet Gynecol* 1971, 110:467–469.

25. Green BE, et al: Uterine cryosurgery in baboons. *Advances in Female Sterilization Techniques*, Sciarra JJ, Droegemueller W, Speidel JJ, (eds), Hagerstown, Md, Harper & Row, 1976, pp 231–239.
26. Shenker JG, Polishuk WZ: Regeneration of rabbit endometrium after cryosurgery. *Obstet Gynecol* 1972, 40:638–645.
27. Burke L, Rubin HW, Kim I: Uterine abscess formation secondary to endometrial cryosurgery. *Obstet Gynecol* 1973, 41:224–226.
28. Hartman CG: Regeneration of the monkey uterus after surgical removal of the endometrium and accidental endometriosis. *West J Surg Obstet Gynecol* 1944, 52:87–102.
29. Shenker JG, Polishuk WZ: Regeneration of rabbit endometrium following intrauterine instillation of chemical agents. *Gynecol Invest* 1973, 4:1–13.
30. Polishuk WZ, Shenker JG: Induction of intrauterine adhesions in the rabbit with autogenous fibroblast implants. *Am J Obstet Gynecol* 1973, 115:789–794.
31. Shenker JG, et al: An in vitro fibroblast-enriched sponge preparation for induction of intrauterine adhesions. *Isr J Med Sci* 1975, 11:849–851.
32. Polishuk WZ: Endometrial regeneration and adhesion formation. *S Afr Med J* 1975, 49:440–442.
33. Henriques FC Jr, Moritz AR: Studies of thermal injury; conduction of heat to and through skin and temperatures attained therein; theoretical and experimental investigation. *Am J Pathol* 1947, 23:531–549.
34. Artz CP, Moncreif JA, Pruitt BA: *Burns: A Team Approach*. Philadelphia, WB Saunders, 1979, pp 23–25.
35. Yoon IB, Wheeless CR, King TM: A preliminary report on a new laparoscopic sterilization approach: The silicone rubber band technique. *Am J Obstet Gynecol* 1974, 120:132–136.
36. Loffer FD (personal communication).
37. Blondy JB: *Transurethral Resection*. London, University Park Press, 1971, pp 92–93.
38. Lapides J: *Fundamentals of Urology* Philadelphia, WB Saunders, 1976, p 335.
39. Lamano JM: Dragging technique versus blanching technique for endometrial ablation with the Nd:YAG laser in the treatment of chronic menorrhagia. *Am J Obstet Gynecol* 1988; 159:152–155.
40. Daniell J, Tosh R, Meisels S: Photodynamic ablation of the endometrium with the Nd:YAG laser hysteroscopically as a treatment of menorrhagia. *Colpos Gynecol Laser Surg* 1986; 2:43–46.
41. Baggish MS, Baltoyannia P: New techniques for laser ablation of the endometrium in high risk patients. *Obstet Gynecol* 1988; 159:287–292.
42. Gimpleson RJ: Hysteroscopic Nd:YAG laser ablation of the endometrium. *J Reprod Med* 1988; 33:872–876.
43. Loffer FD: Laser ablation of the endometrium. *Obstet Gynecol Clin North Am* 1988; 15:77–89.
44. Polishuk WZ, Sadovsky E: A syndrome of recurrent intrauterine adhesions. *Am J Obstet Gynecol* 1975, 123:151–158.

Chapter 8

# Laser Surgery of the Fallopian Tube

Robert W. Kelly, M.D.

## HISTORICAL REVIEW

In the constant struggle to improve the outcome of tubal reconstructive procedures over the years, physicians have used many different approaches. Overall, however, the thrust has been to devise methods that allow the outcome to approximate the normal as closely as possible. The difficulty arises when the seemingly good anatomic result at the end of an operative procedure does not remain after the healing process has occurred. Even in the best examples, fibrosis, constriction, and adherence to surrounding structures take their toll. In procedures where extensive damage has required prolonged dissection and subsequent reconstruction, postoperative scarring has had an even more devastating effect. To further confuse the issue, the same procedure performed by the same surgeon under the same conditions on two different patients not uncommonly results in totally different outcomes, with one patient healing to virtually normal anatomy while the other patient develops massive adhesions. This invariably leads to the conclusion that there is no common denominator upon which we can concentrate our efforts to solve the problem of postoperative scarring.

For these reasons, a lengthy list of adjuvant drugs, instruments, techniques, sutures, irrigations, and second-look laparoscopies has arisen. Few, if any, have been shown by scientific examination to give dramatically better results than any of the others. The lack of applicability of animal studies to human outcome and the moral restraints on human experimentation are stumbling blocks to allowing firm proof of one method's superiority. Thus, the situation is relegated to a series of observational studies by different authors. Very few randomized studies such as those by Tulandi[1–4] are available to give us a better understanding of the status of any of these techniques, including the laser, in tubal surgery. At the present time, these studies cover only a few of the variables involved in tubal surgery.

The major development of the past 2 decades in the surgical treatment of tubal disease has been the introduction of microsurgery. Microsurgery became increasingly popular during the 1970s because the macrosurgical techniques reported in the 1950s[5] and in the 1960s[6] yielded poor pregnancy rates.

In 1967, Swolin,[7] in accordance with the experience of otolaryngologists, reasoned that decreasing the amount of tissue damage through the use of magnification would improve outcome. However, infertility often persists, and patients continue to form adhesions even with microsurgical techniques. Tubes still scar and some still become obstructed as a result of the healing process. Also, it is frequently difficult even with microsurgery to free ovaries bound to the sidewall. The tube that is densely bound to the ovary is difficult to dissect free without disruption of the ovarian capsule or tubal serosa. Even with extension devices for the microcautery, precise dissection deep in the cul-de-sac is cumbersome. These technical problems, along with less-than-acceptable pregnancy rates with adhesiolysis and neosalpingostomy, were a good part of the impetus to adapt the carbon dioxide laser to microsurgery of the fallopian tube.

Thus, in 1974, Bellina, hoping to take advantage of this desirable feature, adapted the carbon dioxide ($CO_2$) laser for use in tubal reconstructive surgery.[8] His early work had led him to believe that the laser offered other advantages, including a reduction in operating time, very fine hemostatic incisions, minimal damage lateral to the incision site, and reduction in postoperative adhesion formation. He found that the micromanipulator, with which the beam was directed, allowed very precise application of the laser. The beam could be applied deep within the cul-de-sac with the same ease as to structures near the anterior abdominal wall. Reflection of the beam off a mirrored surface allowed dissection behind the ovaries and in other generally inaccessible areas. Thus began the process of determining whether the advantages offered by the laser, as an adjunctive tool for the microsurgeon, could indeed improve procedures both technically and in terms of pregnancy rates.

To date, the $CO_2$ laser has been used by various microsurgeons for treating virtually all surgically correctable disorders of the fallopian tube. Tubal obstruction secondary to sterilization procedures can occur at the cornu (e.g., unipolar cautery), at mid-tube (e.g., loops, clips, resections), or in the distal tube (e.g., fimbriectomy). Inflammatory disorders can obstruct the tube either proximally or distally. The tube can be rendered nonfunctional by encasing adhesions from previous surgery, infection, or endometriosis. The infundibulum can likewise be scarred severely by these same culprits. Another major tubal problem that has been approached by laser technique is the conservative management of ectopic pregnancy by linear salpingostomy or segmental resection.

Prior to discussing the clinical applicability of the laser in these situations, it is imperative that certain properties of the $CO_2$ laser as it interacts with these tissues be understood. The technical capabilities of the energy form and its limitations offer the theoretical basis for its rational use as a microsurgical tool. Without this understanding, one is almost certain to attain a poor surgical result. Unfortunately, the blame for a poor result will be attributed to the laser rather than to the surgeon who in reality caused the poor outcome.

## LASER PHYSICS AND TUBAL SURGERY

An important feature of this wave form is based on its strong absorption by the water molecule. The absorption is so complete that cellular necrosis is limited to 70 μm[9] lateral to the impact site. Cellular damage may extend another 200 μm, but healing of this area occurs rapidly.[10] Thus, with a beam that is 200 μm in diameter, the surgeon is capable of making a 350-μm incision. This is not possible by other techniques. The microcautery, for example, may make an incision of less than 1 mm, but the area of thermal necrosis extends about 1 mm deeper than the incision base and 1 mm lateral on each side. This results in incisions that approximate 2 to 3 mm in width. For vessels less than 0.5 to 1.0 mm in diameter, hemostasis is probably equivalent with the two methods. For larger vessels, cautery is undoubtedly superior and will damage far less tissue in accomplishing the end result.

In choosing a laser for tubal microsurgery, certain desirable features should be available in a given instrument. The first item of importance is the unit's Transverse Electromagnetic Mode (TEM). For the precise dissection with minimal damage required for tubal surgery, the unit must be able to deliver a small spot size, generally from 1 mm to 200 μm. For this to be possible, the beam must have a Gaussian distribution or $TEM_{oo}$ mode. Fortunately, most currently available surgical lasers have a $TEM_{oo}$ mode. Thus, power densities far in excess of 100,000 watts/cm$^2$ can be achieved. These power densities are much higher than generally needed in tubal surgery but make the lasers available for multidisciplinary use, which is more cost-effective for most institutions. The author generally works in the range of 3,000 to 20,000 watts/cm$^2$, although some techniques to be described use more or less than these limits.

The spot size for the laser needs to be variable. No single spot size can accomplish all the tasks that are necessary. For very precise dissection, a spot size of 125 to 200 μm appears to be ideal. For vaporizing large areas of surface adhesions or for everting the mucosa during neosalpingostomy, a spot size of 2 to 4 mm is helpful. Most $TEM_{oo}$ surgical lasers can provide spot sizes in this general range by virtue of their variable spot size adaptors.

Because there are no fiberoptic systems available for the $CO_2$ beam for surgical purposes, we must continue to use the articulated arms that transmit the beam with mirrors. For our purposes, the arm must be long enough to reach the surgical site without the laser unit compromising the sterile field. To attain this length, we must suffer the problem of power reduction which occurs as the result of multiple mirrors not being 100% reflective. Mirrors are also notorious for getting out of alignment so that the $TEM_{oo}$ mode is lost, resulting in power loss and the inability to achieve small spot sizes. Because of recent technological advances in laser instrumentation (i.e., permanently aligned mirrors and mirrors of higher reflective capability), these problems are less commonly encountered but still exist. The ideal situation would involve fiberoptic transmission of the $TEM_{oo}$ mode without power loss so that the laser unit could be located outside the operating room. Major engineering difficulties still exist so that it may be some time before these systems are available, if at all.

## Laser Instrumentation

A major consideration in the decision of which $CO_2$ laser to select is how easy it is to use and care for in the surgical suite. Does the unit require frequent mirror adjustments? Can it be moved from one room to another with ease and without compromising the unit's performance? How often does it require maintenance? If the system goes down, how long will it take to get it serviced? Can the system be checked out and set up by the regular operating-room personnel or does it require the attention of a bioengineer? What is the cost of a service contract and are there any restrictions imposed by the service contract? If the unit has a direct current (dc) stimulated plasma tube (which most units currently do), is a source of the gas mixture readily available in your area or does the gas have to be shipped in? What is the expected lifetime in hours of the plasma tube in a closed system? All of these questions need answers before a purchase of any unit is finalized. Do not accept a salesperson's verbal commitment; get it in writing. Reputable laser companies are more than happy to back their product in writing.

Another factor that must be considered before deciding on a given laser is the quality and adaptability of the micromanipulator. There are two major schools of thought on how best to use a laser with a microscope. The first is to use the hand-held laser scalpel and view through the microscope much like one would do using a microcautery needle for standard microsurgery. The proponents of this technique feel that the smaller spot size (125 μm) allows higher power densities and, by allowing less dwell time, decreases thermal damage. This is true, but the depth of focus for this system is much less, a factor that may well offset the proposed advantage. The focal length for the hand-held scalpel is only 125 mm. If one is out of the focal plane by only 5 mm, the power density is decreased by 83%, leaving only 17% of the calculated power density. Consider transection of a 1-cm fallopian tube. The beam will be in focus on the near surface but will rapidly go out of focus as the tube is cut. On the other hand, the ability to defocus the hand-held system at will during the procedure is a distinct advantage (Figs 8–1 and 8–2). By simply moving the laser scalpel back from the tissue, the spot size is increased and the power density is reduced. This is useful in working with adhesions and during neosalpingostomy. However, working deep in the cul-de-sac is cumbersome with the hand-held scalpel, and the focal distance again becomes a problem. The beam cannot be applied in the surgeon's line of sight with the hand-held scalpel. It must be brought in from an angle, thereby increasing the risk that normal tissues may come between the hand-held scalpel and the preferred target. This is especially true when operating at high magnification where the visible operating field is very small. Also, when the hand-held scalpel is not actively being used, it must be held in a place that assures safety for the patient and personnel in the operating room. This requires that someone hold it, usually in a wet towel or similarly protective environment.

In contrast to the hand-held system is the micromanipulator attached to a microscope (Fig 8–3). This system may have a focal length of 250 to 400 mm, but many systems can still give a spot size of 200 μm. Because a 300-mm working distance provides adequate distance between the microscope and the operative site, most laser surgeons appear to prefer it. With this greater focal length, the depth of focus is greater. Being out of focus by

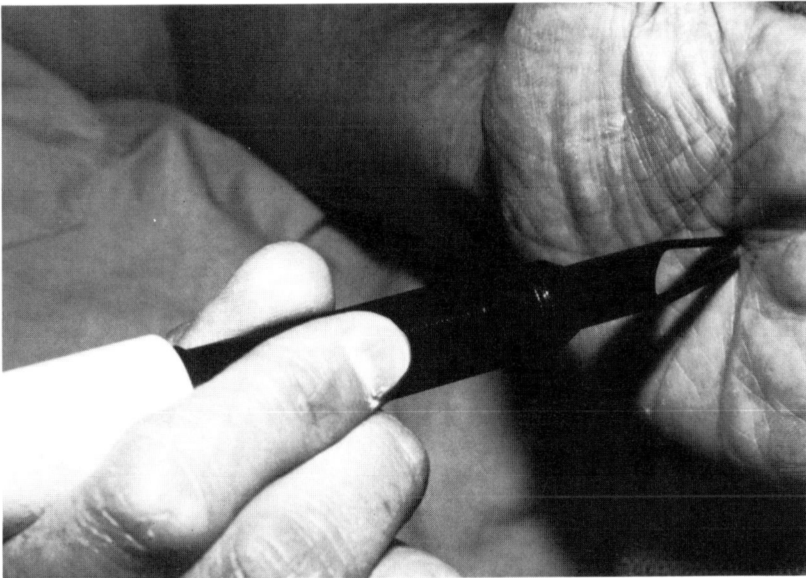

**FIG 8–1.**
Carbon dioxide handpiece with focused beam.

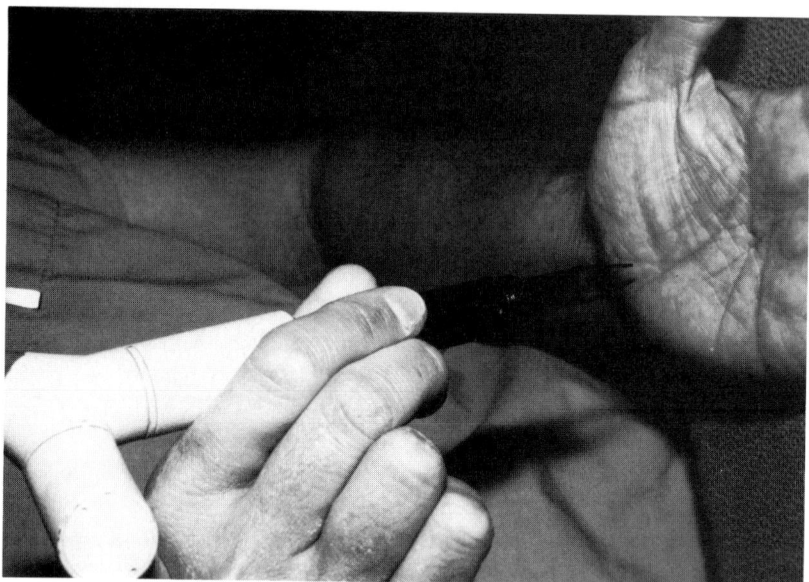

**FIG 8–2.**
Carbon dioxide handpiece with defocused beam.

only 5 mm reduces the power density of a 250-mm focal length system by 47%, as compared to 83% for the 125-mm hand-held system. However, to defocus this system requires manipulation of the adaptor lens. This is generally easily done in a matter of 2 or 3 seconds, but it still does not allow the very large spot size that can be attained by defocusing with the hand scalpel. The beam is delivered in the surgeon's line of vision so that it is improbable that tissue, instruments, or the assistant's fingers can be struck inadvertently

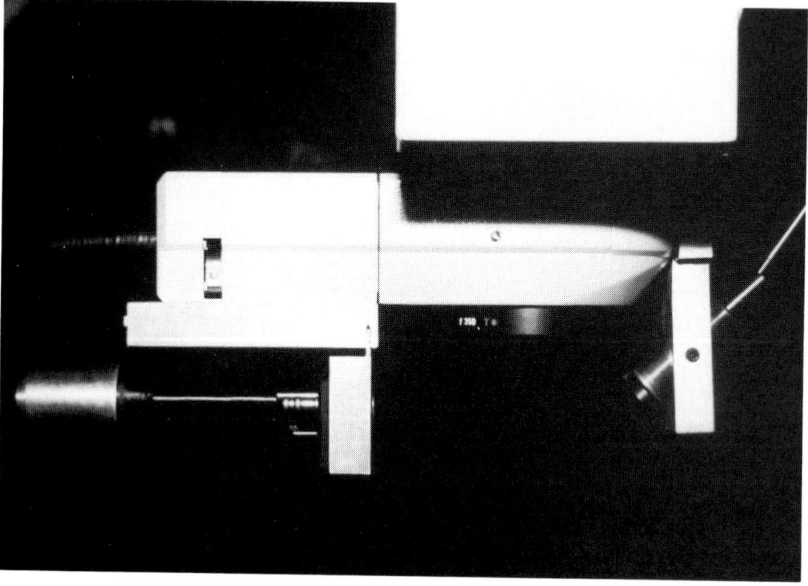

**FIG 8–3.**
Micromanipulator attached to microscope.

by the beam. Another major advantage of the micromanipulator is the precise control it offers over the hand scalpel. Usually, there is a 7 to 1 ratio between the movement of the "joystick" and the movement of the beam in the field (i.e., if one moves the joystick 7 mm, the beam moves only 1 mm). This quality virtually eliminates the effect of any tremor the surgeon may have and offers a degree of control heretofore unknown in the field of microsurgery. Most micromanipulators can be adapted for right- or left-handed use, but those with this feature are not all of the same quality. Some are flimsily constructed of poor quality materials and do not withstand the usual wear and tear of an operating suite. The freedom of movement of the joystick is quite variable. Some joysticks move freely and smoothly in all directions, whereas others cannot be moved smoothly along the diagonal. Some adaptors block a portion of the surgeon's optical field, adding to fatigue and frustration. Frequently, the optical field and the laser field do not coincide and necessitate movement of the microscope.

Another consideration to be weighed before purchase is the beam profile. To attain the small spot sizes (125 to 200 μm) discussed, either a large raw beam diameter on exit from the plasma tube is needed or the raw beam must be expanded by a lens before being focused. According to physical law, the smallest diameter spot size attainable from a laser is equal to the wavelength of the laser (e.g., for $CO_2$ that is 10.6 μm). How closely this may be approximated is dependent upon how much the beam can be expanded prior to focusing, which is a function of the diameter of the lens system. To achieve a spot size of 125 μm at a focal distance of 300 mm, one would need a lens of 3 to 4 cm in diameter. Not only is this difficult from an engineering standpoint, it would be prohibitively expensive to produce.

An item of major importance in laser microsurgery of the fallopian tube is obviously the operating microscope. Most microscopes can be fitted with a micromanipulator or already have standard fittings for the adaptor. Some of the more elaborate and expensive microscopes require minor modifications of the light source to prevent a loss of light intensity when the micromanipulator is attached. The microscope focal length and the laser focal length must be exactly the same; one simply cannot assume that because the adaptor fits the microscope, the two focal points are exact. Otherwise, one will not be able to achieve the predicted spot size. Also, if the surgeon wears glasses, it is necessary to know the diopter correction and set this on the eyepiece before focusing the system at the time of each procedure or the surgeon must wear the glasses during the procedure. Here again, if this is not done, the laser will not be in focus when the microscope is in focus, and the spot size will not be as predicted. Another problem not readily correctable occurs when the microscope is not parfocal at different magnifications. The only definitive answer to this is to use a different microscope. Where that is not possible, the surgeon can sometimes compensate by using the system at the magnification where the laser and microscope have the same focal distance or by living with the larger spot size.

## Accessories

A multitude of accessory instruments are marketed by laser and instrument companies. For the most part, these make procedures technically easier but few are essential and all are expensive.

The most useful tool is the quartz or Pyrex rod (Fig 8–4). These are used as tissue manipulators and as backstops to absorb the laser energy as it passes through tissue so as to protect underlying structures. Used carefully, little risk of breakage exists, and the smooth surface does not abrade tissue. These rods become fatigued with laser impact and should be discarded as subsurface fracture lines appear in significant numbers (Fig 8–5).

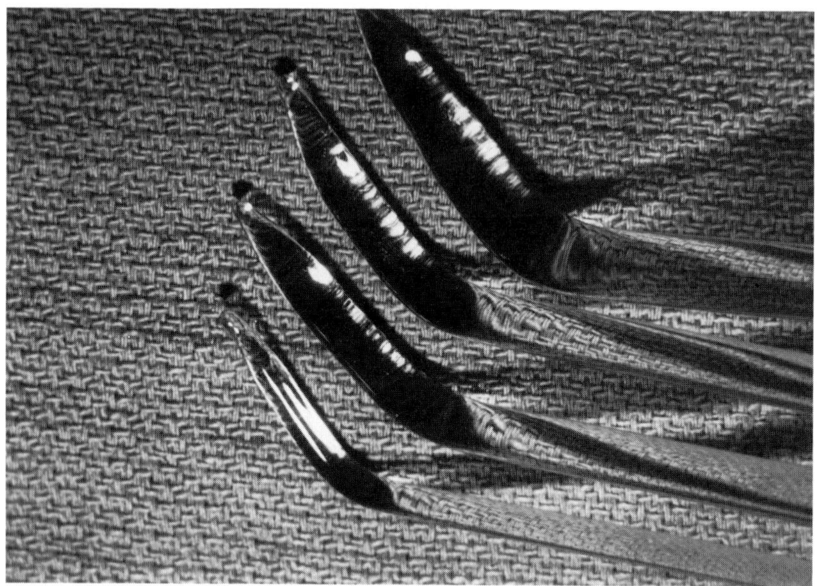

**FIG 8–4.**
Unused pyrex rods of various sizes.

Most rods will last for 2 to 3 procedures. Rods less than 6 mm in diameter appear to have an increased risk of breakage and should be used with caution. Because they do not have the strength of metal retractors, the surgeon and assistant must remember that these rods are backstops and not retractors. The most commonly used rods are 15 to 18 cm long with a 2.0 to 2.5 cm right angle at one end, but any length or configuration that the surgeon finds useful is acceptable. Quartz or crystal rods are more durable but significantly

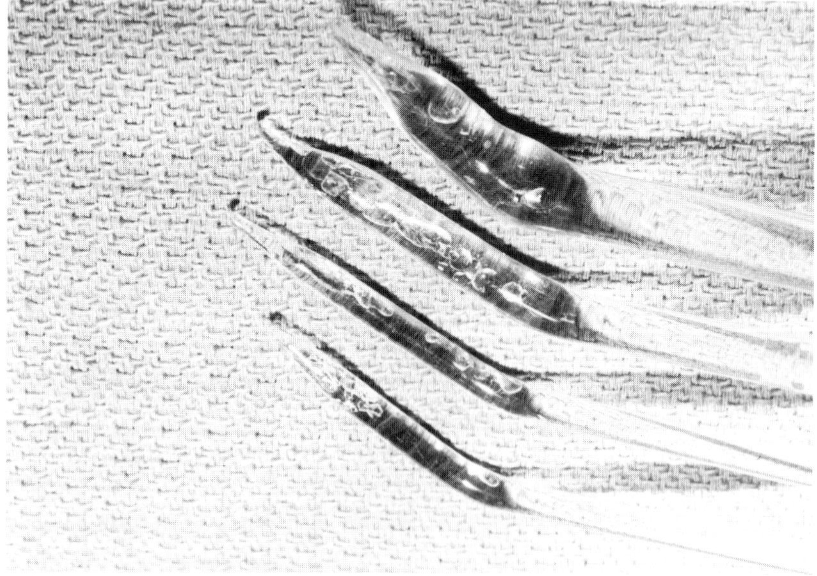

**FIG 8–5.**
Used pyrex rods with subsurface fractures.

more expensive; a full year's supply of Pyrex can be purchased for the same price as one commercially available quartz rod.

Backstops of other materials are available (e.g., titanium, anodized stainless steel), but if they are sufficiently rough to completely avoid reflection of the beam, the risk of tissue abrasion must be considered. One cardinal rule to be observed in the use of any of the backstops is that they should be held slightly away from the tissue being lasered, if possible. This maneuver prevents the heat that is created in them from causing thermal damage to the tissue, a problem that would defeat the purpose of the laser. A simple alternative to all of the backstops mentioned so far is wet Telfa. This material can be cut to any size or shape, and it holds water well. It performs extremely well in protecting adjacent or underlying structures and it is inexpensive, readily available, nonabrasive, and disposable.

In the course of any laser procedure, a considerable volume of smoke is generated. This must be removed efficiently lest the surgeon and assistants breathe it. Although the laser plume of the continuous-wave $CO_2$ has been shown to be free of viable cells and nuclear proteins,[11] no similar definitive studies exist for either the chopped-wave or pulsed-wave applications. Until these data are available, the risk of laser plume inhalation must be considered significant. This issue is less critical when vaporizing nonmalignant intra-abdominal tissues than when treating premalignant or warty disorders of the lower genital tract. Various smoke evacuators are commercially available, but most are cumbersome and noisy. A simple method of removal is to use the standard wall suction equipment (Fig 8–6) available in the operating room with an appropriate in-line filter positioned between the suction bottles and the wall receptacle (Fig 8–7). Anecdotal reports record entire hospital suction systems being rendered nonfunctional by the smoke residue when these filters were not used.

Because the laser follows the laws of physics governing light transmission, it can be reflected off mirrored surfaces. This can be a hazard if it is reflected off an instrument and damages surrounding tissues; however, this has rarely been reported as a complication. Moreover, this characteristic can be put to use in that the laser can be intentionally reflected with accuracy to otherwise inaccessible areas. Either polished stainless steel or a silver-fronted mirror, available through dental suppliers, can be used for this purpose (Fig 8–8). The laser is focused on the image in the mirror, and the surgeon operates on the image. A brief amount of practice with the mirror will usually suffice for mastery of the technique.

Anodized instruments have been touted as essential for use with the laser. These instruments are expensive and are not necessary if the surgeon uses a reasonable amount of care and concentration.

Without a doubt the laser surgeon's best ally in intra-abdominal surgery is irrigation. Because laser energy is entirely absorbed by 1 mm or less of water, flooding those areas surrounding the operative site offers total protection. This also prevents the drying of exposed tissues, a problem thought by most to increase the formation of adhesions. However, the tissue to be dissected must not be covered with solution. The tissue surface can be kept moist by frequent irrigation and excess solution can be removed from the area of dissection by suction prior to applying the laser.

## ANIMAL STUDIES

A number of animal studies have been published about the outcome of tubal surgery performed with the $CO_2$ laser under experimental conditions. Choe, et al., looked at the effect of the $CO_2$ laser on adhesion formation after microsurgical reanastomosis of the li-

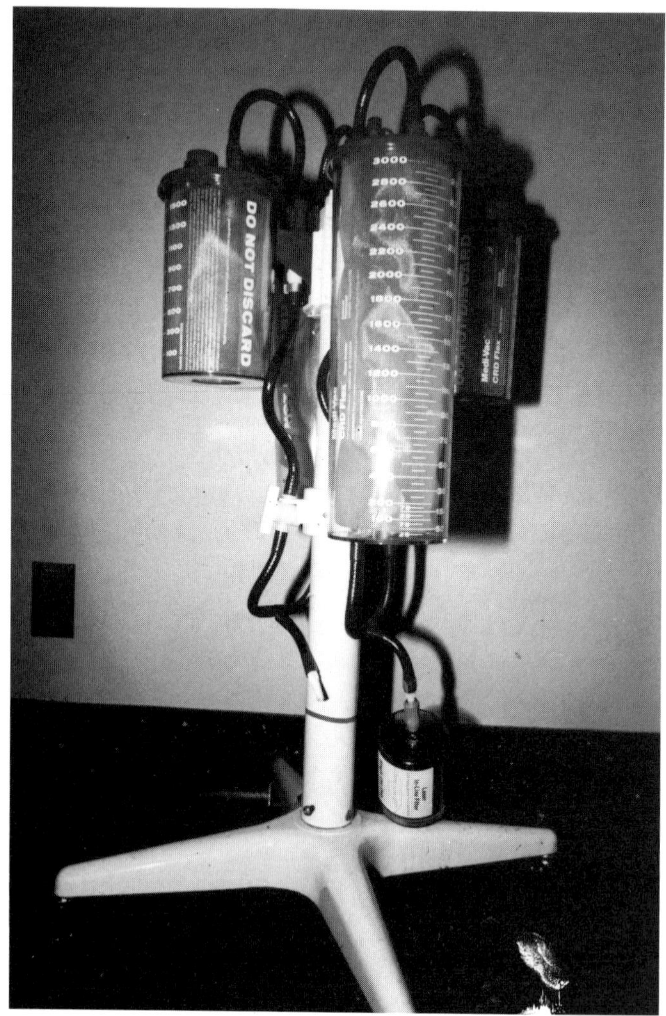


**FIG 8–6.**
Suction cannisters with proper placement of the filter between the cannister and wall suction outlet.

gated uterine horn in the rabbit and compared their results to a control group done with standard microsurgery.[12] Fourteen rabbits had ligation and division of both uterine horns. Four weeks later seven rabbits had conventional microsurgical resection of the ligated stumps and reanastomosis; the other seven rabbits had laser resection of the ligated stumps followed by reanastomosis. Interestingly, they used a laser $TEM_{01}$ mode and a spot size of 2 mm with power densities ranging from 637 to 796 watts/$cm^2$. In view of our previous discussions, the laser conditions these researchers used were not optimal, based on theoretical considerations. However, they still showed a reduction in adhesion formation at 6 weeks postoperatively in the laser group that was significant at the level of $P < 0.001$. Further study along these same lines, using larger numbers of animals, smaller spot sizes, and higher power densities, should be interesting. Unfortunately, Choe et al. did not breed these animals to evaluate pregnancy rates between the two groups.

Martin, et al., performed tubal incision and anastomosis in 18 virgin Sprague-Dawley rats at the time of a laparotomy.[13] They used three different incisional modes: 1,000

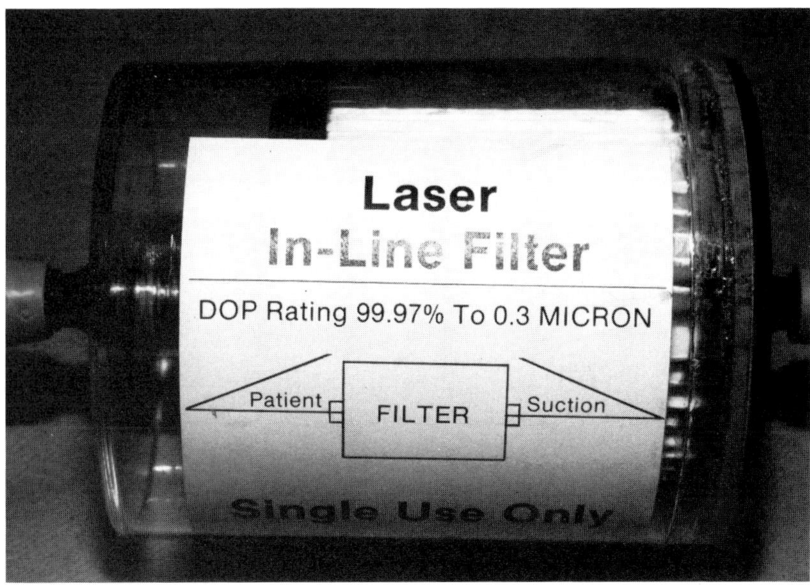


**FIG 8–7.**
In-line filter.

watts/cm$^2$, 12,000 watts/cm$^2$, and sharp incision. Their spot size for the laser was 0.8 to 1.0 mm. They noted no difference in the percentage or severity of adhesion formation among the three groups of animals.

Klink, et al., working with rabbits, excised a 0.5-cm portion of tube near the cornua bilaterally.[14] They then performed end-to-end anastomosis, using only the $CO_2$ laser, by precisely aligning the tubes and coagulating the doubled serosa in a circumferential fash-

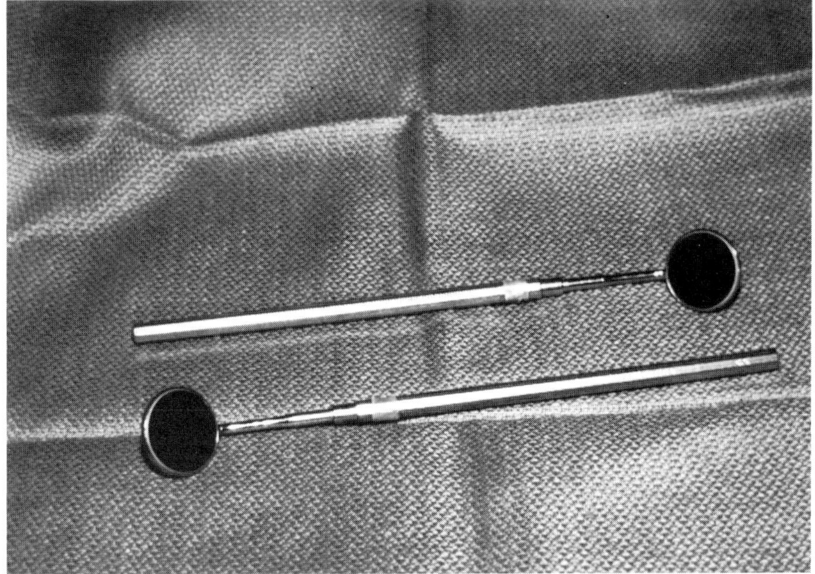

**FIG 8–8.**
Rhodium-surfaced, angled dental mirrors.

ion. They found that "welding" was best carried out using 64 watts/cm$^2$; this gave sufficient coagulation necrosis for stability but no alteration of the deep tissue layers. They used a power of 8 watts for 0.2 seconds, giving a total energy per impact of 1.6 joules. They considered as success nothing short of term pregnancy, which occurred in 70% of the animals in this group. When higher or lower power densities were used in other groups, no pregnancies resulted. In the pregnant animals, post-pregnancy hysterosalpingography and histology showed the formation of very little cicatrix tissue and no stenosis.

Work is also under way in several laboratories evaluating tissue welding with the $CO_2$ laser using powers in the milliwatt range. These studies are looking primarily at vascular anastomosis of small vessels, but may give some insight into the possibility of using similar techniques in the fallopian tube. However, because of its relatively large size, such welding may not be feasible in the tube.

## CLINICAL USES

The $CO_2$ laser is used in various ways to treat tubal disease. Most involve differences in the use of the micromanipulator, the hand scalpel, different spot sizes, or varying power densities. Depending upon his personal preference and surgical skills, with time, each laser surgeon will develop his own technique. Most surgeons find that experience with the laser allows them to operate at progressively higher power densities. There is a move away from the interrupted modes of application (single or repeat pulse), and a greater percentage of the surgery is now done in the continuous delivery mode. It is important to remember that exposing tissue to the laser for the shortest time possible to achieve the desired effect is probably best. Thus, rapid movement of a high power density beam will give the same surgical result as a more prolonged exposure to a lower power density beam, and the thermal damage to the tissue will be much less. Most experts believe a surgeon should operate at the highest power density that can comfortably and safely be controlled in a given situation.

### Adhesiolysis

Removing adhesions with the $CO_2$ laser is possibly the most rewarding use of the technique. Filmy adhesions are excised by holding them with forceps and vaporizing both ends. The 6-mm Pyrex rods are very useful here (Fig 8–9). The rod, as previously mentioned, is held slightly away from the tissue to be lasered, if possible; this prevents transmission of heat from the Pyrex to the tissue. This transmission is easily detected when the rod is in contact with the tissue because the tissue will fuse to the rod. If this occurs, irrigation along with gentle traction is usually sufficient to separate the surfaces. The adhesions are transected immediately adjacent to the serosal surface of the involved organ. If this is carried out properly, there should be no blanching or other detectable change of the organ surface. Power densities in the range of 3,000 to 5,000 watts/cm$^2$ are usually adequate for this type of dissection, although higher power densities are also appropriate. Lower power densities probably increase the risk of thermal damage because increased dwell time is required to achieve the same result. A small spot size is preferable here, usually 200 μm to 800 μm in diameter. This procedure usually proceeds rapidly and is facilitated by flooding surrounding areas with irrigation to avoid constant concern about underlying structures.

Thick fibrous adhesions between surfaces require more tedious dissection but can fre-

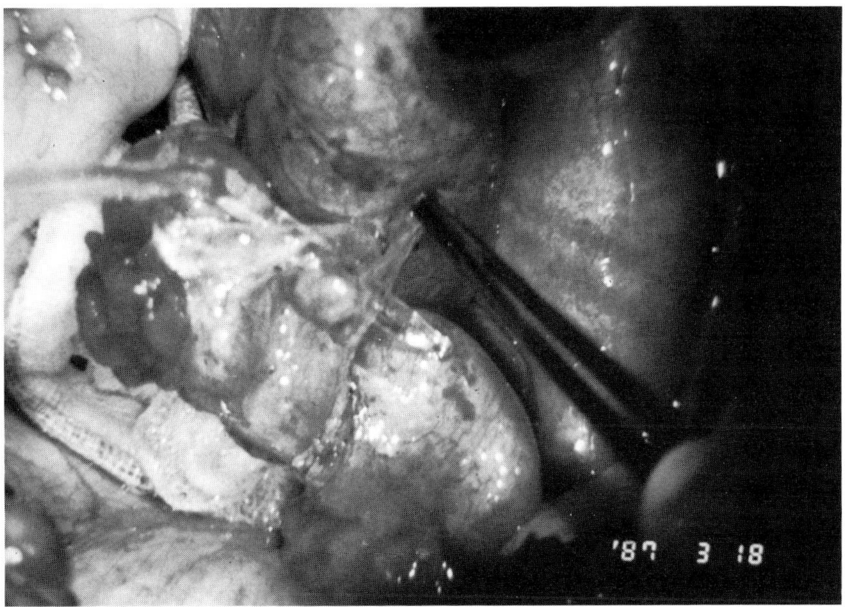


**FIG 8–9.**
Pyrex rod positioned behind peritubal adhesions.

quently result in an excellent anatomic outcome. If the beam can be applied parallel to the axis of the adhesive plane (e.g., bowel densely adherent to the back of the uterus), a small spot size with a high power density seems to work best. If the beam must be applied tangentially (e.g., a tube densely adherent to ovary), it is sometimes necessary to use a larger spot size (1 to 2 mm) with a lower power density. This allows separation of the surfaces with gentle traction and avoids actual incision of the tubal serosa or ovarian capsule. The beam is applied at the leading edge of the adherent surface in a sweeping motion so that the adhesive fibers are vaporized. Traction facilitates removal of the underlying normal tissue from the path of the beam and exposes a fresh supply of adhesive fibers. Traction is best applied with opposing finger pressure or pressure from the Pyrex rods. Clamps and pickups should be avoided if possible and used only on tissue that is to be excised. As the surgeon begins to appreciate the precise way in which the laser can be applied, he soon becomes comfortable operating with the laser beam close to gloved fingers or other vital structures. In situations where the structures are not accessible by direct line of vision, mirrored surfaces become essential to the laser surgeon. The author prefers a silver-fronted dental mirror that is at a 45-degree angle to the handle, which should be of an appropriate length for optimal control. The mirror should be heated to body temperature by warm irrigating solution prior to use; rewarming is generally necessary at frequent intervals. The surface of the mirror must be dried before laser impact lest the water on the surface boil. It must also be kept free of vapor and cellular debris during the dissection. If the mirror surface becomes coated with liquid, dried blood, or debris, it will rapidly become pitted and unsuitable for further use. Since the laser plume is predominantly water vapor, it must be suctioned off before it coats the mirror. Usually placement of the suction tip immediately adjacent to the mirror is sufficient to accomplish this purpose.

One frequently encounters relatively large surface areas (e.g., the ovary, the back of the uterus) that are covered with adhesions that are not amenable to excision. Using a spot size of 2 mm or more with power densities in the range of 500 to 1,000 watts/cm$^2$, these areas can be vaporized. A gentle sweeping motion to cover the involved areas works well and avoids capsular or serosal disruption, although slight serosal blanching may occur. Raw surfaces can be treated in a similar fashion to prevent capillary oozing. Although many feel this maneuver decreases the likelihood of postoperative adherence of neighboring structures, this effect remains to be proven. Again, the large spot with lower power densities is preferable for this action. After surface adhesions are vaporized, a significant amount of carbonized debris can be present on the surface. Some feel this should be removed by debriding with wet cotton swabs; however, this type of removal is traumatic and often leads to bleeding. Copious irrigation of the surfaces is preferable instead. All of the carbonized debris may not be removed by irrigation but, at second-look laparoscopy, little or no carbon is usually visible,[15] it having been removed by the normal activity of peritoneal macrophages.

## Fimbrioplasty

Fimbrial adhesions can present in a variety of ways. Bridging of mucosal fronds can cause the infundibulum to appear constricted. These can be excised with a small spot size and high power density over a Pyrex rod. Many of these structures have blood vessels in excess of 1 mm in them and occasionally require bipolar cautery prior to laser incision. More dense adhesions across the infundibulum are similarly incised while exercising care not to damage the underlying tubal mucosa. Constrictive fibrotic bands that encircle the infundibulum and restrict the size of the ostium can be incised at strategic, avascular points along their circumference. This usually results in restoration of reasonable anatomy.

## Destruction of Paratubal Cysts

It is not uncommon to find cysts located in the mesosalpinx. For the most part, these are small and require no attention. Occasionally, there is a cyst 2 cm or more in diameter that appears capable of altering tubal mobility. These cysts can be excised by opening the mesosalpinx and dissecting them free. An alternative approach is to effectively marsupialize them by creating a window in both the peritoneum and the cyst wall that is of sufficient size that it will not close as healing occurs. The laser fuses the cyst wall to the peritoneum in most cases and no sutures are required. In the author's experience, this technique works well and no incidence of cyst recurrence has been noted at the time of second-look laparoscopy.

## Neosalpingostomy

Treatment of the hydrosalpinx has historically resulted in poor pregnancy rates, regardless of what surgical technique has been used. This poor response has been felt to be related to the damaged mucosa's inability to regenerate to normal, although significant regeneration has been documented.[16] The validity of damaged mucosa as a cause of poor outcome is supported by the reports of high patency rates and poor intrauterine pregnancy rates after neosalpingostomy.[15] If the mucosa is in fact the limiting factor, the addition of the laser to surgical techniques will likely have a less-than-dramatic effect on pregnancy rates for patients with this disorder. Because the vast majority of hydrosalpinges are associated with significant adnexal adhesions, the major benefit of the laser may be in adhesion removal prior to neosalpingostomy.

The technique of neosalpingostomy using laser microsurgery is similar to that of using the needle cautery. The tube is freed from the surrounding adhesions and distended slightly with dye solution. Under moderate magnification, an attempt is made to define the areas of radial scarring that can be used as guides for the incisions. Using a small spot size and power densities from 5,000 to 15,000 watts/cm$^2$, the initial incisions are outlined. One incision is then carried down until dye is encountered and the tube decompresses. The inside of the tube becomes visible as the incision is extended. With care to avoid the mucosa, gentle traction with microsurgical pickups is exerted on the incisional margins. Operating from the inside out, further incisions can then be made between any existing mucosal folds. A sufficient number of radial incisions are made to allow adequate eversion of mucosa and development of a reasonable size stoma. Using power densities in the range of 200 to 500 watts/cm$^2$, the spot size is then enlarged to 2 to 4 mm and the serosal surface is lasered. This causes contraction of the serosa and maintains the eversion.[17] The surgeon should avoid charring of the surface. It is usually sufficient just to cause blanching of the serosa to obtain the desired effect.

This technique of neosalpingostomy is best learned in the laboratory using a canine gallbladder as a model. Thick-walled tubes or the wall of a very large hydrosalpinx will frequently require suturing to maintain the eversion; however, most hydrosalpinges can be kept open by laser technique alone. Patency rates remain high[15] with this technique. Observation of the treated area at a second-look laparoscopy usually reveals well-everted mucosa with no circumferential constriction of the lasered portion of the tube. The area may be slightly pale compared to surrounding tissues but is generally quite pliable. It is rare for adhesions to surrounding structures to involve this area when only laser treatment is used to maintain the eversion.

## Tubal Reanastomosis

Reanastomosis of previously ligated uterine tubes currently enjoys the highest success rate of all tubal reconstructive procedures, but the percentages vary widely depending on the anatomic location of the anastomotic site. Midtubal anastomosis rates are reported to be as high as 80%,[18] whereas cornual anastomosis rates are somewhat lower,[19] 68% or less. The laser's role in tubal anastomosis lies in the preparation of the tubal segments. Using a 200 μm spot size and power densities from 10,000 to 60,000 watts/cm$^2$, the obstructive cap on both proximal and distal segments is quickly and hemostatically resected.

"Superpulse" modes may also find their greatest application in this area because their extremely high peak power densities (e.g., $10^6$ watts/cm$^2$) and reduced tissue exposure time will allow relatively hemostatic incisions with an absolute minimum of tissue damage. The surgeon may find that the reduced hemostasis of the "superpulse" mode can be compensated for by pre-incisional injection of a dilute solution of vasopressin. This injection is virtually mandatory when working on the cornua, regardless of whether one uses the continuous-wave form or "superpulse" applications, because of the rich vascular supply of this portion of the tube.

The laser is used to cut through all three tubal layers (Plates 9 and 10). Some have expressed concern at cutting mucosa with the laser because of thermal damage and because the laser can seal the isthmic or cornual lumen as the incision is made. However, there will be minimal damage to the mucosa if one uses the small spot size and high power density so the incision can be made quickly. The mucosa remains lush and pink and will bleed quite easily upon manipulation with instruments. Luminal patency can be maintained by incising the mucosa while insufflating the tube with indigo carmine in saline infused under gentle pressure. The column of fluid in the tubal lumen stops the laser, dissipates the heat, and assures that the tube wall will not constrict. This technique is particularly important in working on the intramural portion of the tube, which can on occasion be as small as 300 μm in diameter.

Large spot sizes and low power densities are completely inappropriate for incisional work in this area of the tube but can be used for sculpturing away uterine tissue around the lumen. This sculpturing capability of the laser allows hemostatic and anatomically precise preparation of the proximal stoma. It avoids the repeated thin sectioning of the uterine cornu that so frequently ends up as a large raw surface that cannot be covered by the available tubal serosa around the distal segment. When one has a small proximal lumen to which the ampulla must be anastomosed, the ampullary opening can be custom-tailored to the desired size by using a small spot size with the laser. Anastomoses are carried out in the usual fashion using fine suture with magnification to assure good anatomic approximation.

Occasional comments are made about "tubal welding" with the laser, but there are still no published reports of merit on human subjects addressing this topic in a convincing fashion. It will be interesting to watch for this development in the next several years as lasers with differing tissue effects are developed and "tubal welding" becomes a reality.

Resection of diseased segments of tubes with subsequent reanastomosis is also readily carried out with the $CO_2$ laser. This obstruction usually occurs in the isthmus or intramural tube. On occasion, the isthmus may be nothing more than a fibrotic cord. Histologic evaluation frequently reveals endometriosis or salpingitis isthmica nodosa to be the cause of the damage, but it is equally common that no etiology can be determined. The key to successful management of this type of obstruction, if it is approached surgically, is to be certain that all the abnormal tissue is resected. Just as with preparing the segments of previously ligated tubes, one must use a small spot size, high power density, and constant pressure on the dye insufflation system. After each incision, the mucosa and muscularis should be examined carefully for evidence of normalcy. At this point in the procedure, merely demonstrating tubal patency is not sufficient. Once the mucosa and muscularis are determined to be normal under high magnification with the operating microscope (i.e., normal mucosal folds and normal vascular pattern and texture), the resection can cease. It is not uncommon to find that one has resected all of the isthmus and a good portion of the intramural tube. Ampullary-intramural anastomosis is carried out in the standard fashion.

## Linear Salpingostomy for Ectopic Pregnancy

Conservative surgical management of the unruptured ectopic pregnancy can be difficult if trophoblasts have invaded the rich vascular supply coursing in the mesosalpinx. A rather small benign-looking ampullary ectopic can become a hemorrhagic disaster with little warning once the tube is incised. Attempts to control hemorrhage by injecting the tube with vasopressin, ligating vessels in the mesosalpinx, and using occlusive vascular clamps meet with general success but are still inadequate in many instances. It has been this author's experience on more than one occasion that linear salpingostomy made with the laser or cautery and followed by gentle removal of the products of conception is followed by profuse hemorrhage from the implantation site. Fine mattress sutures, vasoconstrictors, vessel ligation, pressure, and cautery have at times failed to control bleeding. This situation requires resection of the bleeding tubal segment and is followed by reanastomosis, or simple ligation with anastomosis at a subsequent laparotomy. This author has found anastomosis done at the time, if possible, to be most satisfactory. This is in agreement with information by other investigators in their series on conservative surgical management of ectopic pregnancy.[20, 21] The laser used in combination with the bipolar cautery is useful for performing the linear salpingostomy or tubal transection, but this author has not found it useful in achieving hemostasis at the implantation site. The main problem is that the laser is not effective in the presence of significant hemorrhage because of the high water content of blood.

### Tubal Reimplantation

Tubal reimplantation procedures have had a wide variation in reported pregnancy rates over the years. In 1977, Peterson, Behrman, and Musich described a technique of reimplantation that achieved a 50% pregnancy rate.[22] In 1983, Peterson reported the superiority of microsurgical cornual anastomosis over that of reimplantation technique in his hands.[23] Other authors have reported pregnancy rates as low as 15% for reimplantation.[24]

The $CO_2$ laser would seem to offer a distinct advantage over standard techniques for this purpose. The uterine opening can be made perfectly cylindrical and of the precise diameter of the tubal segment to be implanted. Such a procedure using the laser has been described by Bellina.[25] He used the hand scalpel with a small spot size and power densities of 50,000 watts/cm$^2$ to fashion a cylindrical opening on the myometrium. He injected the uterine wall with vasopressin (Pitressin) and kept the vessels in the wall compressed, using a transcervical dye insufflation system that allowed significant intrauterine pressure to be generated. With this technique, he was able to form the opening rapidly and hemostatically. No follow-up has yet been published on a significantly large number of patients to allow meaningful comparison with earlier techniques. This author has attempted this procedure and found it somewhat more difficult than originally described, but that may only represent lack of experience. The microsurgical anastomosis previously described appears to be superior technically and much simpler in my hands.

## CLINICAL RESULTS

Since 1982, a number of clinical studies have been published on the results achieved with the $CO_2$ laser in infertility surgery and on comparisons of laser and microelectrocautery. Pittaway, et al., using a rabbit model to compare standardized injuries created by either the $CO_2$ laser or microelectrocautery, found no significant differences in the degree of adhesion formation.[26] In a prospective, randomized human study, Tulandi compared the result of salpingovariolysis using the $CO_2$ laser and the microdiathermy needle;[1] the pregnancy rate was the same in both groups after 2 years. Although the surgery-to-conception interval tended to be shorter in the laser group, the difference did not achieve statistical significance. In a later paper, the same question was addressed, but adhesion reformation and tubal patency were used as points of comparison.[2] Still no difference could be shown in the two techniques. Tulandi also looked at pregnancy rates and surgery-to-conception intervals in hydrosalpinx repairs with laser surgery and electrosurgery. In his initial article on this subject, he found that the pregnancy rates were similar but that the surgery-to-conception interval was shorter in the laser surgery group after a 1-year follow-up.[3] His subsequent report of the patients with a 2-year follow-up showed that the difference in the surgery-to-conception interval had disappeared.[4] He thus concluded, based on pregnancy rate and surgery-to-conception interval, that the laser offered no advantage over electromicrosurgery. In a 1986 observation study, Daniell, et al., found repair of hydrosalpinges with $CO_2$ laser microsurgery to offer similar pregnancy rates to those reported with conventional techniques.[27] They observed a shorter surgery-to-conception interval than other published series using conventional techniques. Mage and Bruhat compared outcomes of hydrosalpinx repair in sequential groups of patients.[28] The first group (January 1977 through December 1978) was treated by electrosurgical salpingostomy and the second group (January 1979 through January 1981) was treated by $CO_2$ laser salpingostomy. They found no statistically significant difference between the results achieved in the two groups. Bellina, in 1983, reported a series of 230 cases of laser microsurgery of the fallopian tube; 75% of the patients in this series had had previous pelvic laparotomies.[29] The overall pregnancy rate of this study was 39.6%. In patients with bipolar tubal disease Bellina achieved an intrauterine pregnancy rate of 36%, and in sterilization reversals, 71%. Mage and Bruhat[30] reported 123 cases of laser microsurgeries in 1987 concluding, as did Bellina,[29] that the results compared favorably with conventional techniques and that the laser had a place in the armamentarium of the microsurgeon.

This author's own series of $CO_2$ laser microsurgeries now exceeds 600 cases with the initial 69 patients having been reported in 1983.[31] Out of more than 200 patients currently with a minimum follow-up of 2 years, 70 patients underwent adhesiolysis or fimbrioplasty, or both, with an overall pregnancy rate of 54.3% (38 pregnancies). Patients were subgrouped according to Hulka's 1978 adhesion classification,[32] which rates severity by the amount of ovarian surface that is visible and the density/vascularity of the adhesions. Patients with minimal (I-A) adhesions had an 80% overall pregnancy rate, whereas patients with the most severe disease (IV-B) had a 44.4% overall pregnancy rate. Six ectopic pregnancies (8.6% of patients) occurred in this group.

In the 73 patients having repair of hydrosalpinges, 88% had at least one tube or their only remaining tube patent on follow-up hysterosalpingogram or laparoscopy. The overall pregnancy rate was 31.5%. In the patients who were followed at least 5 years, the overall pregnancy rate was 39.3% and the term pregnancy rate was 28.6%. The ectopic rate in this entire group of 73 patients was 9.6% of patients (7 cases).

Thirty-nine patients had reversal of sterilization. Twenty-one of 25 (84%) patients having tube-tube anastomosis and 10 of 14 (71.4%) having tube-uterus anastomosis had intrauterine pregnancies. Two spontaneous abortions, but no ectopic pregnancies, occurred.

Of 20 patients who had segmental resection and reanastomosis for pathologic proximal obstruction, eight (40%) conceived. One spontaneously aborted and one was ectopic for a term rate of 30%.

In the process of assigning patients into either laser microsurgery or electromicrosurgery groups over the last 3 years, this author has had multiple opportunities to view the surgical results from both laser microsurgery and electromicrosurgery at second-look laparoscopy. The individual healing characteristics of each patient seem to predominate, and it is not always possible to determine which technique was used. Currently, this author is collecting objective data at early second-look laparoscopy on adhesion formation after each of the techniques.

## ADVANTAGES OF LASER SURGERY OF THE FALLOPIAN TUBES

In the clinical evaluation of the $CO_2$ laser as a tool in microsurgery of the fallopian tube, one has only to use it for its technical advantages and limitations to become apparent. It is initially cumbersome until one becomes accustomed to the "no-touch" nature of laser surgery. Even with the needle cautery, there is a sense of pressure perceived as one contacts the tissue with the cautery tip. With the laser, all proprioceptive feedback is from the joystick of the micromanipulator or from the hand scalpel that is pointing at the tissue. An entirely new set of hand-eye coordination signals must be established by the surgeon through practice and experience. The beauty of no-touch surgery, however, becomes apparent as the surgeon begins to realize how much less traumatic it is not to have to physically manipulate the tissue to make an incision. For most, this carries over and results in a general improvement in their overall microsurgical technique (i.e., minimal tissue handling).

Although the incidence of pelvic infection after tubal reconstructive procedures is low, the laser widens the margin of safety by its inherent property of sterilizing the impact zone. Any bacteria or viruses in the line of the beam will be vaporized or incinerated instantly. Although this may be only a theoretical advantage in most cases, it is comforting.

The other technical advantages of the laser in microsurgery have already been alluded to but deserve repetition for emphasis. They include the shortened operating time, the improved hemostasis, an increased precision of application, and the decreased tissue damage. The laser's ability to be reflected off mirrored surfaces improves access to difficult areas. The construction of the micromanipulator decreases the significance of extraneous movements by the surgeon.

The major technical disadvantage of the $CO_2$ laser is its poor coagulating ability in comparison to either electrocautery or the argon, KTP, or Nd:YAG lasers. This author is not aware, however, of any reports in the literature on the use of these lasers for tubal microsurgery. They are all characterized by an increase in the amount of thermal necrosis they cause when compared to the $CO_2$. This may limit their overall usefulness for tubal microsurgery.

## COMPLICATIONS

Complications from the use of the $CO_2$ laser for intra-abdominal procedures have not been well addressed in the literature. The primary reason for this is the lack of reportable complications from laser surgery. This author has personally performed over 600 laparotomies with the laser without a laser-related complication. Common sense is the best guide for avoiding problems with the laser. Cloth or paper drapes that can be ignited by the beam should be moistened or kept from the beam path. Flammable liquids or adhesive plastic drapes should not be used on the skin if the laser is to be used to incise the skin. Always keep areas surrounding the dissection flooded or covered with wet packs. Use Pyrex or quartz rods behind adhesions or other tissues that are being lasered. If the target area is not clearly visible or the beam path not free of obstructions (i.e., fingers, bowel, instruments), then do not fire the laser. The most certain way to avoid operative complications is to be knowledgeable in the operation of the laser and well trained in the type of surgery in which it will be used.

## TRAINING

Training of the gynecologic surgeon in the use of the $CO_2$ laser for microsurgery should begin with a basic course in standard microsurgery. Once the surgeon has gained sufficient skill through practice on inanimate objects and animal models, a preceptorship with an established microsurgeon should follow. The surgeon can then gain individual clinical skills and experience by appropriate application of the techniques on judiciously selected patients. The time this process takes and the number of cases required will depend primarily on the skill of the individual involved. Only when one is comfortable with the standard microsurgical techniques should the laser be added to the cadre of microsurgical tools. The training sequence then starts over with a basic course in laser physics and tissue interaction, followed by appropriate practice in the animal lab. The surgeon should then spend time practicing on inanimate objects, tissue specimens, and animal models, to develop the hand-eye coordination necessary to apply the laser to human use. As previously mentioned, the no-touch aspect of the laser takes some getting used to. At this point, one should be ready for another preceptorship and, finally, for individual clinical application. One simply does not go from macrosurgery to laser microsurgery and omit everything in between.

Along with learning surgical techniques and laser physics, it is also important to learn to troubleshoot your own laser. Nothing is more frustrating and embarrassing than to have the laser go down in the middle of a laparotomy and not be able to get it working again quickly. The surgeon should know more about the operation of the laser than anyone else in the operating room (with the possible exception of the bioengineer who probably will not be readily available). Being able to change a fuse or attach a gas tank with the proper laser mixture can be invaluable talents when one is dealing with an ectopic pregnancy in the middle of the night.

Another incentive for the surgeon to understand the operation and care of the laser is the cost of a given unit. In 1988, $CO_2$ lasers for use in tubal microsurgery ranged in cost from $40,000 to $125,000, and this does not include the cost of the microscope or accessory instruments. Something as simple as using the wrong material to clean the mirror in the micromanipulator or bumping the articulated arm against the wall can render an instrument useless until replacement parts can be obtained. The laser should be handled with the same care as the tissue upon which the microsurgeon intends to use it.

## SUMMARY AND CONCLUSIONS

Since the first reported use of the $CO_2$ laser in tubal microsurgery in 1974, its use has grown rapidly. It has shown great technical advantages in its precision of application, hemostatic abilities, and decreased tissue damage. Most users agree that it makes the treatment of certain cases technically easier because of the way it can be controlled and the way it can be used with mirrored surfaces. It is attractive because of its no-touch characteristic and because it frequently shortens operative procedures. As of this writing, the addition of the laser to tubal microsurgery has not been shown to improve pregnancy rates. This does not represent a negative statement about the laser, but rather the basic lack of patient numbers and follow-up time to make any intelligent judgements.

The question of whether the addition of a laser to microsurgical techniques is a cost-efficient move is difficult to answer. If the laser can be shown to result in higher pregnancy rates, its emotional impact on infertility patients with tubal disease will make cost effectiveness a moot point except for academic discussions because patients will demand its use, whatever the cost. Actual economic considerations must be individualized by each institution. Answers will need to be calculated, based upon whether or not that hospital's admissions for tubal procedures increased as a result of laser use, on whether hospital stay was shortened for tubal surgery patients, on whether transfusions decreased in relative number in patients treated with the laser, and on a multitude of other factors. It quickly becomes apparent that the original question will remain very difficult to answer for the health-care system as a whole.

The use of the $CO_2$ laser as an adjunctive tool in tubal microsurgery will ultimately find its proper place. For that process to occur, the instrument must be used wisely by those in the field. It must be looked upon as an aid to improving the technical aspects of tubal surgery procedures. It must be evaluated carefully for its impact on pregnancy rates. It cannot be viewed as the ultimate savior of patients with tubal disease. It will not compensate for poor surgical technique or poor patient selection. Those who use the laser now or who will use it in the future must act responsibly to see that it is evaluated fairly and completely.

## REFERENCES


1. Tulandi T: Salpingo-ovariolysis: A comparison between laser surgery and electrocautery. *Fertil Steril* 1986; 45:489–491.
2. Tulandi T: Adhesion reformation after reproductive surgery with and without the carbon dioxide laser. *Fertil Steril* 1987; 47:704–706.
3. Tulandi T, Farag R, McInnis RA, et al: Reconstructive surgery of hydrosalpinx with and without the carbon dioxide laser. *Fertil Steril* 1984; 42:839–842.
4. Tulandi T, Vilos GA: A comparison between laser surgery and electrosurgery for bilateral hydrosalpinx: A two-year follow-up. *Fertil Steril* 1985, 44:846–848.
5. Siegler AM, Hellman LM: Tubal plastic surgery: Report of a survey. *Fertil Steril* 1956; 7:170–177.
6. O'Brien JR, Arronet CH, Eduljee SY: Operative treatment of fallopian tube pathology in human fertility. *Am J Obstet Gynecol* 1969; 103:520–531.
7. Swolin K: Fifty fertility operations: Literature and methods. *Acta Obstet Gynecol Scand* 1967; 46:234–250.
8. Bellina JH: Gynecology and the laser. *Contemp Ob/Gyn* 1974; 4:24–34.
9. Baggish MS: High power-density carbon dioxide laser therapy for early cervical neoplasia. *Am J Obstet Gynecol* 1980; 136:117–125.
10. Bellina JH: Carbon dioxide microsurgery in gynecology. *Int Adv Surg Onc* 1978; 1:227–236.
11. Bellina JH, Stjernholm RL, Kurpel JE: Analysis of plume emission after Papovirus irradiation with the $CO_2$ laser. *J Reprod Med* 1982; 27:268–270.
12. Choe JK, Dawood MY, Andrews AH: Conventional versus laser reanastomosis of rabbit ligated uterine horns. *Obstet Gynecol* 1983; 61:689–964.
13. Martin DC, McCoy TD, Poston WM: Comparative study of reanastomosis following laser incision and sharp incision of the rat uterine horn. Presented at the First World Conference: Fallopian tube in health disease, Miami Beach, Florida, May 1983.
14. Klink F, Grosspietszech R, Von Klitzing L, et al: Animal in vivo studies and in vitro experiments with human tubes for end-to-end anastomotic operation by a $CO_2$ laser technique. *Fertil Steril* 1978; 30:100–102.
15. Kelly RW, Roberts DK: Experience with the $CO_2$ laser in gynecologic microsurgery. *Am J Obstet Gynecol* 1983; 146:285–588 (updated by personal communication).
16. Brenner RM: The biology of oviductal culia, in Hafez ESE, Blandau RJ (eds): *The Mammalian Oviduct*. Chicago, University of Chicago Press, 1969, Chapter 8.
17. Bruhat MA, Mage G, Pouly JL: The use of the $CO_2$ laser in neosalpingostomy: *Proceeding of the Third International Congress for Laser Surgery*, 1979; 271–273.
18. Gomel V: Microsurgical reversal of female sterilization: A reappraisal. *Fertil Steril* 1980; 33:587–597.
19. Winston RML: Microsurgical tubocornual anastomosis for reversal of sterilization. *Lancet* 1977; 1:284–285.

20. Ansari AH, Ulbrich P: Conservative operative procedures for management of tubal pregnancy. *Int J Fertil* 1983; 28:30.
21. Marik JJ: Pregnancy outcome following conservative management of tubal pregnancy. *Int J Fertil* 1983; 28:33.
22. Peterson EP, Musich JR, Behrman SJ: Uterotubal implantation and obstetric outcome after previous sterilization. *Am J Obstet Gynecol* 1977; 128:662–667.
23. Peterson EP: Uterotubal implantation—A reappraisal. *Int J Fertil* 1983; 28:26.
24. Williams GFJ: Tubo-uterine implantation. *Lancet* 1969; 1:825.
25. Bellina JH: Reconstructive microsurgery of the fallopian tube with the carbon dioxide laser - procedures and preliminary results. *J Reprod Med* 1981; 5:1–7.
26. Pittaway DE, Maxson WS, Daniell JF: A comparison of the $CO_2$ laser and electrocautery on postoperative intraperitoneal adhesion formation in rabbits. *Fertil Steril* 1983; 40:366–368.
27. Daniell JF, Diamond MP, McLaughlin DS, et al: Clinical results of terminal salpingostomy with the use of the $CO_2$ laser: Report of the Intraabdominal Laser Study Group. *Fertil Steril* 1986; 45:175–178.
28. Mage G, Bruhat MA: Pregnancy following salpingostomy: Comparison between $CO_2$ laser and electrosurgery procedures. *Fertil Steril* 1983; 40:472–475.
29. Bellina JH: Microsurgery of the fallopian tube with the carbon dioxide laser: Analysis of 230 cases with a two-year follow-up. *Lasers Surg Med* 1983; 3:255–260.
30. Mage G, Pouly JL, Canis M, et al: $CO_2$ laser microsurgery: Five years experience with long-term results. *Microsurgery* 1987; 8:89–91.
31. Kelly RW, Roberts DK: Experience with the $CO_2$ laser in gynecologic microsurgery. *Am J Obstet Gynecol* 1983; 146:285–288 (updated by personal communication).
32. Hulka JF, Omran K, Berger GS: Classification of adnexal adhesions: A proposal and evaluation of its prognostic value. *Fertil Steril* 1978; 30:661–665.

# Chapter 9

# Laser Laparoscopy: $CO_2$

Joseph Feste, M.D.

Endoscopic use of the laser is not new in medicine, since laser endoscopy has already been used in otolaryngology, gastroenterology, orthopedics, urology, and gynecology. This chapter reviews all aspects of the clinical uses of the laparoscopic attachments that allow intraperitoneal endoscopic use of the carbon dioxide ($CO_2$) laser.

The advent of the $CO_2$ laser raises two pertinent questions: (1) how often would one use the laser laparoscope if it were available for every diagnostic laparoscopy; and (2) what are its advantages over conventional techniques and lasers of other wavelengths?

The first question may be answered in part by my own experience. An earlier study reported use of the laser laparoscope in 423 consecutive patients scheduled for diagnostic laparoscopy for infertility or pelvic pain.[1] The laser laparoscope was used in 202 cases (48%). In each instance, the condition diagnosed during the laparoscopy was completely treated at the time of diagnosis, so that no further surgical or medical therapy was required. The 221 patients (52%) in whom the laser laparoscope was not used had conditions that were either inoperable or were too extensive to be treated at laparoscopy. A continuation of this study, from 1982 to the present, shows a cumulative increase in use up to 57%. The indications for the use of the laser at laparoscopy in this period are listed in Table 9–1. From March 1987 to March 1988 there was a 67% utilization of the $CO_2$ laser at laparoscopy. This fact suggests that using lasers at operative laparoscopy tends to increase as one's technical skills and confidence in the laser increase.

The second question basically concerns a comparison of $CO_2$ laser surgery to microsurgery or electrocoagulation, as well as to laser surgery of other wavelengths. There are at least two theoretical advantages of $CO_2$ laser laparoscopy over conventional operative laparoscopy: (1) precise destruction of tissue and (2) the ability to provide excellent hemostasis with minimal damage to the adjacent normal tissue. The $CO_2$ laser provides "what you see is what you get" destruction of tissue. The amount of thermal effect can easily be demonstrated on the surface of an egg white (Fig 9–1). The bottom line of thermal burns are the result of coagulation with an Easley-Keplinger forcep and microneedle. In contrast, the top line of thermal burns were achieved with the $CO_2$ laser using continuous, repeat pulse, and superpulse. The effect on the egg white is clearly demonstrated to be more discrete and precise in the area of the thermal effect than in the zone affected by the electrical coagulation technique.

Because of its precision cutting ability, the $CO_2$ laser produces a thermal effect limited to a 0.1 mm depth of tissue; the normal adjacent tissue is spared any significant thermal effect. The zone of necrosis reflects the maximum depth of destruction, and the zone

**TABLE 9–1.**
Indications for Use of $CO_2$ Laser at Laparoscopy in 611 Patients Between 1982 and 1988

| | | |
|---|---|---|
| Non-infertility | | 205 |
| Endometriosis only | | 75 |
| Stage I | 48 | |
| Stage II | 18 | |
| Stage III | 8 | |
| Stage IV | 1 | |
| Endometriosis with adhesions | | 44 |
| Stage I | 25 | |
| Stage II | 13 | |
| Stage III | 2 | |
| Stage IV | 4 | |
| Adhesions only | | 46 |
| Mild | 23 | |
| Moderate | 16 | |
| Severe | 7 | |
| Dysmenorrhea | | 136 |
| Ectopic pregnancy | | 1 |
| Hydrosalpinx | | 4 |
| Leiomyomata | | 10 |
| Infertility | | 406 |
| Endometriosis only | | 238 |
| Stage I | 178 | |
| Stage II | 50 | |
| Stage III | 9 | |
| Stage IV | 1 | |
| Endometriosis with adhesions | | 91 |
| Stage I | 48 | |
| Stage II | 30 | |
| Stage III | 12 | |
| Stage IV | 1 | |
| Adhesions only | | 53 |
| Mild | 30 | |
| Moderate | 19 | |
| Severe | 4 | |
| Dysmenorrhea | | 102 |
| Ectopic pregnancy | | 8 |
| Hydrosalpinx | | 13 |
| Leiomyomata | | 33 |

of thermal conductivity and repair determines the damage to the adjacent normal tissues. When the $CO_2$ laser is in a single-pulse, repeat-pulse, or superpulse mode, both of these layers are thinner than when the argon, KTP, or YAG lasers are used in a non-contact fashion and are significantly thinner than when electric coagulation is used. Whether these reduced effects will result in improved pregnancy rates is yet to be determined. Encouragingly, in preliminary studies, pregnancy rates and relief of symptoms have proved to be at least as good as those performed with the more conventional techniques.[2]

## DEVELOPMENT OF PROTOTYPES FOR CARBON DIOXIDE LASER LAPAROSCOPY

Prototype instruments for $CO_2$ laser laparoscopy and investigations of their use began independently on three continents, with reports by Bruhat, Mage, and Manhes (1979) from

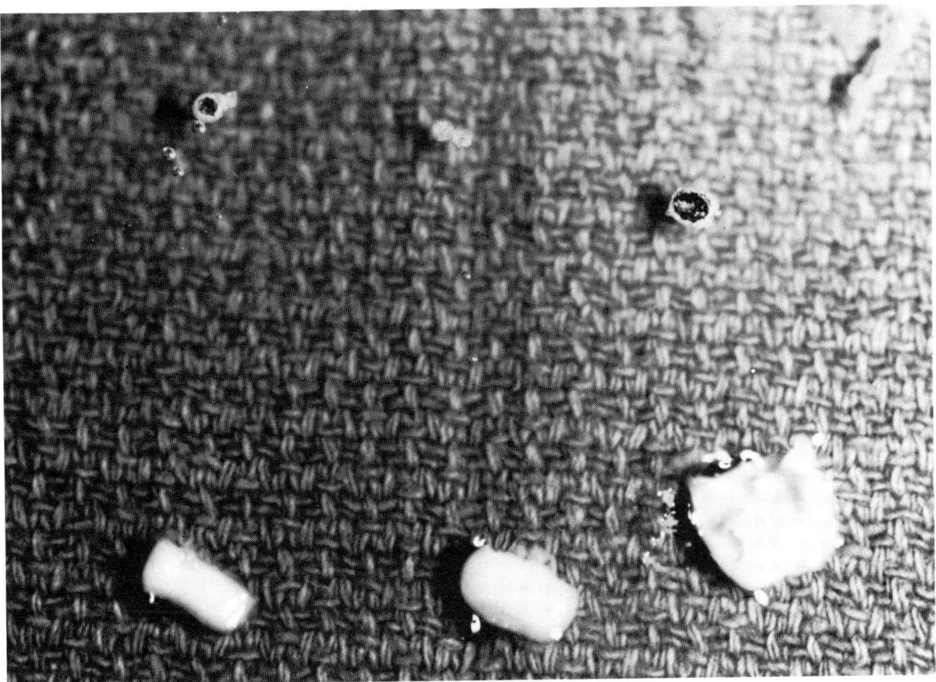

**FIG 9–1.**
Thermal effect on egg white, comparing coagulation with an Easly-Keplinger forcep (bottom line of burns) with the $CO_2$ laser, using repeat-pulse, superpulse, and continuous pulse.

France,[3] Tadir and colleagues (1981) from Israel,[4] and Daniell and Brown (1982) in North America.[2] It was not until 1980 that animal studies and clinical trials were begun in the United States, using a prototype laparoscope designed jointly by Eder Instrument Company (Chicago, Illinois) and Advanced Surgical Technologies, Inc. (Schaumburg, Illinois), that would allow articulation of a focusing lens to the surgical arm of the Sharplan 733 $CO_2$ laser. This early system made it possible to aim and fire the focused $CO_2$ beam through the 5-mm operative channel of the laparoscope.

In the first evaluations in animals and humans, this prototype laser laparoscope was found to be impractical and unusable, because of the poor optics and the operator's inability to keep the $CO_2$ beam from reflecting off the walls of the operative channel of the laparoscope, through which the beam had to pass in order to affect the tissue.

Similarly, the first prototype for a second-puncture laparoscopic probe to introduce the $CO_2$ laser beam intraperitoneally proved to be cumbersome to use and inadequate because of the loss of the carbon dioxide, the accumulation of intraperitoneal smoke, and the difficulty in keeping the beam focused in the center of the channel.

The use of a second-puncture instrument to introduce the laser beam into the pelvis did, however, make it possible to use a standard laparoscope and solved the problem of inadequate visibility. Unfortunately, in addition to the continuing problem of poor beam alignment, there was a loss of the pneumoperitoneum, as a result of the lack of airtight articulations, and visibility was still poor because of the intraperitoneal smoke. In addition, the introduction of the $CO_2$ laser beam through an accessory trocar site made the procedure more cumbersome. This development also led to a "clashing of swords" as the intraperitoneal ends of the instruments collided during the manipulations necessary to align the laparoscope, the laser probe, and the accessory instruments needed for traction, suction of smoke, or as backstops for the beam. In some procedures, four or five instruments, and therefore four or five incisions, were occasionally needed. This system was unwieldy and clinically unacceptable.

Fortunately, with the development of new laparoscopic instrumentation for $CO_2$ laser use, most technical problems have been overcome. This has been accomplished for the most part by close cooperation between the laparoscope and laser manufacturers and the investigators who evaluate each new modification in animal models.

## PRESENT SYSTEMS FOR USE OF THE CARBON DIOXIDE LASER LAPAROSCOPE

Although modifications of the $CO_2$ laser laparoscope delivery systems continue, the systems now available are suitable for clinical application by the laparoscopist who is comfortable with the advanced techniques of laparoscopic surgery and who is also well versed in the physics of the intra-abdominal use of the $CO_2$ laser.

### Single-Puncture Laser Laparoscopy

At present, single-puncture operative laparoscopes for laser laparoscopy are either 12.7 mm in diameter with a 6-mm operative channel or 10.5 mm in diameter with a 5-mm

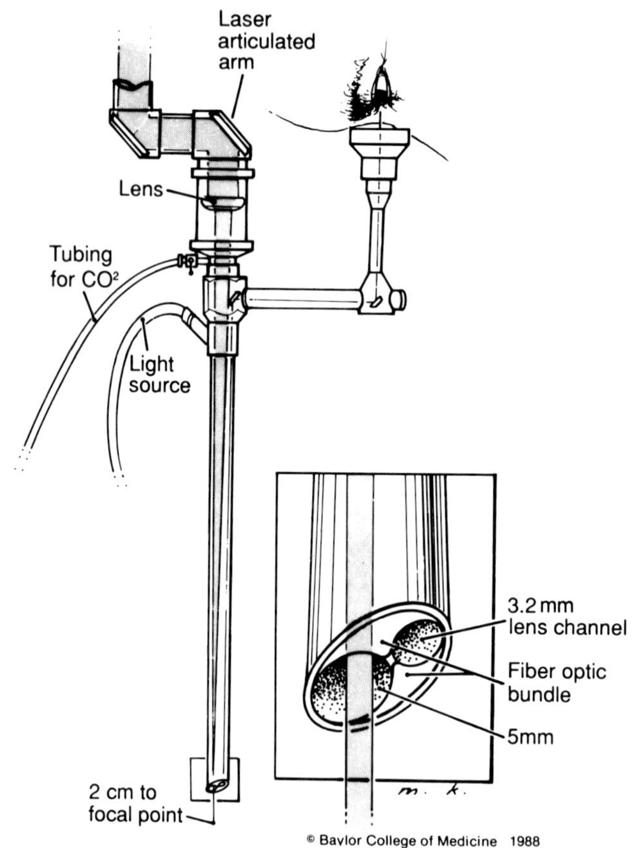


**FIG 9–2.**
Parallel operative laser laparoscopy with a 5-mm operating channel.

operative channel. The instrument can be used as either a standard operative laparoscope with 5-mm accessory forceps or as a laser laparoscope. Once the decision has been made to use the $CO_2$ laser through the laparoscope, the operator simply swings the articulated arm of the laser over the operative field and attaches a direct coupler or a special mirror and focusing lens, in their sealed housing, to the operative channel of the laparoscope (Figs 9–2 and 9–3). The lens and mirror allow final focusing and correct alignment of the beam that passes through the operative channel of the laparoscope to vaporize the tissue. The operator must then attach the $CO_2$ insufflation tubing to this channel, distal to the mirror attachment, which allows a flow of fresh carbon dioxide down the beam channel. The flow of carbon dioxide from the insufflator keeps the warm intraperitoneal carbon dioxide from fogging the mirror and lens in the housing and also displaces smoke from the laser channel. This displacement is extremely important because smoke can reduce the power of the beam as it emerges from the laser channel.

The laparoscope is then test-fired. A moist tongue depressor is used to check the alignment of the helium:neon optical aiming beam and, if necessary, to center the beam down the operative channel of the laparoscope with the alignment mirror. As long as the mirrors in the articulating arm are all in proper alignment, the direct couplers are more convenient and preferable.

The laparoscope is then reintroduced into the abdomen, and the red aiming beam is

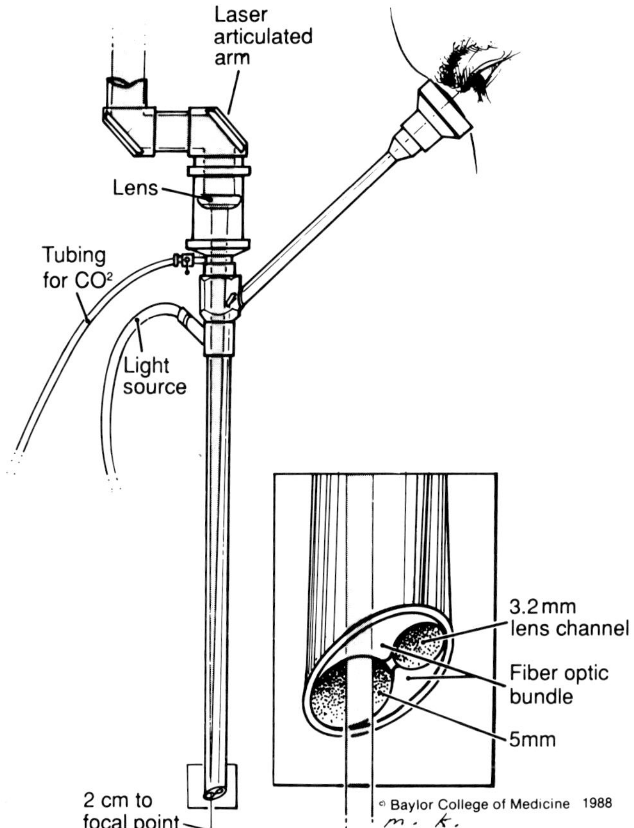


**FIG 9–3.**
Off-set 45° laser laparoscopy with a 5-mm operating channel.

sighted before the firing. It is necessary to pass a second puncture instrument into the pelvis to manipulate pelvic structures and to vent off the smoke that occurs with vaporization. The operator must keep the suction probe close to the site of impact of the laser beam and must immediately suction off the smoke to avoid operating through a dense fog (Fig 9–4). This technique will allow the assistant not only to maintain a clear field by evacuating the laser plume but also to aspirate the irrigating fluid as well. In this manner, the surgeon can concentrate on operating the laser and manipulating the pelvic viscera.[5]

## Double-Puncture Laser Laparoscopy

The second-puncture probe currently used with the $CO_2$ laser laparoscope is a double-ring probe that measures 8 mm in external diameter (Fig 9–5). The probe attaches to the same lens and mirror, or direct coupler, that is used with the operative laparoscope. As with the operative laparoscope, the carbon dioxide insufflation tubing is attached to the probe so that the carbon dioxide can flow down the channel. The smoke of vaporization is drawn out through the outer ring channel of the probe and is controlled by a valve that allows the intraperitoneal smoke to pass into the suction tubing and filter system.

A separate, double-barreled, second-puncture probe with a specially designed backstop is also available for use in vaporizing adhesions (see Fig 9–5). This accessory instrument, with its backstop, eliminates the risk of inadvertent injury to the intraperitoneal structures caused if the beam passes through tissue being treated and comes in contact with the underlying structures.

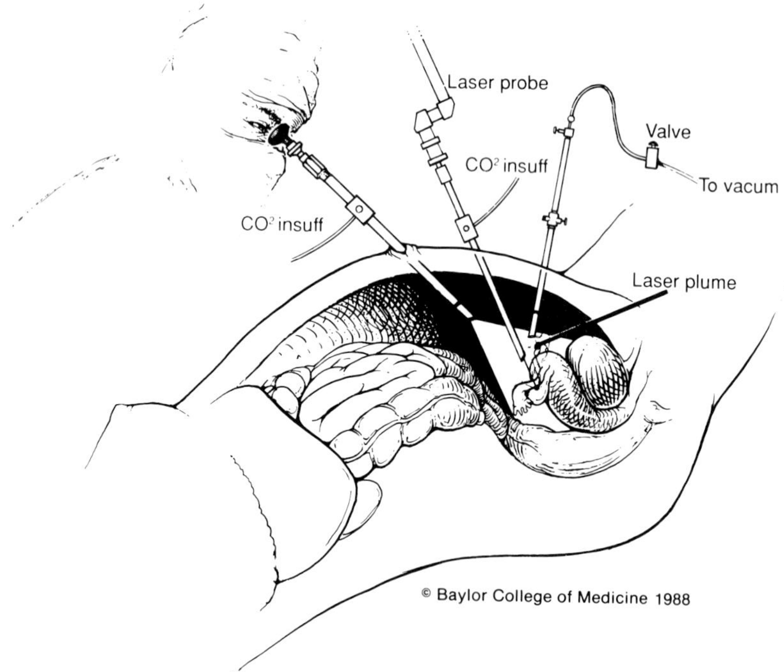


**FIG 9–4.**
A three-puncture technique for removing the laser plume with a suction probe and an abdominal suction valve to prevent the excessive laser plume from obscuring the view of the pelvis (Surgimedics, Houston, Texas).

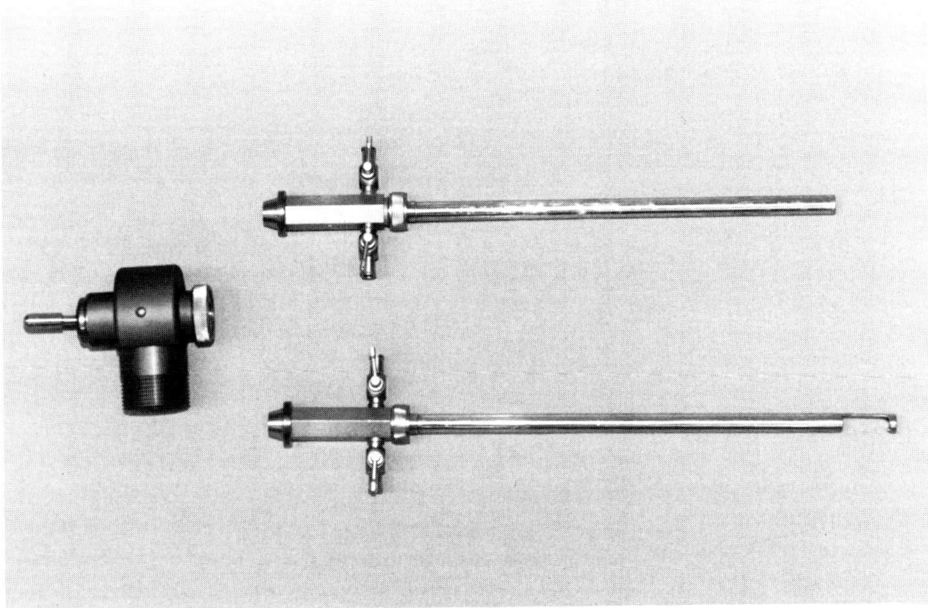

**FIG 9–5.**
Two second-puncture probes with a double ring. Internal diameter of 6 mm and external diameter of 8 mm, one with and one without a backstop.

## Alternative Probes and Lenses

The focusing lens for the standard $CO_2$ laser laparoscope is 300 to 315 mm, with its focal point 2 cm from the end of either the operative laparoscope or the second-puncture probe. This long focal length produces a spot diameter of approximately 0.5 mm, which is greater than that obtained with a shorter lens. This long focal lens also makes it difficult to defocus the laser by pulling the laparoscope away from the tissue. These factors also limit the range of power densities obtainable with this system. The length of the second-puncture system results in an instrument that is uncomfortably long for use with multiple puncture techniques.

Because of these problems, a lens and mirror attachment is available that provides two focal lengths: 250 mm and 300 mm. This feature gives the system greater flexibility. Use of the 250-mm lens with a shorter second-puncture probe (230 mm) will result in an instrument that is less cumbersome. This lens will also allow higher power densities and a focused beam of a smaller diameter. Conversely, the 250-mm lens, when aimed and fired through the longer operative channel of the laser laparoscope, will result in a substantially defocused beam and lower power density. These differences in power density can only be appreciated in connection with the different clinical uses that are currently obtainable with the $CO_2$ laser laparoscope. The main disadvantage of this system is that it requires three separate punctures. One of the instruments must be held by an assistant or a mechanical laparoscopy holder. In both instances, this merely complicates the procedure. In reality, most of these procedures can be performed with the single operative laparoscope, and the problems with multiple punctures can be eliminated. The more difficult treatment of endometriosis, adhesions, or salpingostomies may require a multiple puncture approach.

### $CO_2$ Laser Fibers and Wave Guides

Attempts to develop a flexible fiber for the $CO_2$ laser have met with multiple difficulties in the last several years because of the wavelength of this laser and because of the toxicity of the materials used to make the fibers. With the shorter wavelength lasers, quartz can be used as a transmitting medium, but this is not true with the $CO_2$ laser. Consequently, rigid wave guides have been developed to pass the $CO_2$ energy through a small diameter channel and, at the same time, provide a focusing system at the tip of the instrument (Fig 9–6). These rigid wave guides couple directly to the articulating arm of the $CO_2$ laser and are introduced through either the operating channel of a single-puncture operating laparoscope or through a suprapubic incision (see Fig 9–6). They are then advanced until they almost touch the tissue. This system gives a better feeling of control of the laser beam and eliminates the need to align the beam down the operating channel. The ability to focus and defocus over a distance of 2 cm or less has been useful. The inflexibility of the wave-guide delivery system is not a problem in laparoscopy. Even with the short wavelength lasers (YAG, argon, and KTP), the fibers are passed through a rigid instrument for better stability. Therefore, the flexibility of the fiber is not used at laparoscopy. In contrast, the need for flexibility of the fiber for hysteroscopy is more apparent. In the next few years, several clinical trials will be performed with these wave guides to prove their efficiency at laparoscopy. In the meantime, the search will continue for a truly flexible fiber through which the carbon dioxide wavelength can pass.

## CLINICAL APPLICATIONS

To date, several procedures have been carried out successfully with the $CO_2$ laser laparoscope. These procedures include the following:

1. Vaporization of endometriosis.
2. Uterosacral ligament ablation (laser neurectomy).
3. Terminal neosalpingostomy.
4. Pelvic adhesiolysis.
5. Excision of ectopic pregnancies.
6. Laparoscopic treatment of polycystic ovaries.
7. Vaporization of small uterine fibroids.
8. Ovarian cystectomies.
9. Excision of hydatid cysts of Morgagni.

The clinical role of the $CO_2$ laser laparoscope becomes more evident as use by experienced laparoscopists increases. Techniques for using the $CO_2$ laser are outlined in detail in the following pages.

### Pelvic Endometriosis: Technique and Early Results

One of the diseases most amenable to treatment by laser laparoscopy is pelvic endometriosis. Because endometriosis is basically a disease of the peritoneal surface, it is easily treated with the laser. In the beginning, a surgeon's use of the laser laparoscope should be limited to treating only minimal and mild cases of endometriosis (Stages I and II). With experience, the laser laparoscopist can safely and successfully treat moderate (Stage III)

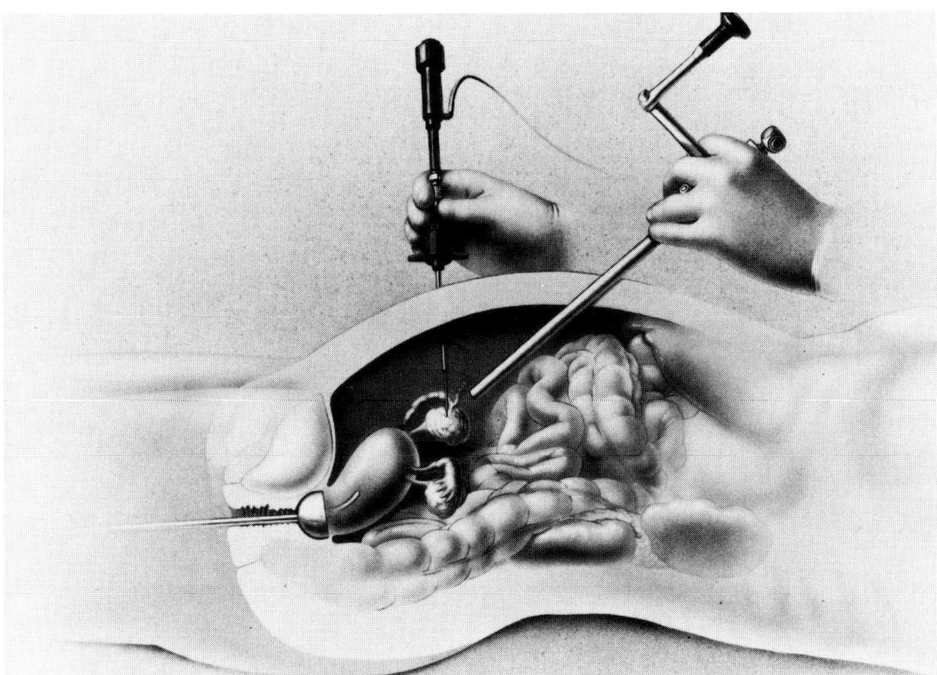

**FIG 9–6.**
$CO_2$ laser wave-guide (Infra-guide™ by Haereus Lasersonics).

and some severe (Stage IV) endometriosis with the laser laparoscope. Eventually, with careful use of either the operative laparoscope or the second-puncture probe, one can safely and adequately vaporize most visible endometriotic implants. Ideally, endometriosis diagnosed at laparoscopy performed for the evaluation of infertility or pelvic pain can be vaporized at that time, thus decreasing the need for long-term medical therapy or subsequent major surgery.

Vaporization with the $CO_2$ laser laparoscope offers several advantages over cautery of endometriotic implants. With cauterization, one is unable to control the "star burst" effect of the unipolar or the bipolar cautery. In addition, there is no way to evaluate the depth of cauterization, and thus, no way to know at the time whether the lesion has been completely destroyed. However, with the $CO_2$ laser, the process of vaporization allows visualization of the three-dimensional boundaries of the lesion, thereby permitting its complete destruction and removal.

In general, power densities between 2,500 and 5,000 W/cm$^2$ are used. Debulking endometriotic implants is best performed by using a continuous firing mode. But for lesions overlying a vital structure (the ureter, urinary bladder, colon, or larger blood vessels), single- or repeat-pulse modes of 0.05 to 0.1 second in duration provide safer vaporization. This duration allows a 100- to 200-mm depth of vaporization, thus substantially limiting the depth of penetration. In addition, the intermittent blast of the laser decreases heat transfer and prevents damage to the underlying tissue and injury to vital structures. Single- or repeat-pulse modes are generally a safer modality for the beginning $CO_2$ laser laparoscopist.

The lesions of endometriosis are basically avascular and therefore, hemostasis is a concern only in the underlying normal tissues. When vaporizing an endometriotic implant, one first sees the bubbling of old blood, followed by a curdy, white material that represents vaporization of the stromal layer. After the entire endometriotic lesion has been vaporized, retroperitoneal fat is encountered, and the appearance of the "bubbling of water" confirms the complete vaporization of the lesion (Fig 9–7). The absorption of the $CO_2$ laser by water prevents deeper penetration of the laser beam for a few seconds after the endometriotic implant is vaporized.

Small endometriomas of the ovaries can be vaporized with continuous-mode application, depending upon the size of the lesion and the presence of follicles containing fluid, which act as an excellent medium for the absorption of the laser beam. It is best to fire the laser at the surface of the implant, allowing the chocolate-colored material to drain from the lesion, and then to continue to vaporize the lesion down to the visually normal tissue. Small implants on the fallopian tube should be vaporized using single-pulse modes, because of the decreased thickness and absence of fat in the tube, as well as its marked vascularity. Lesions overlying the bladder, colon, or ureter should be treated in a similar fashion. Occasional irrigation is helpful throughout the procedure to wash off debris and to better expose the site of laser impact.

The choice between the operative laser laparoscope and the laser second-puncture probe basically depends upon the number and location of endometriotic lesions. A few small, scattered implants, less than 1 cm in diameter, can be quickly and efficiently vaporized with the operative laser laparoscope. This technique does not require a second puncture and can be performed in a few minutes. If multiple lesions are encountered, a second-puncture probe can be used to manipulate the pelvic organs as well as to aspirate the smoke of vaporization. Lateral wall lesions may be treated by the laser probe through a third puncture site, which allows a more perpendicular vaporization of the implants. Figure 9–4 illustrates this three-puncture technique. However, most procedures can be performed easily with the operative laparoscope.

As a safety measure, irrigation fluid can be introduced into the pelvis to protect the

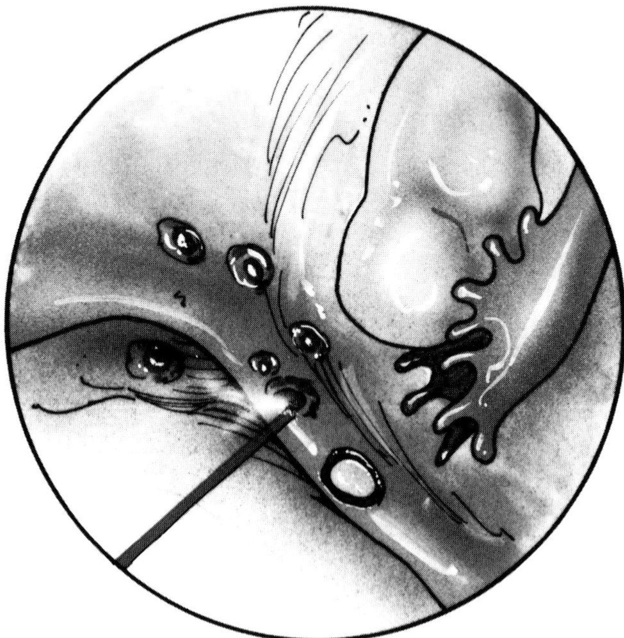

**FIG 9–7.**
Vaporization of endometriosis by $CO_2$ laser laparoscope.

**TABLE 9–2.**
Pregnancy Rates and Outcome After Laparoscopic Laser Surgery for Endometriosis (N = 178) by Stage of Disease

| Stage | Total Patients | Total Pregnant | Pregnancy Outcome: Term | Abortion | Ectopic |
|---|---|---|---|---|---|
| I | 127 | 93(73.2%) | 75 | 16 | 2 |
| II | 45 | 34(75.6%) | 31 | 3 | 0 |
| III | 6 | 4(66.7%) | 2 | 0 | 2 |
| IV | 0 | 0 (0%) | 0 | 0 | 0 |
| | 178 | 131 (73.6%) | 108 (82.4%) | 19 (14.5%) | 4 (3.1%) |

bowel and pelvic sidewalls from the inadvertent reflection of the laser beam off an instrument. It is also of major importance that the tip of the laser probe always be kept in view so that the fallopian tubes, ovaries, or bowel cannot get between the end of the laser probe and the lesion being vaporized. Following vaporization of the lesion, the base is irrigated well with heparinized Ringer's solution to remove all of the excess carbonized particles. At the end of the procedure and after removing the blood from the cul-de-sac, 100 to 200 cc of 32% dextran 70 (Hyskon) may be instilled into the pelvis to aid in the prevention of postoperative adhesions.

In a series of 301 of our patients with Stages I to IV endometrioses, 178 have been followed for a minimum of 1 year; of these, 131 became pregnant (73.6%). The pregnancy rates for each stage are listed in Table 9–2. Almost 48% of those who conceived became pregnant within 6 months of their surgery (Table 9–3). If one includes only those patients who had endometriosis as the sole known cause of their infertility, the overall pregnancy rate was 74.2% (Table 9–4). Life table analysis projected an 82% cumulative pregnancy rate at 41 months (Fig 9–8) for this patient subgroup. For those patients with significant male or other female factors also contributing to their infertility, the pregnancy rate was 66.4% (Table 9–5). These pregnancy rates are well above those reported for the 361 patients treated with electrocautery (average pregnancy rate of 45%) (Table 9–6). Martin has recently reported a gross pregnancy rate of 32 (61%) in 64 patients treated for endometriosis by laser laparoscopy.[14] Of those who conceived, 86% had term pregnancies, 12% had spontaneous abortions, and 4% had ectopic pregnancies. Keye, et al. have reported on 92 patients treated with the argon laser, and Lomano reported on patients treated with the YAG laser for ablation of endometriosis.[15, 16] Both reports had pregnancy rates comparable to those in Martin's series.

**TABLE 9–3.**
Length of Time From Surgery to Conception in Patients Who Achieved Pregnancy Following Laser Laparoscopy for Endometriosis by Stage of Disease

| Stage | Total Pregnancies | Time to Conception: <6 Months | 6 to 12 Months | >12 Months |
|---|---|---|---|---|
| I | 93 | 47 | 20 | 26 |
| II | 34 | 14 | 11 | 9 |
| III | 4 | 2 | 0 | 2 |
| IV | 0 | 0 | 0 | 0 |
| | 131 | 63 (48%) | 31 (24%) | 37 (28%) |

**TABLE 9–4.**

Pregnancies Following Laser Laparoscopy for Endometriosis in Patients Without Male or Additional Female Factors by Stage of Disease

| Stage | Total | Pregnancies |
|---|---|---|
| I | 48 | 33 (68.8%) |
| II | 14 | 14(100.0%) |
| III | 4 | 2 (50.0%) |
| IV | 0 | 0 (0%) |
| | 66 | 49 (74.2%) |

**TABLE 9–5.**

Pregnancies Following Laser Laparoscopy for Endometriosis in Patients With Male or Other Female Factors by Stage of Disease

| Stage | Number of Patients | Number Pregnant |
|---|---|---|
| I | 88 | 58 (65.9%) |
| II | 31 | 21 (67.7%) |
| III | 3 | 2 (66.7%) |
| IV | 0 | 0 (0%) |
| | 122 | 81 (66.4%) |

While it appears that higher pregnancy rates can be achieved with $CO_2$ laser laparoscopy than by electrocautery, a comparison of pregnancy rates from one center to those of other centers is of questionable validity because of the inability of the investigators to match subjects for such confounding variables as age, duration of infertility, presence of other infertility factors, treatment of other infertility factors, previous treatment failures, and skill of the operator. A valid comparison of the $CO_2$ laser with electrocautery or other laser wavelengths will require a randomized, controlled study by a single surgeon or team of surgeons.

A subsequent review of 882 of our patients with endometriosis treated by the $CO_2$ laser at laparoscopy reveals pregnancy rates of 58% for all stages. If endometriosis was the only infertility factor evaluated, the pregnancy rate averaged 70% for 380 patients. At

**TABLE 9–6.**

Pregnancies After Laparoscopic Coagulation and Excision*

| Author | Year | Patients | Follow-up | Pregnancies |
|---|---|---|---|---|
| Eward[6] | 1978 | 25 | 1–2 Years | 14 (56.0%) |
| Hasson[7] | 1979 | 8 | 1–4 Years | 6 (75.0%) |
| Mettler, et al[8] | 1979 | 90 | 1–6 Years | 22 (24.0%) |
| Sulewski, et al[9] | 1980 | 100 | 1–5 Years | 40 (40.0%) |
| Daniell and Christianson[10] | 1981 | 60 | 1–2 Years | 34 (57.0%) |
| Seiler, et al[11] | 1985 | 45 | 7 Months | 22 (49.0%) |
| Reich and McGlynn[12] | 1986 | 20† | 1–7 Years | 12 (60.0%) |
| Reich and McGlynn[13] | 1986 | 13‡ | 1–7 Years | 12 (92.0%) |
| | | 361 | | 162 (45.0%) |

*Data from references 6–13.
†Endometriomas greater than 2 cm.
‡Endometriomas greater than 2 cm, endometriosis as an isolated factor.

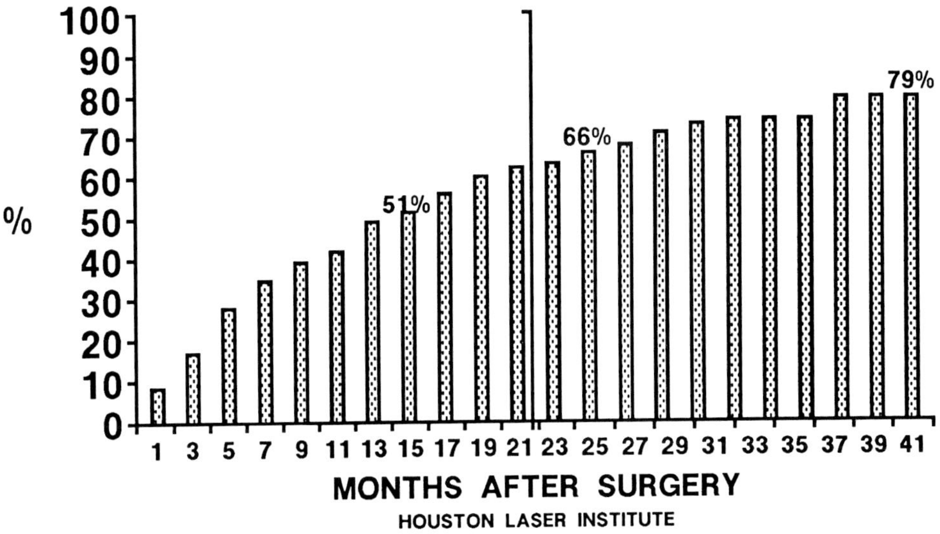


**FIG 9–8.**
Life-table analysis of patients treated for endometriosis by laparoscopy after 2 years of follow-up.

present, there are not enough data to evaluate the treatment of advanced (Stage IV) endometriosis by laser laparoscopy.[17]

## Ablation of the Uterosacral Ligament for Dysmenorrhea (Laser Neurectomy)

The excision of the uterosacral ligaments adjacent to the cervix has been used as a treatment for dysmenorrhea, but little has been reported concerning the efficacy of this procedure. Laser vaporization of the ligament at its attachment to the posterior portion of the cervix destroys the sensory nerve fibers to the cervix and lower uterine segment in an atraumatic, bloodless fashion. Anatomic studies have shown a concentration of nerves from the utero-vaginal plexus to this area. It has been suggested that the severance or removal of these nerves often provides relief in cases of primary or secondary dysmenorrhea. Doyle, who first described this procedure using standard techniques of surgical dissection, approached this procedure both vaginally and abdominally. He reported relief of dysmenorrhea in 86% of 235 patients.[18] However, the vaporization of the uterosacral ligaments at their attachment to the back of the cervix is a simple and rapid alternative procedure using the operative laser laparoscope or laser probe. Its use with the $CO_2$ laser was first described in 1983.[1] An area 1 to 2 cm long and 1 cm in depth is vaporized over the avascular portion of the ligament (Fig 9–9). It is important to vaporize more medially than laterally, however, because of vessels located just lateral to the uterosacral ligament attachment. This technique essentially severs the uterosacral ligaments as well as vaporizes the secondary ganglia within the ligaments. The procedure can be performed in less than 5 minutes. Early results in a combined series of 50 patients treated by another investigator and this author with laser neurectomy have shown complete relief of symptoms or only mild recurrence of dysmenorrhea in 30 of those treated (60%). There were no complications in this first series of patients. In a continuation of this series over a period of 5 years, a total of 146 patients have been treated; 98 cases were associated with endometriosis and 48 cases were associated with primary dysmenorrhea. Of the 98 patients with endometriosis that were followed, 44% had complete relief of symptoms, 24% had significant relief, 11% had moderate relief, and 22% had no relief. Of the 48 patients with primary dysmen-

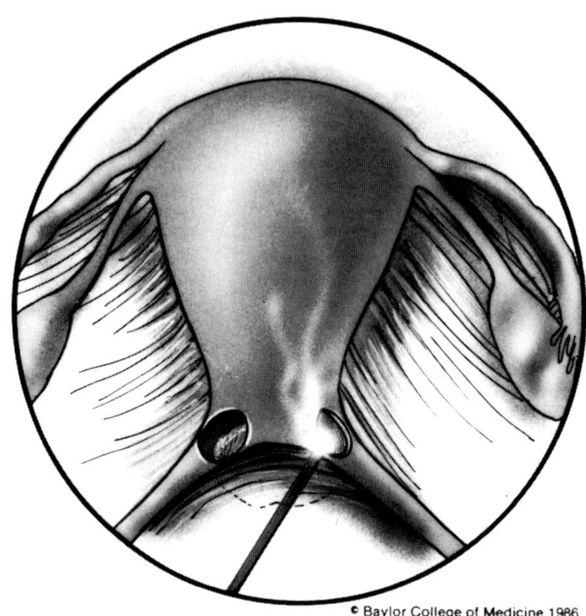


**FIG 9–9.**
Laser neurectomy—vaporization of the uterosacral ligaments at their attachment to the cervix using the $CO_2$ laser. (From Feste JR: The laser in gynecologic procedures: Advantages and pitfalls *Female Patient* 1989; 14:69–83. Used by permission.)

orrhea that were followed, 59% had complete relief of symptoms, 21% had significant relief, 6% had moderate relief, and 14% had no relief. There have been no complications in the larger series of patients.

On the basis of these preliminary studies, it appears that in the absence of any demonstrable disease, relief of symptoms can be accomplished in many patients by this simple technique. On several occasions, patients subsequently underwent laparoscopic laser neurectomy or had a laparoscopy or laparotomy performed for other reasons. This allowed examination of the neurectomy site and revealed re-peritonealization without any significant adhesion formation.

Further investigation of this rapid, safe, and apparently effective operative procedure is continuing in several centers. Keye and his co-workers at the University of Utah have also reported similar results with the argon laser laparoscope (personal communication).

A recent study by Lichten and Bombard, the only randomized and controlled study to date, reported that uterosacral ablation is effective in the relief of dysmenorrhea.[19] They reported that a study was devised to evaluate the effectiveness of a laparoscopic technique for the interruption of the uterosacral nerves. In a double-blind study of 21 patients with primary dysmenorrhea, 81% (9 of 11) reported significant relief from menstrual pain after the surgery. None of those patients who underwent laparoscopy alone reported pain relief. Half of the treated women reported continued relief of menstrual pain at 12 months. These results suggest that uterosacral nerve interruption may prove an effective alternative treatment for this menstrual disorder.

## Laparoscopic Treatment of Polycystic Ovarian Disease

In the past, polycystic ovaries have been treated laparoscopically by cautery and multiple ovarian biopsies with good results.[20] The $CO_2$, argon, YAG, and KTP lasers have been used to treat clomiphene citrate resistant polycystic ovaries by vaporizing multiple defects in the capsule of each ovary. A power of 20 to 25 watts is used to create approximately 15 defects in each ovary (Fig 9–10). The results have been excellent, with 60% of patients experiencing spontaneous ovulation and the other 40% responding to clomiphene citrate. The pregnancy rates vary from 50% to 69%.[21] Since January of 1984 when we began using this procedure, none of our patients with polycystic ovarian disease have required gonadotropins for injection (Pergonal). The procedure is considered temporary, with most patients reverting to an anovulatory state within 9 months to 1 year if they do not conceive. There have been no complications, and in those patients who have had a second-look procedure, there has been no evidence of any significant adhesion formation on the ovaries. This operation may be an excellent alternative to injected gonadotropins (Pergonal) therapy or to a laparotomy and wedge resection for patients who do not respond to clomiphene citrate in doses of 250 mg or for patients who have responded but have not conceived and require a laparoscopy for other reasons.

## Terminal Salpingostomy

The results of conventional microsurgical tuboplasty performed at laparotomy for hydrosalpinx are notoriously poor, with most series reporting no better than a 20% to 30% term pregnancy rate.[22, 23] Laparoscopic salpingostomy using conventional techniques of operative laparoscopy has been performed by Gomel, who reported several pregnancies occurring in the small number of patients studied.[24] Daniell and Fayez reported similar results in a large series of $CO_2$ laser salpingostomies performed at laparotomy.[25–28]

In light of these poor results, $CO_2$ laser laparoscopic salpingostomy seemed to be a reasonable alternative in selected patients who desired pregnancy but who did not wish to undergo a major surgical procedure for hydrosalpinx. This interest led Daniell to begin

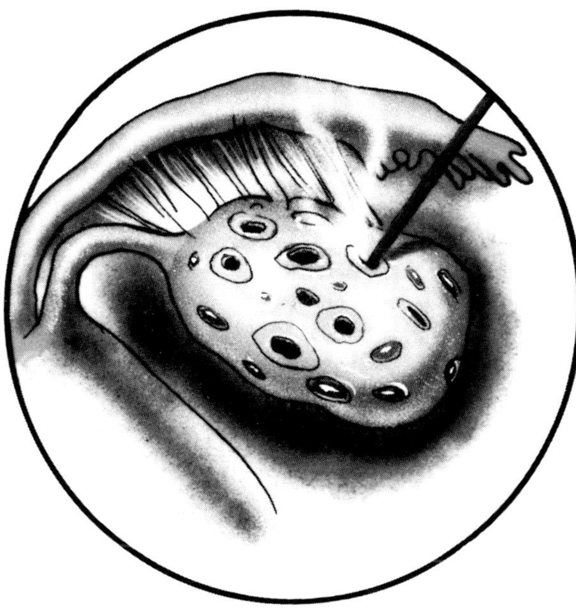

**FIG 9–10.**
Vaporizing defects in the cortex of the ovary with the $CO_2$ laser for treatment of polycystic ovarian disease. (From Feste JR: The laser in gynecologic procedures: Advantages and pitfalls. *Female Patient* 1989; 14:69–83. Used by permission.)

selective recruitment of patients who, on review of their medical records, were thought to be probable candidates for $CO_2$ laser laparoscopic salpingostomy.[26]

At laparoscopy, the fallopian tube and ovary are assessed for adhesions or other important pelvic disease. Adhesiolysis of the tubes and ovaries is performed first. A transcervical instillation is used to distend the fallopian tube with indigo-carmine dye. If the distal tube is free and distended well with dye, an attempt is made to open the tube. A linear incision is made with the finely focused $CO_2$ beam set at the high power density of at least 10,000 W/cm$^2$. A superpulse may also be used with an average power of 5 to 15 watts. When the blue dye begins to spill through the open tube, the incised ends of the tube are carefully grasped with accessory forceps. Two grasping forceps are used; a 5-mm atraumatic forceps is passed through the operative channel of the laparoscope, and a 5-mm alligator forceps is used through a third-puncture trocar for gentle countertraction on the tubal opening. A second incision is then made with the high power density laser beam at a 90-degree angle to the first linear incision in the end of the hydrosalpinx, creating “four flaps.” If the hydrosalpinx is thin-walled, the “Bruhat maneuver” may be used to reduce the chance of postoperative closure of the distal tubes. The $CO_2$ laser power is reduced to 3 to 5 watts (power density between 200 and 300 W/cm$^2$), or the beam can be defocused by selecting a shorter focusing lens, i.e., 250 mm. The beam is aimed at the peritoneum of the hydrosalpinx, a few millimeters proximal to the incised edges. With the firing of this defocused beam at a lower power density, the peritoneum will constrict slowly and evert the edges of the hydrosalpinx (Fig 9–11). This eversion will cause the newly constructed fimbria to “flower back” or “Bruhat maneuver” and maintain an opening of the ampullary portion of the tube. After copious irrigation with heparinized Ringer's solution, chromopertubation is carried out. The fluid is suctioned from the pelvic cavity, and 200 cc of 32% dextran 70 or heparinized Ringer's lactate can be instilled intraperitoneally before the laparoscopy is completed.

In Daniell's initial series of 22 patients, he achieved an 8-week postoperative patency

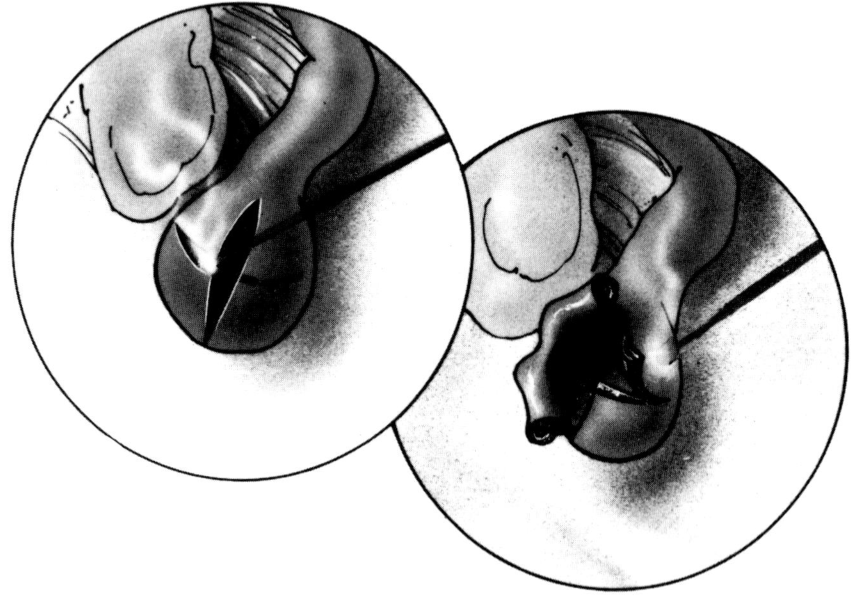

**FIG 9–11.**
Neosalpingostomy utilizing the $CO_2$ laser by laparoscopy. (From Feste JR: The laser in gynecologic procedures: Advantages and pitfalls. *Female Patient* 1989; 14:69–83. Used by permission.)

rate of 75%. The pregnancy rates were similar to those achieved with conventional open intra-abdominal microsurgery, with three intrauterine pregnancies, one ectopic pregnancy, and one spontaneous abortion. All patients undergoing laparoscopic salpingostomy were discharged 24 hours postoperatively, and there were no complications in this series. In an expanded series reported by Daniell, 120 patients were treated with neosalpingostomy; 106 of these were followed for at least one year.[27] The patency rate was 82%, and the total pregnancy rate was 34%. There were 22 term and 14 ectopic pregnancies. The benefits of this procedure included decreased cost, less time off from work or routine activities, and less postoperative discomfort. Although additional follow-up on these patients is necessary before drawing any firm conclusions, it appears that the technique of laser laparoscopic salpingostomy may be of benefit to selected patients.

## Adhesiolysis

In many patients, postoperative or postinfectious adhesions are amenable to vaporization by laser laparoscopy. Whether the standard technique with cautery is used or the laparoscope scissors or blunt dissection, there is probably no difference in the outcome when the adhesions are small and avascular. With more vascular adhesions or particularly with thick, bulky peritubular and periovarian adhesions, however, the $CO_2$ laser allows more precise destruction of the adhesions with minimal injury to the adjacent normal tissue. Using power densities between 1,500 and 3,000 W/cm$^2$, adhesions can be both coagulated and incised. Filmy peritubular and periovarian adhesions are easily vaporized with the operative laser laparoscope or the laser probe with its backstop. A second- or third-puncture probe can be used to insert a 5-mm titanium rod, which acts as a backstop to the laser beam. Care must be taken to place the trocar sheath in the position that will provide the best location for the titanium rod behind the adhesions being vaporized (Fig 9–12). In many instances, a laser probe with a "firing platform" on the end (see Figure 9–5) may eliminate the need for titanium rods. When this probe is used, the adhesion is placed

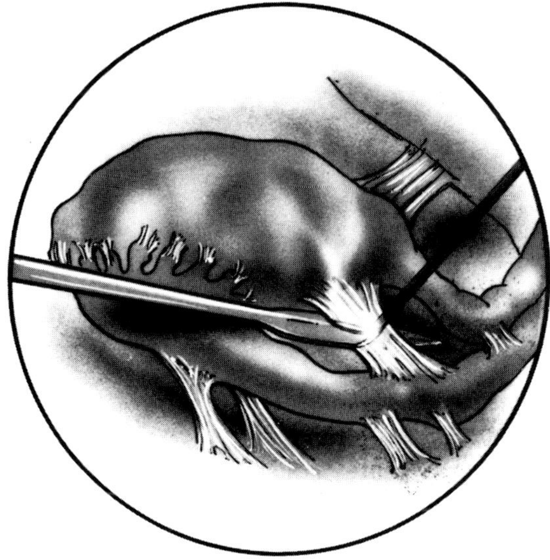

**FIG 9–12.**
Titanium rod used as a backstop while adhesiolysis is performed with the $CO_2$ laser. A laser probe with a built-in firing platform can be used. (From Feste JR: The laser in gynecologic procedures: Advantages and pitfalls. *Female Patient* 1989; 14:69–83. Used by permission.)

across the platform and the laser is fired to vaporize the band. By moving the laser probe across the adhesion slowly, the surgeon can completely vaporize the lesion with ease and total safety, because the backstop always "catches" the beam.

In general, single- and repeat-pulse modes or a superpulse with an average power of 5 to 15 watts is used for laser vaporization of adhesions. Short exposure times of 0.05 or 0.1 second are usually adequate to vaporize the adhesions around the fallopian tubes and ovaries and will prevent the laser beam from penetrating more than 100 to 200 micrometers. The more dense the adhesions, the longer the duration of laser energy pulse that can be used safely. Using the continuous mode can be dangerous, however, since one has little control over the depth of penetration of the laser beam if it is not constantly moved. Dense adhesions of the ovary or fallopian tube to the lateral pelvic wall are best treated by open intra-abdominal surgery. Further clinical experience with the laser laparoscope will be necessary to determine which types of adhesions can be treated safely by this new technique. The use of traction on the adhesion via alligator grasping forceps at a third puncture site has been quite helpful in the vaporization of adhesions. One must be careful not to apply too much traction to avoid tearing the adhesion at the point of its attachment and causing bleeding that defeats the purpose of hemostatic surgery.

During procedures in which three or four punctures are required, it is helpful to use a laparoscopic teaching attachment or video camera, thus allowing the participation of an assistant. The assistant can manipulate the pelvic viscera or aspirate the smoke of vaporization.

## Salpingostomy for Ectopic Pregnancy

The advent of sensitive beta-hCG assays and the early use of ultrasound have allowed physicians to diagnose early unruptured ectopic pregnancies more frequently than has been possible in the past. The physician with a high index of suspicion combined with training in laparoscopic laser technique has an excellent opportunity to diagnose and treat an ectopic pregnancy before it can rupture. Our practice is to consider all patients who have had previous tubal surgery as having a high risk of an ectopic pregnancy. A high index of suspicion must be given to those patients who have had previous tubal anastomosis and neosalpingostomies.

If an unruptured ectopic pregnancy is suspected and the patient desires preservation of childbearing, a preoperative consultation and discussion should be carried out in great detail with the patient and her family. Specifically, she should be warned that a laparotomy may be necessary although every effort will first be made to repair the tube laparoscopically.

We use a three-puncture technique with either the $CO_2$, argon, or KTP laser. Once the laparoscopy is done and an ectopic pregnancy confirmed, the tube is inspected and chromotubation is performed to determine whether the ectopic pregnancy can be flushed through the distal tube to remove the need for making an incision in the tube. If this is not possible, dilute vasopressin (Pitressin), 1 ampule in 20 cc saline, may be injected with a spinal needle transabdominally just beneath the cornua of the uterus into the mesosalpinx just beneath the ectopic pregnancy. A portion of the solution may be injected into the antimesenteric serosa of the ectopic pregnancy as well. The area of the ectopic pregnancy is grasped, and a linear incision is made on the antimesenteric border over the thinnest portion of the tube (Fig 9–13).

Because fiberoptic lasers cut with less bleeding, we prefer to use them. However, the

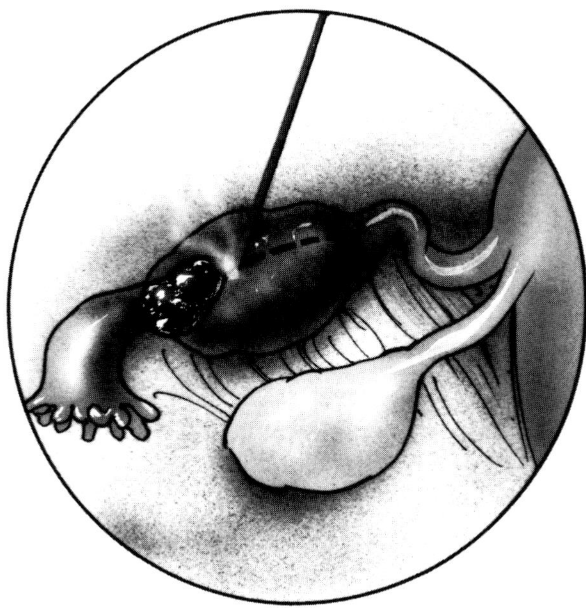

**FIG 9–13.**
Laparoscopic linear salpingostomy with $CO_2$ laser for unruptured ectopic pregnancy. (From Feste JR: The laser in gynecolgic procedures: Advantages and pitfalls. *Female Patient* 1989; 14:69–83. Used by permission.)

procedure can be accomplished either with the $CO_2$ or with a needle electrode if the short wavelength lasers are not available. In France, Bruhat has reported excellent results in treating a large series of patients with ectopic pregnancies in this fashion.[29] Once the incision is made in the tube, the gestational tissue is milked out through the tube and then the linear incision is irrigated copiously and chromotubation done to flush out any tissue remaining in the tube. If any bleeding occurs, it is treated by point coagulation or pressure with a grasping forceps. Follow-up with beta-hCGs is important so that the occult retention of ectopic pregnancy tissue will not be missed. A personal communication with James Daniell of Westside Hospital, Nashville, Tennessee, reports 28 patients treated by laparoscopy, with 3 lost to follow-up. Follow-up hysterosalpingograms were performed in 20 patients, 18 of whom had a patent tube. Of 25 who attempted to conceive after the conservative treatment of their ectopic pregnancies, 6 had intrauterine pregnancies and 3 had repeat tubal pregnancies. The results are similar to those in the 15 patients reported by Johns and the 6 patients reported by Voros.[30, 31]

In the last 2 years, we have had few instances of tubal occlusion in patients treated by laparoscopic laser procedures. We have had a 15% repeat ectopic rate and a 25% intrauterine pregnancy rate.

## Miscellaneous Uses

In addition to the previously discussed indications for laser laparoscopy, the controlled destruction of tissue with the properly focused $CO_2$ laser beam is possible in other situations. Small uterine fibroids and ovarian fibromas can be ablated easily with a moderately defocused beam. These lesions can be completely destroyed without injury to the adjacent underlying healthy tissue. Hydatid cysts can likewise be vaporized with ease. Additionally, the laser can be used to perform bloodless drainage of small benign ovarian cysts without difficulty.

## CONCLUSIONS

Despite continuing development of new instrumentation for the $CO_2$ laser via laparoscopy, there are still problems with the system. The expense of the surgical laser is no small item ($50,000 or more). The system requires specialized equipment that needs competent ongoing biomedical maintenance plus specialized technical care in the operating room. It is still somewhat cumbersome, with problems of intraperitoneal smoke accumulation, gas leakage, and maintenance of proper beam alignment. In addition, it is necessary for the physician to acquire proper training in the safe use of this new surgical tool.

In spite of the problems associated with the application of the $CO_2$ laser to intraperitoneal pelvic pathology, there are certain potential advantages. The system allows precise bloodless destruction of diseased tissue under the illuminated magnification of the laparoscope. It eliminates the risks of cautery in the destruction of endometriotic implants, selected pelvic adhesions, ectopic pregnancies, and uterosacral ligament transection. Laser laparoscopy appears to allow for successful correction of distal tubal obstruction, in some cases without major surgery. In the hands of a careful, experienced laparoscopist who is familiar with the biophysics of the $CO_2$ laser and its interaction with intraperitoneal tissue, it appears safe and effective in early clinical trials. Finally, its use has extended our ability to perform operative laparoscopy, thus decreasing the need to perform laparotomy with its greater morbidity and cost.

Although it is not for every laparoscopist, the $CO_2$ laser laparoscope offers the potential for correcting certain pelvic abnormalities that were not previously correctable by operative laparoscopy. The judicious use of these techniques, combined with carefully planned further investigations by adequately trained and experienced laparoscopists and continuing improvements in the delivery systems, will soon answer the question of the true efficacy of the $CO_2$ laser laparoscope.

## REFERENCES


1. Feste JR: Utilization of the $CO_2$ laser laparoscope. *J Reprod Med* 1985; 30:413.
2. Daniell JF, Brown DH: Carbon dioxide laser laparoscopy: Initial experience in experimental animals and humans. *Obstet Gynecol* 1982; 59:761.
3. Bruhat M, Mage G, Manhes M: Use of the $CO_2$ laser in laparoscopy, in Kaplan I (ed): *Proceedings of the Third International Society for Laser Surgery*, September 1979, pp 274-276.
4. Tadir Y, Ovadia J, Zuckerman Z: Laparoscopic applications of the $CO_2$ laser, in Atsumi K and Nimsakul N (eds): *Proceedings of the Fourth Congress of the International Society for Laser Surgery*, September 1981, pp 25–26.
5. Feste JR, Lloyd JM: A new valving system for removal of laser plume during pelvic laser endoscopic procedures. *Obstet Gynecol* 1987; 69:669.
6. Eward RD: Cauterization of Stage I and II endometriosis and resulting pregnancy rate, in Phillips JM (ed): *Endoscopy and Gynecology*. Downey, California, American Association of Gynecologic Laparoscopists, 1978, pp 276–278.
7. Hasson HM: Electrocoagulation of pelvic endometriotic lesions with laparoscopic control. *Am J Obstet Gynecol* 1979; 132:115.
8. Mettler L, Giesel H, Semm K: Treatment of female infertility due to obstruction by operative laparoscopy. *Fertil Steril* 1979; 32:384.

9. Sulewski JM, Crucia FD, Brenitskey C, et al: The treatment of endometriosis at laparoscopy for infertility. *Am J Obstet Gynecol* 1980; 138:128.
10. Daniell JF, Christianson C: Combined laparoscopy surgery and danazol therapy for pelvic endometriosis. *Fertil Steril* 1981; 35:521.
11. Seiler JC, Ballard LA, Gadwani C: Laparoscopic cauterization of moderate endometriosis for fertility: A controlled study. Presented at the Forty-First Annual Meeting of the American Fertility Society, Chicago, 1985 (Abstract).
12. Reich H, McGlynn F: Treatment of ovarian endometriosis using laparoscopic surgical techniques. *J Reprod Med* 1986; 31:557.
13. Reich H, McGlynn F: Laparoscopic oophorectomy and salpingo-oophorectomy in the treatment of benign tubo-ovarian disease. *J Reprod Med* 1986; 31:609.
14. Martin DC: $CO_2$ laser laparoscopy for endometriosis associated with infertility. *J Reprod Med* 1986; 31:1089.
15. Keye WR, Hanson LW, Astin MT, et al: Argon laser therapy of endometriosis: Review of 92 consecutive cases. *Fertil Steril* 1987; 47:208.
16. Lomano JM: Photocoagulation of early pelvic endometriosis with Nd:YAG laser through the laparoscope. *J Reprod Med* 1985; 30:77.
17. Nezhat C, Cromway SR: Surgical treatment of endometriosis via laser laparoscopy. *Fertil Steril* 1986; 45:778.
18. Doyle JB: Paracervical uterine denervation for relief of pelvic pain. *Clin Obstet Gynecol* 1963; 6:742.
19. Lichten EM, Bombard J: Surgical treatment of primary dysmenorrhea with laparoscopic uterine nerve ablation. *J Reprod Med* 1987; 32:37.
20. Gjonnaess H: Polycystic ovarian syndrome treated by ovarian electrocautery through the laparoscope. *Fertil Steril* 1984; 41:20.
21. Daniell JF: Unpublished data. Presented at the American Society of Lasers in Surgery and Medicine, Dallas, Texas, May 1988.
22. Tulandi T, Faray R, McInnes RA, et al: Reconstructive surgery of the hydrosalpinx with or without the carbon dioxide laser. *Fertil Steril* 1984; 42:839.
23. Daniell JF, Diamond MP, McLaughlin MD, et al: Clinical results of terminal salpingostomy with the use of the $CO_2$ laser: Report of the Intra-abdominal Laser Study Group. *Fertil Steril* 1986; 45:175.
24. Gomel V: Salpingostomy by laparoscopy. *J Reprod Med* 1977; 18:265.
25. Daniell JF: Laparoscopic salpingostomy: Early clinical results. *Lasers Surg Med* 1983; 3:161.
26. Daniell JF, Pittaway DE, Manson WS: The role of laparoscopic adhesiolysis in the in-vitro fertilization program. *Fertil Steril* 1983; 40:49.
27. Daniell JF, Herbert CM: Laparoscopic salpingostomy utilizing the $CO_2$ laser. *Fertil Steril* 1984; 41:558.
28. Fayez T: Assessment of the role of operative laparoscopy in tuboplasty. *Fertil Steril* 1983; 39:476.
29. Bruhat MA, Manhes H, Mage G, et al: Treatment of ectopic pregnancy by means of laparoscopy. *Fertil Steril* 1980; 33:411.
30. Johns DA, Hardie RP: Management of unruptured ectopic pregnancy with laparoscopic carbon dioxide laser. *Fertil Steril* 1986; 46:703.
31. Voros JI, Bellina JH, Moorehead ME, et al: Management of ectopic pregnancy by carbon dioxide laser. *Lasers Surg Med* 1983; 135:9.

# Chapter 10

# Laser Laparoscopy: Argon

William R. Keye, Jr., M.D.

Gregory R. McArthur, Ph.M.

In the past 15 years, lasers have become increasingly important in most surgical specialties. To the surgeon, the laser has made it possible to dissect or destroy tissue with greater control and precision than ever before. However, the hope that this precision and control will lead to dramatically better clinical results has not yet been realized. As a result, skeptics and critics alike have labeled the laser as nothing more than a "very expensive electrocautery device." Indeed, lasers currently used in gynecology coagulate, vaporize, and cut tissue by heating the tissue much like electrocautery. Therefore, the clinical results of current laser surgery are not the result of the inherent properties of the laser but are the direct result of the skill and precision with which the surgeon directs the beam of laser light.

Delivering the laser energy into the pelvis through a laparoscope has involved using an articulated arm for the carbon dioxide ($CO_2$) laser. These arms require a gas-tight fit at each articulation to maintain a pneumoperitoneum; they also require the perfect alignment of all the mirrors located at each articulation to facilitate delivery of the laser beam. For many surgeons this system is cumbersome and frustrating to use. As a result, there have been several attempts to develop a flexible fiber for the $CO_2$ laser to overcome these problems. However, the optical absorption characteristics of the flexible fiber materials currently available for the $CO_2$ laser have made delivery of this wavelength through fiberoptic materials impractical.

There are several wavelengths of laser energy in the visible and near infrared portion of the electromagnetic spectrum that can be passed through fiber optics. These include the 1064 nm Nd:YAG, the 2940 nm Er:YAG, the frequency-doubled Nd:YAG at 532 nm, the copper vapor laser at 511 or 578 nm, the gold vapor laser at 628 nm, and the argon laser. However, each of these has its own set of limitations and problems. For example, the depth of penetration of the near infrared lasers makes them difficult to control and use safely. The metal vapor lasers require temperatures that jeopardize the materials used to contain the metal vapor; additionally, they cannot be operated in a continuous mode but must be pulsed. Finally, the technology of frequency doubling is difficult to incorporate into a mass-produced machine. In contrast, the argon laser is available commercially, has desirable tissue interaction characteristics, and can be delivered through small diameter fiberoptics. In addition, the visible light lasers (those with wavelengths between 390 and 690 nm, such as the argon laser) are more than just tools for cutting or vaporizing, properties that are dependent on the photothermal effects of laser light. They also have the ability to destroy pathologic tissue through the photochemical effects of laser light that are dependent upon the color or chemical composition of tissue. As a result, they can selectively destroy pathologic tissue while causing minimal effects to normal tissue.

Recognizing the principle of selective absorption of laser light by some tissues, we investigated the use of the argon laser for treating endometriosis. Theoretically, the argon laser was an ideal laser for treating this disease because the wavelength of light generated by the argon laser (488 and 514.5 nm) is preferentially absorbed by red pigments such as hemoglobin and hemosiderin, both of which are present in abundant amounts in endometriotic lesions. Fortunately, this has proven to be one of those rare situations where the application has been nearly as good as the theory.

## INSTRUMENTATION

The argon laser is a gas discharge laser. Argon atoms within the argon laser tube are excited by passing an electric current along the length of the tube. Much like a fluorescent light, this electric current excites the argon molecules within the bore. In a fluorescent tube, the excited gas molecules return to the ground state and emit photons spontaneously. However, in the argon laser, the laser tube has mirrors on either end that reflect a portion of the light back through the laser tube to stimulate the emission of photons that create laser light.

The power output of gas lasers, such as the argon laser, is proportional to the square of the tube current density and the length of the laser tube. In addition, the tube current density can be controlled by measuring the power output of the laser tube with a photodiode and by feeding the electrical output from the diode to a feedback circuit which regulates the tube current density. This type of control is unique to gas discharge lasers. In contrast, solid state lasers, such as the Nd:YAG and the frequency-doubled Nd:YAG, must be run at maximum output because they are excited by a flash lamp. Flash lamp–excited lasers run continuously at maximum power, and output is controlled by mechanically attenuating the beam. As a result, the tube life of the argon laser is significantly longer than the Nd:YAG and the frequency-doubled Nd:YAG lasers.

The argon laser tube is composed of mirrors and optics that stimulate emission. The efficiency of the gas discharge lasers is enhanced by placing the tube in an axial magnetic field. As a result of this magnetic field, which surrounds the laser tube, any argon ion within the tube that is traveling toward the sides of the laser tube will spiral back into the center of the tube where the stimulated emission of radiation can occur.

The only argon laser currently approved for marketing by the Federal Drug Administration for gynecologic procedures is manufactured by HGM Medical Laser Systems, Inc., in Salt Lake City, Utah (Fig 10–1). The laser is available with a maximum output of 6 watts (Model 8[tm]) or 16 watts (Model 20[tm]). The Model 8 is 16.25 × 8 × 31.5 inches, is water cooled (3 gallons per minute), and requires a 208 to 240 volt, 50 amp, single-phase electrical source. The Model 20 is larger at 16.25 × 8 × 40 inches, is water cooled (3 gallons per minute), and requires a 208 to 240 volt, 50 amp, three-phase electrical source identical to that required by many Nd:YAG lasers. The Model 20 is generally favored by most gynecologists because it is more powerful, thus making it possible to more easily vaporize the uterosacral ligaments and to lyse thick adhesions more quickly and, therefore, more safely than with the lower-powered model.

The energy from the argon laser is delivered through a flexible optical fiber with either

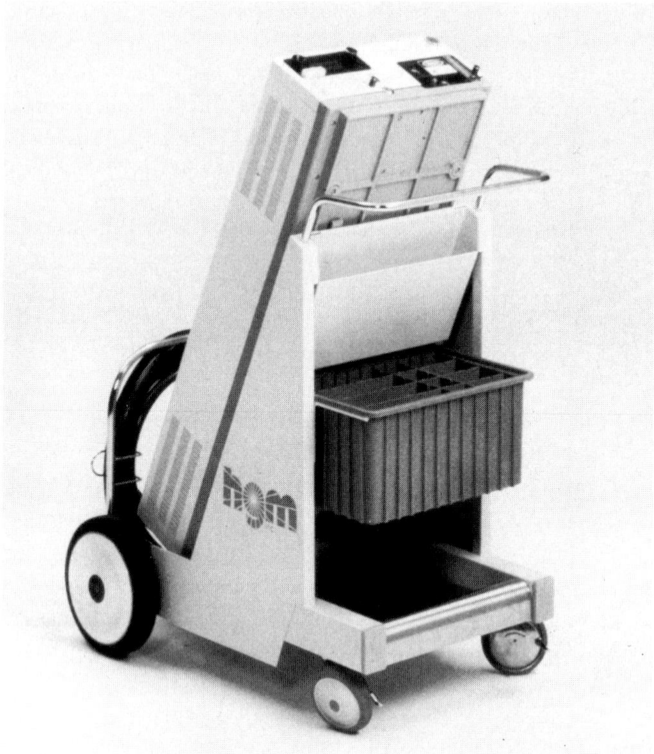


**FIG 10–1.**
The Model 20 argon laser manufactured by HGM Medical Laser Systems, Inc. (Courtesy of HGM Medical Laser Systems, Inc.)

a 300- or a 600-micron core diameter (660- and 1,010-micron outside diameters, respectively) (Fig 10–2). This fiber is extremely efficient and delivers over 85% of the output from the laser tube to the tissue. The fiber is composed of a central core of silica that is surrounded by a quartz cladding and a protective polytetrafluroethylene (PTFE) jacket. It is supplied sterile, for single use, but can be cleaved and re-sterilized by gas or liquid agents. The fiber easily passes down the operating channel of any unmodified, single-puncture, operating laparoscope, operative hysteroscope sheath, or any of several accessory suprapubic hollow probes. The fiber is extremely durable and can be bent into a circle with a diameter as small as 0.5 inches without breaking.

The optical fiber used for delivery of the argon laser light transmits the light because of the principle of total internal reflection. Light entering the fiber optic is reflected at the silica core–quartz cladding interface and leaves the fiber at the opposite end with the same angle that it entered. The beam diverges from the end of the fiber at a 7°- to 8°-half-angle. As a result, the spot size increases (Table 10–1) and the power density decreases (Table 10–2) rapidly as the distance between the tip of the fiber and the tissue increases.

Protective safety goggles or eyewear are essential when using the argon laser, for significant retinal damage can occur if the eye is exposed to the unfiltered laser beam (Fig 10–3). The lens of the eyewear has an optical density (OD) of greater than 5 at 488 and 514.5 nm. A filter with an OD of 5 transmits only 0.001% of the argon laser light.

The proposed American National Standards Institute (ANSI) standard (Z136.3) sug-

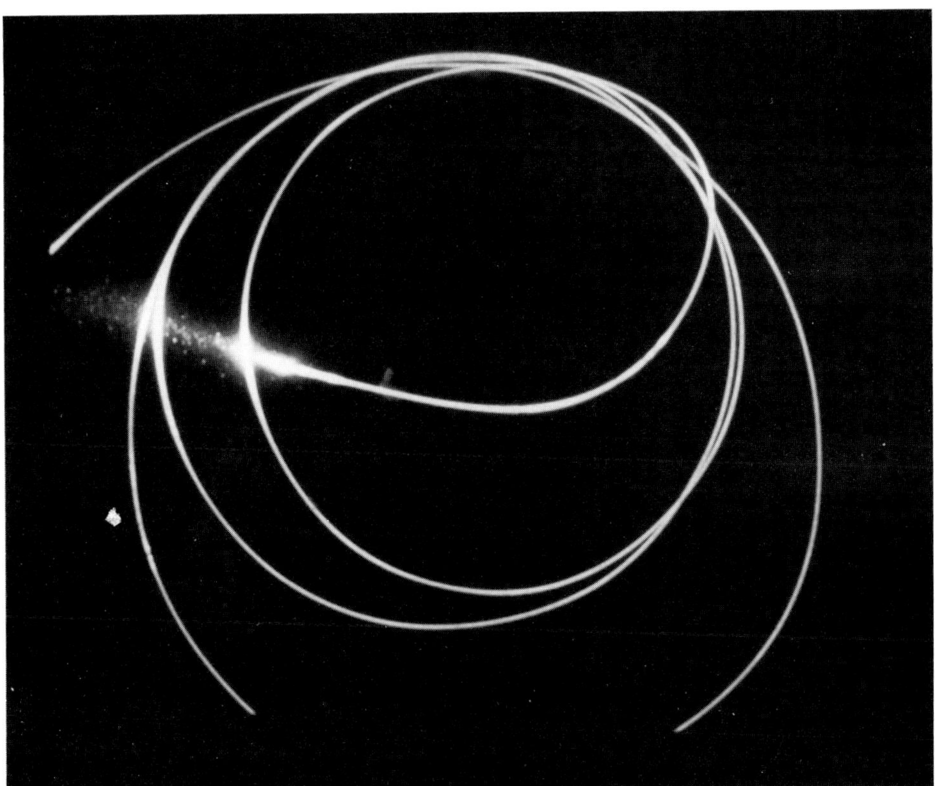

**FIG 10–2.**
A flexible optical fiber used to deliver the argon laser beam.

gests exposure limits and establishes several new concepts for the use of lasers in a hospital environment. Maximum permissible exposure (MPE) is the highest level to which a person may be exposed without hazardous effect or adverse biological changes in the eye or skin; MPE is expressed in terms of power density and varies with exposure time. For a 0.25-second exposure (time of the "blink response"), the MPE for the argon laser is $2.5 \times 10^{-3}$ W/cm$^2$. For a 600-second exposure (approximate time of intentionally viewing a pro-

**TABLE 10–1.**
Distance From the Tip of the Argon Laser Fiber to the Tissue and the Spot Size

| Distance Fiber to Tissue (mm) | Diameter of Spot (mm) | |
|---|---|---|
| | 300 μ Fiber | 600 μ Fiber |
| 0 | 0.30 | 0.60 |
| 1 | 0.49 | 0.79 |
| 2 | 0.69 | 0.99 |
| 3 | 0.88 | 1.18 |
| 4 | 1.07 | 1.37 |
| 5 | 1.26 | 1.56 |
| 10 | 2.23 | 2.53 |

**TABLE 10–2.**
Distance From the Tip of the Argon Laser Fiber and Its Power Density

| Distance Fiber to Tissue (mm) | Power Density (watts/cm²) 10 watts | |
|---|---|---|
| | 300 μ Fiber | 600 μ Fiber |
| 0 | 14,147 | 3,537 |
| 1 | 5,248 | 2,027 |
| 2 | 2,712 | 1,312 |
| 3 | 1,653 | 918 |
| 4 | 1,111 | 678 |
| 5 | 798 | 521 |
| 10 | 257 | 200 |

cedure), the MPE is $16.7 \times 10^{-6}$ W/cm$^2$. The nominal hazard zone (NHZ) is defined as the space within which the level of direct, reflected, or scattered radiation during normal operation of the laser exceeds the applicable MPE. (Exposure levels beyond the NHZ are below the appropriate MPE level.) Nominal ocular hazard distance (NOHD) is the distance along the axis of the unobstructed beam from the laser to the human eye beyond which the

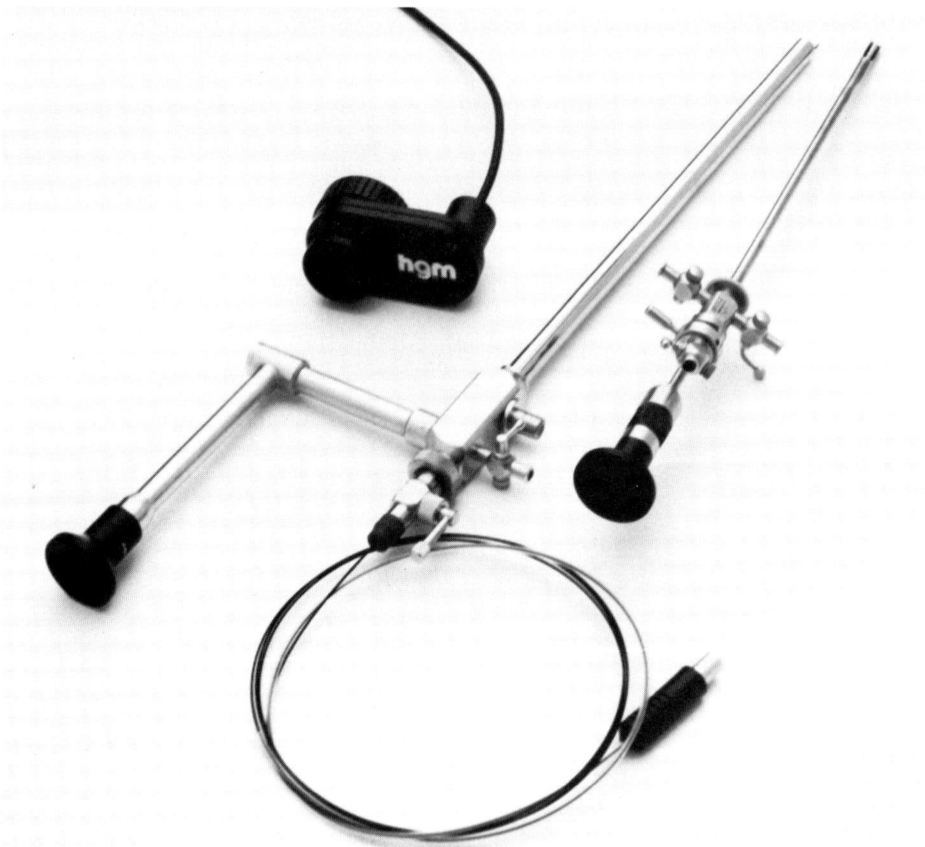


**FIG 10–3.**
An operative laparoscope and protective Monoshutter designed to protect the eye of the laparoscopist.

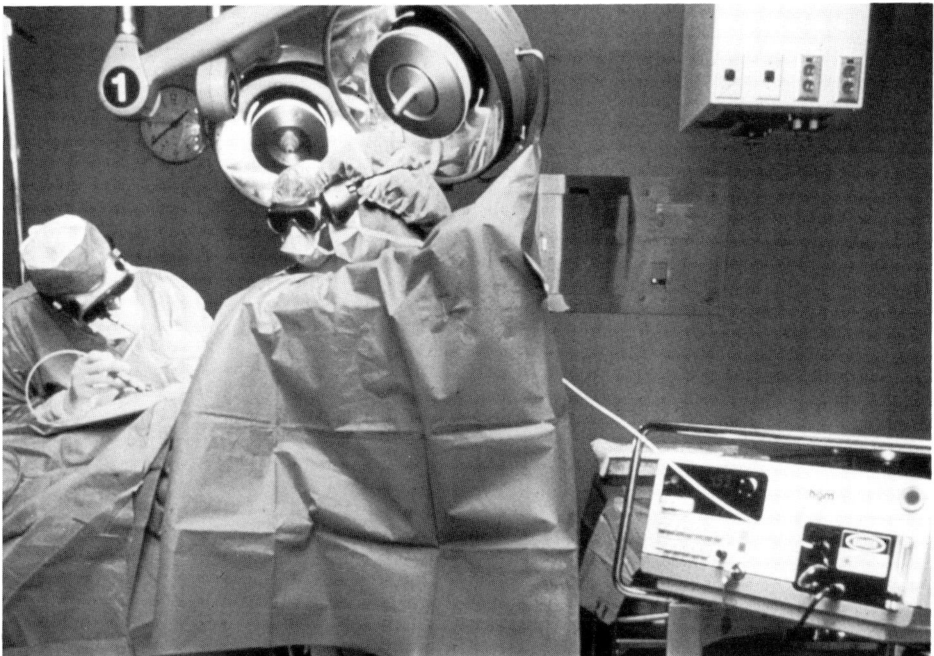

**FIG 10–4.**
The operating room set-up for use of the argon laser.

irradiance or radiant exposure during normal operation is not expected to exceed the appropriate MPE.

Unless shielded by barriers or screens, persons within the NHZ should wear such eye protection as special glasses or goggles. Optical viewing devices, such as laparoscopes, should be equipped with devices that provide adequate protection. A Monoshutter containing a special filter has been developed for the eyepiece of the laparoscope, which eliminates the need for the surgeon to wear protective goggles (Fig 10–4). Proper labeling of eyewear specifies optical density and the laser wavelength for which it is applicable. A raised drape is a common means of protection for anesthesiology personnel. Persons in the operating room watching a procedure on video do not need eye protection if the video monitor is placed so that observers have their backs to the procedure.

The laser is triggered by a footpedal with a protective shroud that eliminates the accidental depression of the pedal by an assistant or by other operating room personnel. The laser pedal should always be placed away from other footpedals such as those for the electrocautery unit or microscope.

## RESULTS OF CLINICAL TRIALS

After animal studies in which the efficacy and safety of the argon laser to treat experimental endometriosis were demonstrated,[1] we began clinical trials with the argon laser for the treatment of human endometriosis. Initially, five women were treated for 31 superficial implants of endometriosis on the uterosacral ligaments, ovaries, fallopian tubes, bladder, and sigmoid colon. They experienced no complications.[2] Using the Model 8, each implant was coagulated with a "no-touch" technique, which involved advancing the fiber through the operating channel of the laparoscope until it emerged into the abdomen to within 1 to 5 mm from the implant. With the laser set at 2 watts power, the aiming beam was directed at each implant and the laser fired until the implants were totally blanched and thus coagulated (1 to 2 seconds).

Two years later, in 1985, we reported performing adhesiolysis and excision of endometriosis or adhesions, as well as vaporization or coagulation of endometriotic implants, using a contact or touch technique in which the tip of the fiber actually contacted the tissue.[3] We used 5.5 watts of power and were able to safely and effectively prepare the pelvis for laparoscopic oocyte collection for in vitro fertilization. We recently reported our experience in 92 consecutive patients who were studied prospectively.[4] Each subject was followed for 6 to 36 months and evaluated for conception and reduction of pain; 67% had already failed to conceive following other therapies. It should be emphasized that all had additional infertility factors (an average of 1.5 additional factors per patient) and had experienced long-standing infertility (average of 4.8 years). In spite of these factors, which would have predicted that the laser would have little effect on fertility, 19 of 56 (34%) of those with infertility became pregnant (average monthly fecundity rate of 2.5%). Nearly two-thirds (64%) conceived within 6 months of therapy. Among a small group of women with infertility of less than 24 months, 63% conceived. These results compare favorably with life table analyses of other treatment modalities.

The most dramatic finding was the reduction of pain (dysmenorrhea, dyspareunia, and other pelvic pain) that occurred in 92% of the 50 women who had complained of preoperative pelvic pain. Similar results have now been achieved in nearly 500 patients treated between 1982 and 1988 (unpublished data).

## SURGICAL TECHNIQUES

### Destruction of Superficial Implants

Implants overlying the uterus, fallopian tubes, ovaries, rectosigmoid, bladder, ureters, broad ligaments, and uterosacral ligaments can be safely treated with the argon laser. Individual implants can be coagulated or vaporized. For lesions overlying a hollow viscus or large vessels, coagulation is preferred. Animal experiments have demonstrated that the pigment in the implant efficiently absorbs the energy of the argon laser and therefore "buffers" the underlying tissue from the thermal effect of the laser (unpublished observation). In rabbit studies in which concentrated hemoglobin was injected just below the serosa, the hemoglobin reduced the depth of the thermal damage to normal tissue by approximately 50%. Thus, implants over the ureter, bladder, fallopian tube, rectosigmoid, and major vessels within the broad ligament can be completely coagulated without clinically significant damage to the underlying structures. Because of the selective absorption of the argon laser light by the hemoglobin and hemosiderin within the implant, the argon laser is an extremely safe laser. The chance of perforating a viscus is extremely low. In nearly 500 cases, we have not perforated a viscus with the argon laser.

To coagulate implants, the 600-micron fiber is delivered into the pelvic cavity through either the operating channel of a single-puncture laparoscope or through the channel of any of a number of suprapubic probes used for smoke evacuation or irrigation. The fiber is advanced until it is within 1 to 5 mm of the lesion (Fig 10–5). While the aiming beam aids in directing the fiber, the fact that the fiber is almost in contact with the lesion renders the use of the aiming beam unnecessary in most cases. The laser power is set at 2 to

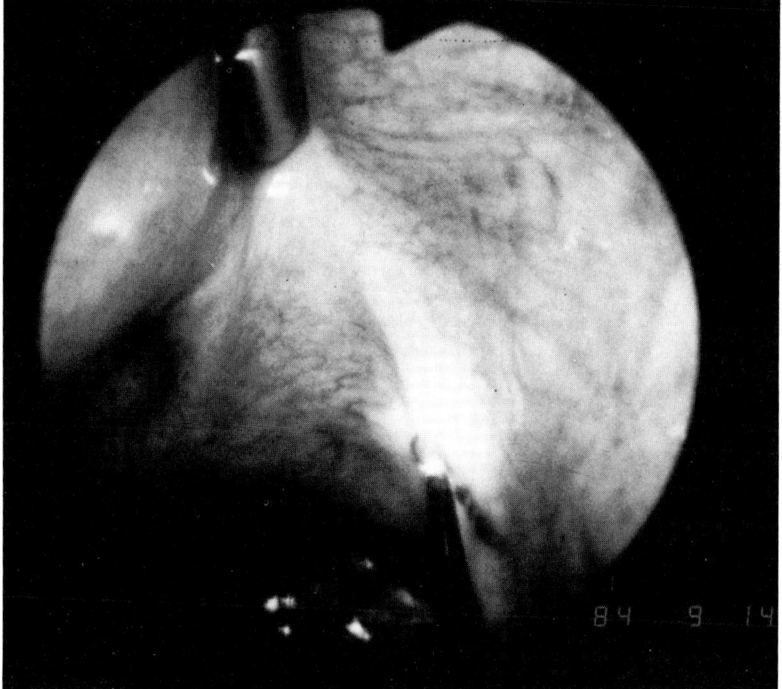


**FIG 10–5.**
The tip of the optical fiber as it is positioned near the peritoneal surface.

5 watts in the continuous mode. Using a foot pedal, the laser is activated and the argon energy delivered to the implant until it either becomes extremely pale, as in the case of lightly pigmented lesions, or the hemoglobin turns black, resembling carbon (Fig 10–6). The operator turns the laser beam off by lifting his foot from the pedal and then moves on to the next implant.

In the case of implants on the uterosacral ligaments, nodules of endometriosis, or non-pigmented endometriosis, vaporization of the implant is preferred. Vaporization is accomplished by touching the tip of the 600-micron fiber to the implant and adjusting the power setting to 5 to 12 watts in the continuous mode. The foot pedal is activated and the implant is vaporized until it is completely gone and the normal subserosal tissue is seen (Figure 10–7). The foot pedal is then released, turning the laser beam off.

## Destruction of Ovarian Endometriomas

The treatment of ovarian endometriomas is a controversial one. Some believe there is no place for the laparoscopic drainage of any ovarian cyst other than small follicular cysts. They argue that a laparoscopist cannot always predict the histology of a cyst by its outward, gross appearance, and that the spill of the contents of mucinous cystadenomas, benign cystic teratomas, or cystic epithelial carcinomas is not only unwise but potentially fraught with long-term complications. Others believe appropriate treatment requires only the simple drainage. Yet others believe it is not only safe but effective to remove or destroy the cyst wall of an ovarian endometrioma at laparoscopy.

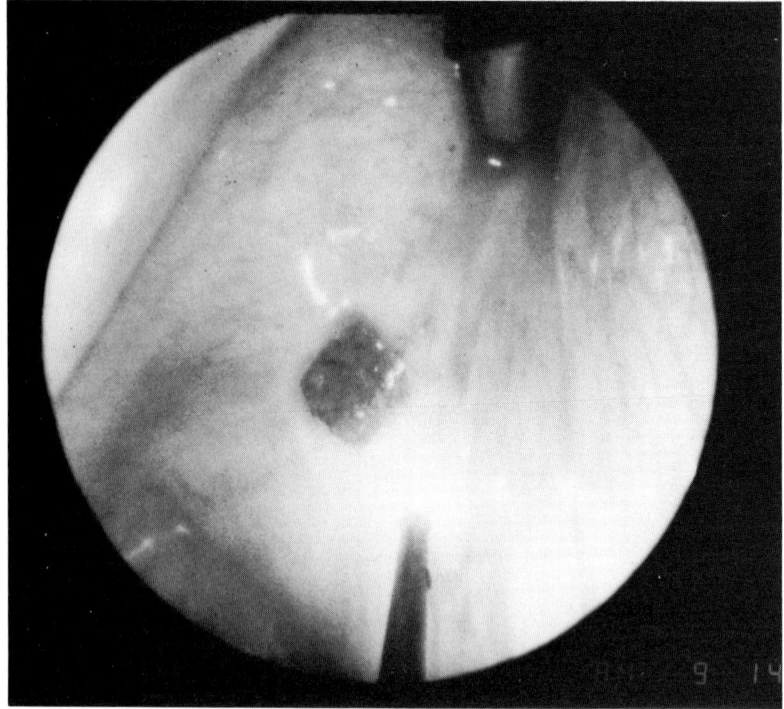

**FIG 10–6.**
The appearance of an endometriotic implant after its coagulation with the argon laser.

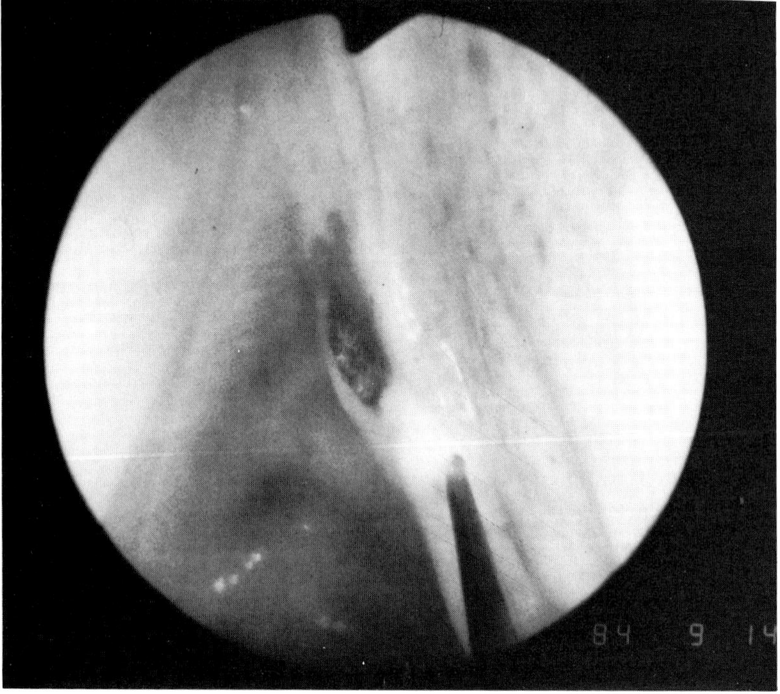


**FIG 10–7.**
The appearance of an endometriotic implant after its vaporization with the argon laser.

When approaching an endometrioma laparoscopically, the goal is to drain the old blood, which often reduces pelvic pain, and to prevent its recurrence. To do this, the quartz fiber is advanced until its tip touches the ovarian capsule at the thinnest part of the endometrioma. Using 10 to 15 watts of power from the argon laser, a linear incision is made in the ovarian capsule and the cyst wall. The bloody contents are then evacuated and the cyst irrigated with heparinized, lactated Ringer's solution. By using one or two forceps introduced into the pelvis through suprapubic sites, the edges of the cyst are held open and the fiber directed into the cyst. Then, using 5 to 10 watts of argon laser power, the inside of the cyst is coagulated or vaporized until it is completely destroyed. The inside of the cyst is then copiously irrigated and the debris suctioned from inside the cyst and the pelvic cavity. The cyst does not bleed when this technique is used, and the defect in the ovary is left open to heal secondarily.

Brosens recently described a new and novel technique using the argon laser and "ovarioscopy."[5] After identifying an ovarian endometrioma, he passes the quartz fiber down through the operating channel of a single-puncture laparoscope. A small defect is then created with the argon laser in the ovarian capsule overlying the endometrioma. Next, he removes the fiber from the laparoscope and replaces it with a salpingoscope modified to include an operation channel. The cyst wall is then punctured with the salpingoscope, and the dark old blood from within the cyst is irrigated. The internal features of the cyst are visualized by distending the endometrioma with normal saline or lactated Ringer's solution, and the fiber from the argon laser is advanced into the cyst through the operating channel of the salpingoscope. Next, the surgeon coagulates and vaporizes the cyst wall under direct vision and coagulates any small varicose veins present at the base of the endometrioma. The salpingoscope is removed from the endometrioma, which is left with only a small puncture wound of several millimeters in diameter. Long-term follow-up is not yet available to demonstrate the superiority of this technique over those just described. Nevertheless, it does have the theoretical advantage of a possible reduced rate of recurrence and fewer postoperative adhesions.

## Adhesiolysis

The introduction of an argon laser capable of delivering between 10 and 16 watts of energy has facilitated adhesiolysis with this wavelength. In addition, the availability of a 300-micron fiber has made it possible to obtain very small spot sizes (300 microns) and high power densities (up to 22,600 $W/cm^2$). This allows most pelvic adhesions to be efficiently removed or incised with the argon laser. The advantages of this system over that of the $CO_2$ laser are the reduction in smoke and the improved hemostasis when vaporizing with the argon laser.

The principles of adhesiolysis are similar to those used with other modalities. The adhesion is isolated, put on traction, and either incised or excised. The advantage of the argon laser's flexible fiberoptic system over the currently available $CO_2$ laser systems is the decreased need for a backstop behind the adhesion. The diverging beam from the argon laser fiber causes a rapid reduction in power density as one moves the tip of the fiber away from the tissue so that structures more than 1 to 2 cm past the fiber tip are generally spared from any significant thermal damage.

The laser is activated just before the fiber tip touches the adhesion, and the fiber tip is then drawn across the adhesion, maintaining direct contact between them. Remember that the laser energy is directed from the end of the fiber optic, not from the side. Therefore, unlike electrocautery, the side of the device does not affect tissue. Once the adhesion is incised, the laser is inactivated. If the laser is inactivated while the fiber is in contact with the tissue, the tissue often sticks to the fiber and increases the chance that the fiber will burn out. The fiber can usually be freed with limited damage by firing the laser again while withdrawing it.

### Neosalpingostomy

If the fallopian tube is freely mobile and the end of the tube easily visualized, incising the dilated terminal portion of the tube can be done easily and the tube made patent with any of several lasers, including the argon laser. With the increasing success of in vitro fertilization and the traditionally poor results of terminal salpingostomy, there is decreasing enthusiasm for subjecting patients to a laparotomy to perform this procedure. Thus, laparoscopic surgery for distal tubal disease has grown in popularity.

To perform a terminal salpingostomy, the tube is first distended with indigo carmine in normal saline and the scarred end of the tube is identified. The tubal mucosa overlying the ampulla is then grasped with a laparoscopic forcep introduced through a suprapubic site. The fiber is then introduced into the pelvis through the operation channel of a single-puncture laparoscope until it touches the end of the tube. Using a power setting of 10 to 12 watts and a 300-micron fiber, the end of the tube is incised in a standard fashion with three or four radial incisions originating at the center of the scarred end of the tube. No backstop is necessary because of the diverging beam.

Once the flaps are made, the power is reduced to 3 to 5 watts and, using a no-touch technique, the serosal surfaces are heated and the flaps are allowed to "flower back," using the technique originally described by Bruhat.[6]

### Ectopic Pregnancy

The argon laser is ideally suited for the conservative management of an unruptured ampullary tubal pregnancy because of its ability to cut and coagulate simultaneously. The fiber can be delivered through either the operating channel of a single-puncture laparoscope or an accessory suprapubic port. After the base of the ectopic pregnancy has been injected with several milliliters of vasopressin (ADH) in normal saline solution (20 units in 20 cc), the tip of the 300- or 600-micron fiber is placed on the antimesenteric edge of the tube and, with a power setting of 10 to 12 watts, a linear incision is made. Generally, the incision is completely free of bleeding. The products of conception are then shelled out and the tube is left to heal without suturing the edges together.

## ADVANTAGES AND DISADVANTAGES

There are several advantages of the argon laser laparoscopic system over other laser systems (Table 10–3). Several of these deserve additional comment. The flexible fiber delivery system is extremely easy to use. It can be introduced either through the operation channel of a single-puncture laparoscope or an accessory suprapubic port. The fiber is either in contact with the tissue or very close, so the tip of the fiber and the path of the laser beam are always in view. No special devices or couplers need to be purchased, aligned, or maintained. No articulating arm hinders the motion of the laparoscope. The laser leaves only a small "footprint" and, while in use, is out of the way of the scrub technicians and assistants. Only the fiber enters the operative field. Its small size and light weight make it very portable. If the fiber tip breaks (rare) or burns out (common), it can be

**TABLE 10–3.**
Advantages of Argon Laser Laparoscopy

1. Simple fiberoptic delivery system.
2. Coagulation, vaporization, and cutting can be achieved with a single wavelength.
3. Color-selective absorption.
4. No special equipment necessary.
5. No need for backstop.
6. No bulky articulated arm.
7. No beam alignment necessary.
8. Coagulates larger diameter blood vessels than the $CO_2$ laser.
9. Portable.
10. Flexible fiber, which makes it possible to direct the fiber into hard-to-reach areas in the pelvis by use of a laparoscopic bridge.
11. Contact and no-contact surgical technique possible using an inexpensive and reusable fiber.
12. Multispecialty applications (decreased cost per case, increased utilization).
13. Spot sizes to 50 microns and power densities to 500,000 W/cm$^2$ can be created with the micromanipulator.

repaired easily and quickly during the surgery. In addition, the technique of using a flexible fiber is remarkably similar to those operative laparoscopic techniques already acquired by most laparoscopists. Therefore, the learning curve is short, and most laparoscopists feel comfortable using this system after practicing with only a few animal procedures.

Vaporization and coagulation can be performed easily and the desired tissue effect can be controlled by varying the distance between the fiber tip and the tissue. Although the tissue effect can be controlled also by the size of the fiber and the power setting, most laparoscopists prefer to leave these constant during most of the operating time and to continuously change instead the distance between the fiber tip and the tissue in order to achieve the desired effect.There is less char and less smoke created with the argon laser than with the $CO_2$ laser, often eliminating the need for a smoke evacuation system during many procedures. The ability of the argon laser to vaporize and coagulate simultaneously makes this a very hemostatic tool.

The argon laser is extremely dependable and requires little maintenance or upkeep. This author has used an argon laser for nearly 250 procedures without interruption for repairs. Only occasional minor adjustments were made between scheduled operating days to maintain its optimal performance.

The major disadvantage of the argon laser (Table 10–4) is the need to wear tinted eye protection. The goggles and glasses are cumbersome when performing endoscopy. In addition to altering the color of tissues at times, they interfere with the ability of the surgeon to identify subtle and lightly pigmented lesions. The electronically controlled Monoshutter that fits over the eyepiece of the laparoscope or hysteroscope largely eliminates this disad-

**TABLE 10–4.**
Disadvantages of the Argon Laser

1. The surgeon must wear tinted, protective eyewear.
2. Laser must be water-cooled.
3. Requires three-phase electrical power source.
4. FDA approval of lower tract disease is pending.

vantage. Until the laser is actually fired, the filter is not in place and does not distort tissue color. By using pulses of 1 to 2 seconds, the surgeon can monitor the tissue effect almost continuously during a procedure. However, the Monoshutter does decrease the size of the field of vision, which does interfere slightly with the surgeon's comfort level. Moreover, this laser also needs running water to cool the machine and a 208- to 240-volt, three-phase electrical system identical to that used by many Nd:YAG lasers. These requirements limit the use of the argon laser to those facilities that supply these water and power requirements. Finally, the Federal Drug Administration has not yet approved the argon laser for lower genital tract applications.

## FUTURE APPLICATIONS

Although the argon laser was originally used in gynecology to coagulate endometriotic implants, it is now used to treat a number of pelvic diseases. For example, energy from the argon laser has been used to traumatize the ovary for treatment of polycystic ovary disease. More recently, the argon laser has been used to cut, coagulate, and vaporize tissue at hysteroscopy for the hysteroscopic resection of uterine septa, and resection of fibroids and polyps. In addition, there is limited use of the argon laser for treating intra-epithelial neoplasia of the cervix.

Recently, clinical trials using the argon laser to perform endometrial ablation have begun. This is accomplished by the hysteroscopic application of argon laser energy to carve the endometrium from the inside of the uterine cavity using a contact technique.

Other experimental applications include using the laser photodynamically to treat endometriotic lesions in monkeys that have been pretreated with hematoporphyrin derivative (HPD). Such innovative applications have established an important role for the argon laser in gynecology.

## CONCLUSIONS

Over the past 5 years the indications for using lasers in gynecology have expanded greatly. Currently, at least three different ranges of wavelengths are used for gynecologic endoscopy (visible, mid-infrared, and near-infrared). Fortunately, the gynecologic pelvic surgeon does not need to purchase or to have access to each of these lasers, for new techniques and delivery systems have made it possible to perform most gynecologic pelvic procedures with any of these wavelengths. Experience has demonstrated that the argon laser is extremely versatile, simple to use, effective, and safe.

## REFERENCES

1. Keye WR, Jr, Matson GA, Dixon J: The use of the argon laser in the treatment of experimental endometriosis. *Fertil Steril* 1983; 39:26.
2. Keye WR, Jr, Dixon J: Photocoagulation of endometriosis by the argon laser through the laparoscope. *Obstet Gynecol* 1983; 62:383.
3. Keye WR, Jr, Poulson AM, Worley RJ: Application of simplified laser laparoscopy to preparation of the pelvis for in vitro fertilization. *J Reprod Med* 1985; 30:418.

4. Keye WR, Jr, Hansen LW, Astin M, et al: Argon laser therapy of endometriosis: A review of 92 consecutive patients. *Fertil Steril* 1987; 47:208.
5. Brosens I: Ovarioscopy. Presented at the First International Symposium on Salpingoscopy. Newport Beach, Calif, November 1987.
6. Bruhat NA, Mage G, Pouly JL: The use of the $CO_2$ laser in neosalpingostomy, in Kapln I (ed): *Proceedings of the Third Interational Congress for Laser Surgery*. Tel Aviv, 1979.

# Chapter 11

# Laser Laparoscopy: KTP

James F. Daniell, M.D.

The potassium-titanyl-phosphate (KTP) laser is the latest laser to be evaluated and clinically approved for laparoscopic surgery in North America. The KTP produces a visible-light laser beam at a wavelength of 532 nm. The pumping energy of the laser is generated from a neodymium:yttrium-aluminum-garnet (Nd:YAG) laser. The Nd:YAG laser beam is then passed through a crystal of potassium titanyl phosphate. This results in a doubling of the frequency by halving the wavelength from 1,064 nm to 532 nm. At various times this laser has been called the frequency-doubled YAG laser, the KTP laser, the 532 nm laser, or the Laserscope laser (the name of the company that produces it). For simplification here, we will call it the KTP laser.

## KTP LASER

This laser is a visible-light laser in the green spectrum and thus has no need for an aiming laser (Figs 11–1, 11–2, and 11–3). Its transmission and absorption characteristics are similar to the argon laser beam. It can be passed through quartz fibers, will transmit through clear fluids, penetrates human tissue to a depth between that of the carbon dioxide ($CO_2$) and the Nd:YAG lasers, and has moderate scatter. It is moderately color-dependent but has an effect on all colored tissues. The delivery system for laparoscopy is through flexible fiberoptic quartz fibers coated with clear plastic. The fibers come in two diameters: 400 micrometers and 600 micrometers. The fibers are passed through the operating channel of the laparoscope or through a special cannula as a second puncture.

The KTP laser requires running water and special electrical connections and thus is less mobile than the $CO_2$ laser. However, the KTP laser can be placed in the corner of the operating room and the fiber brought to the field through a long, protected cable. This gives more space around the operating table for assistants to participate more easily.

The major effect of the KTP laser on tissue is vaporization when the fiber is touching the tissue and coagulation when the fiber is not touching the tissue. Because of the backscatter qualities of the beam caused by its effects on tissue, it is necessary for the physician to use a protective eye filter. For endoscopic surgery, there is a special filter provided that fits over the eyepiece of the laparoscope. The filter only drops into place over the lens when the laser is activated. For safety, the laser cannot be fired when the eye filter is removed or is nonfunctional.

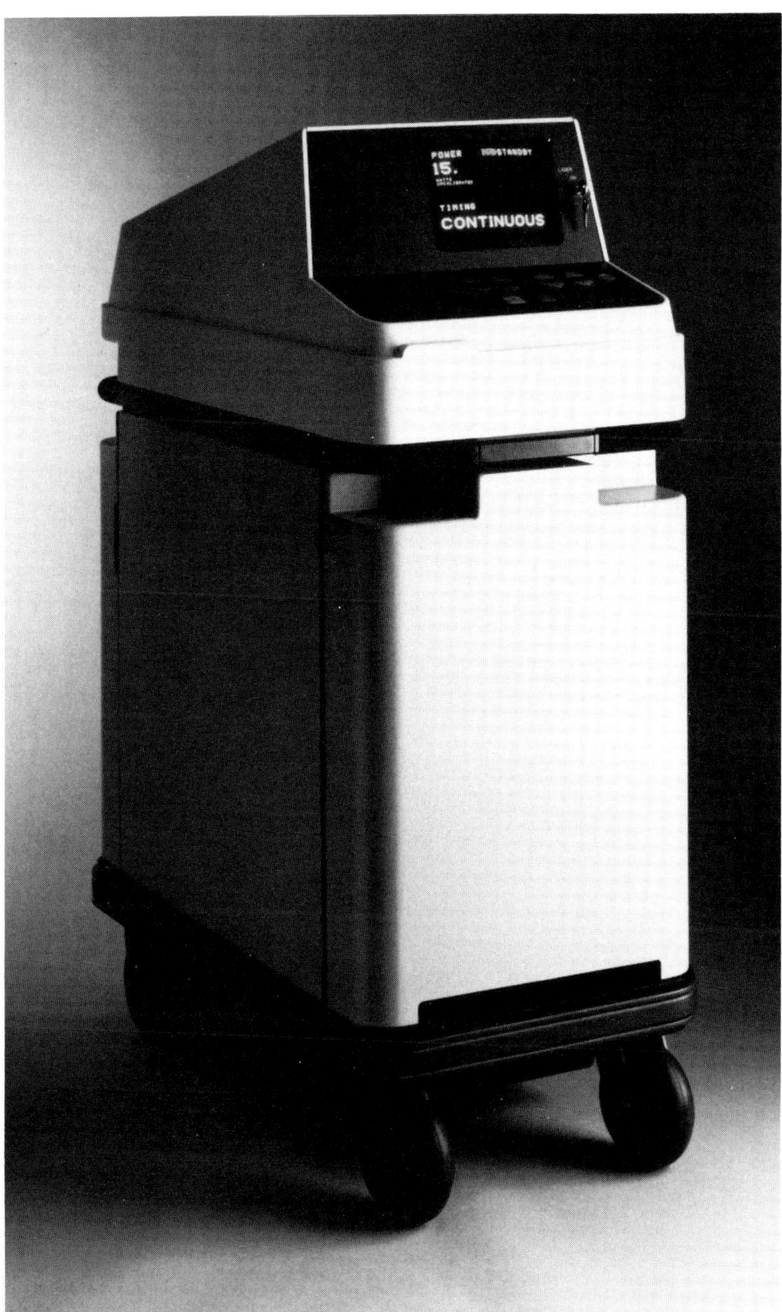


**FIG 11–1.**
A KTP/532 laser.

## INITIAL STUDIES

Laboratory investigations of the KTP laser first began in October 1985, with a series of animal experiments performed with rabbits.[1] Under general anesthesia, immediate tissue effects were evaluated both at open laparotomy and laparoscopy. The results of these animal studies suggested that effective vaporization, incision, and coagulation would be possible under laparoscopic control using a flexible-fiber delivery system. Tissue studies did not demonstrate any thermal damage more than 2 mm from the point of contact of the fiber tip to the bowel, bladder, or peritoneal surface in the rabbit.

## CLINICAL TRIALS

Beginning in November 1985, with an FDA-approved investigative protocol, laparoscopic use of the KTP laser was begun by the author at West Side Hospital in Nashville, Tennessee. The initial conditions treated were endometriosis, pelvic adhesions, distal tubal obstruction, polycystic ovarian disease, ectopic pregnancy, small subserosal uterine fibroids, and laparoscopic transection of uterosacral ligaments for dysmenorrhea.[2] Simultaneously, a clinical trial was also begun of hysteroscopic use of the KTP laser for resec-

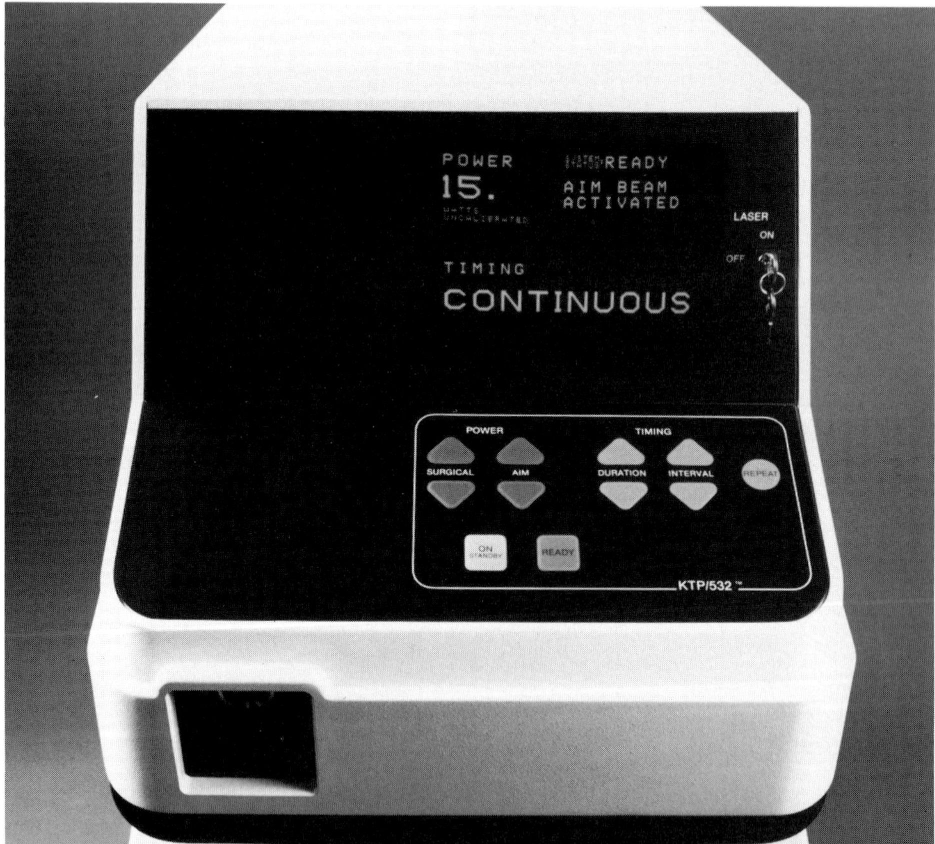


**FIG 11–2.**
The control panel of a KTP/532 laser.

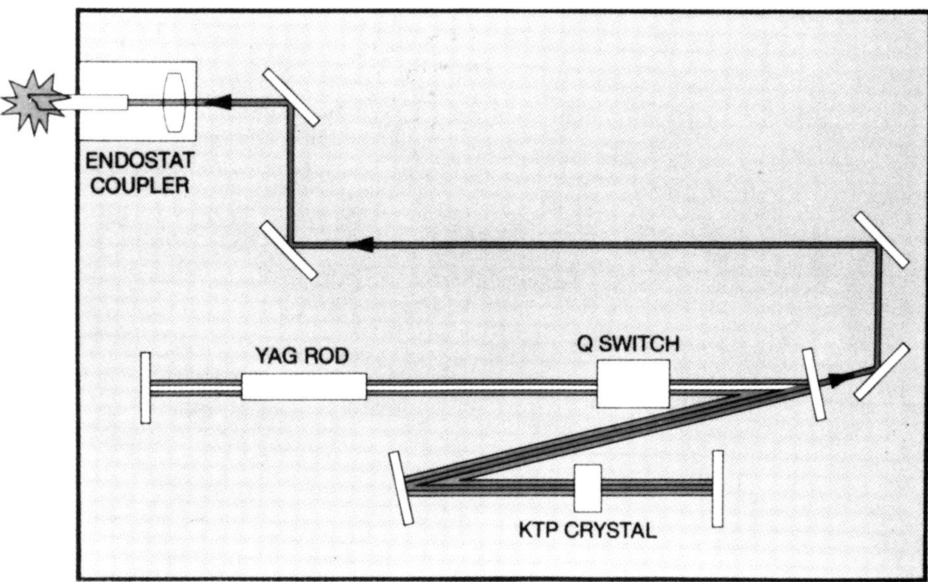


**FIG 11–3.**
A schematic representation of the design of a KTP/532 laser.

tion of uterine septi, vaporization of intrauterine adhesions, and vaporization of small submucosal fibroids.[3]

The clinical results from the early investigations of the KTP laser were excellent. No complications occurred in the more than 100 study patients. Clinical symptoms were evaluated in a retrospective questionnaire to determine whether treatment with the KTP laser resulted in a reduction of pelvic pain in patients presenting with pain and in achievement of pregnancy for patients whose primary indication for laparoscopy was infertility. The results of these early studies, both in patients with endometriosis and those without, have been published in part.[1, 2] The complete results of our clinical experience are presented later in this chapter.

## CLINICAL TECHNIQUES FOR LAPAROSCOPIC USE

We have now performed over 900 procedures of laparoscopic surgery with the KTP laser at West Side Hospital with no complications and have developed a fairly standardized technique that is efficient, effective, and limits the risk to the patient. Unless medical indications require early admission, all patients are treated on an outpatient basis. When possible, surgery is performed during the proliferative phase of the cycle to avoid early pregnancy and the necessity of dissecting around a corpus luteum that might bleed during laparoscopic manipulations.

All procedures are done under video control with a 90/10 beam splitter (Wolf Instrument Company, Rosewood, Illinois) attached to a video recorder with a second video recorder attached. This allows us to make a videotape with sound for the patient, as well as to give us a master copy of interesting and unusual cases or a record for use in potential medical/legal situations. For later patient viewing, a microphone is attached so that the surgeon can selectively talk to the patient during the procedure. We find that this adds tremendously both to the patient's understanding and that of her family. Videotaping for the patient is only done during selected portions of the operation and can be controlled by a remote control switch on the camera attached to the laparoscope. We normally videotape the beginning and end of the procedure and also certain portions of the surgery for the patient's benefit. Other reasons for videotaping include enhanced educational opportunities, increased referrals for surgery, and greater participation by operating room personnel. Two monitors are also used so that the surgeon, a nurse, and assistants can watch the monitors. This enhances assistance by the scrub nurse and resident or fellow who observe the monitor. We use a specially designed, dual-channel, irrigation device (Gynescope, Willoughby, Ohio) to achieve suction and to irrigate the pelvis.

Before the patient arrives in the operating room, the laser coordinator checks the laser, which remains in the corner of the operating room. After the patient is prepped, draped, and in lithotomy position, the laser fiber is brought to the operating field. (A straight catheter has been used to drain the bladder in all cases and a uterine manipulator is generally used for dye injection and for manipulation of the uterus.)

The green light produced by the KTP/532 laser can, under some circumstances, cause irreversible retinal damage. Therefore, the eyes of everyone in the operating room must be protected. For example, the taping of the eyes of the anesthetized patient and the wearing of protective eyewear by all other personnel are advisable. Alternatively, the surgeon may not need to wear protective eyewear if the eyepiece of the laparoscope is equipped with a safety filter. The protective eyewear must be specifically designed for the KTP/532 laser with an optical density of at least 2.3. In addition, signs should be placed at each entrance to the operating room and should warn all who intend to enter the room about what type of laser is being used and what type of eyewear is required. Finally, windows should be covered with a protective sheeting, cloth drape, or window shade.

The fiber can be delivered into the abdomen by various methods. It can be passed through the operating channel of an operating laparoscope, through the central portion of a 3- or 5-mm suction irrigation probe originally designed for $CO_2$ laser laparoscopy, or through a special 5-mm steerable probe designed for ease of use in the pelvis (Gynescope, Willoughby, Ohio). If during a procedure the tip of the fiber melts back slightly, reducing laser transmission, the fiber tip can be cleaved by the circulating nurse, stripped, and recleansed for use within 30 seconds. This can be done rapidly throughout the procedure. One fiber can be used for many procedures, until the length of the fiber is used totally by repeated cleaving. Those in the operating room must be careful not to step on the fiber and break it; they must also avoid stepping on the eyefilter cable.

After evaluating the pelvis for the location and type of disease present, a decision is made about which of the three methods of entry for the laser fiber will be used. When videotaping, a 10-mm diagnostic laparoscope of good quality is used so that the physician can see as well as possible and so that the other observers can also see on the video monitors. For this reason, we usually choose to deliver the fiber either through a 3-mm or a 5-mm probe introduced through a suprapubic incision. The correct placement of the probe can vastly simplify the procedure. For our initial accessory probe for manipulation, we normally place a 5-mm probe in the midline suprapubically. Then, if a third probe is necessary, it is usually brought in 3 or 4 cm lateral to the umbilicus on the side opposite to the major portion of disease. This lateral placement of the accessory third probe reduces clashing the tips of the instruments, which can occur when they are all bunched in the midline.

A final check of the laser setting is made before beginning application of energy. With the eyefilter attached, the laser is placed on ready and the power setting set on 10 watts. (When the laser is fired, the eyefilter drops in front of the eyepiece of the laparoscope and slightly changes the color of the view. This eyefilter only distorts the view minimally for the operator as well as for the television camera.) We usually use the laser on 10 watts with continuous firing and vary the tissue effects by pulling the fiber away from the tissue, thereby eliminating the need to depend on the circulating nurse to change the power setting during a procedure. If a combination of coagulation and vaporization is indicated, the coagulation portions will be performed first to preserve the tip of the fiber and to reduce the need for repeated recleaving. For example, if the patient has implants of endometriosis over the bladder and adhesions to the latter sidewall, we would first photocoagulate the implants by positioning the laser 0.5 cm away from the tissue. Then, to vaporize the adhesions, we would touch the tip of the fiber to them, being careful to monitor ıt is behind the adhesions. The fiber is never advanced more than 1 or 2 cm from the tip of the delivery probe. This reduces the potential for breaking the tip of the fiber and inadvertently losing it in the abdomen. If the probe through which the fiber is passing is also being used for manipulation, which often occurs, the fiber should be retracted during that portion of the procedure.

The scrub nurse stands between the patient's legs and suctions the smoke and irrigates during the procedure as necessary. Irrigation is accomplished with heparinized Ringer's solution with a concentration of 5,000 units of heparin in each liter of lactated Ringer's solution. With the same hand, the nurse can also elevate or depress the uterus by moving the uterine elevator. Thus, one hand is free to hold accessory instruments. In this way, the scrub nurse is a very valuable participant in the operation. Smoke is vented through the Lastech special suction device into disposable floor canisters, which have a biological filter in line before entering the wall suction of the operating room.

Smoke production with the KTP laser is considerably less than with the $CO_2$ laser. For this reason, we use a high-flow insufflator and vent the smoke at the point of accumulation whenever possible. Smoke production can be reduced by irrigating the pelvis and by coagulating instead of vaporizing. We generally use the 600-micrometer fiber; this diameter gives a bigger spot size and therefore can be used to incise and ablate greater surface areas more rapidly. However, when a hydrosalpinx is present or when an ectopic pregnancy requiring linear salpingostomy is encountered, the smaller diameter fiber is used because it gives a narrower and cleaner cut due to its smaller spot size. If during the procedure the transmission of energy through the tip of the fiber decreases, the fiber is removed, its outer covering stripped back, and the tip of the fiber cleaved before continuing.

Small vessels can be prophylactically coagulated before cutting them by positioning the fiber as needed. After the surgery is completed, the pelvis is copiously irrigated with fresh heparinized Ringer's solution, which is then left in the pelvis. The patient is discharged the day of surgery unless she is too uncomfortable or lives too far away. Patients experience the standard postoperative discomfort; we have seen no different sensations in these patients than in those undergoing operative laparoscopy involving other laser or non-laser techniques. Operative times are approximately one-third less compared to the $CO_2$ laser. This reflects the shorter time necessary to prepare for surgery and less need for suctioning smoke and reinsufflation of the peritoneal cavity. Tables 11–1 and 11–2 list some of the short-term clinical results we have obtained in non-controlled studies of laparoscopic laser surgery with the KTP laser.

**TABLE 11–1.**
LUNA* Results With KTP Laser at 6-Month Follow-up

| | Pain Symptoms | | |
|---|---|---|---|
| | Improved | Same | Worse |
| Endometriosis (n = 80) | 60(75%) | 17(21%) | 3( 4%) |
| Primary dysmenorrhea (n = 20) | 12(60%) | 6(30%) | 2(10%) |
| Totals | 72(72%) | 23(23%) | 5( 5%) |

*LUNA = laparoscopic uterosacral nerve ablation.

## ADVANTAGES OF THE KTP LASER FOR LAPAROSCOPIC SURGERY

Compared to other forms of laparoscopic laser surgery, we have found the KTP laser to be advantageous, particularly in procedures in which greater depth of penetration is needed or in which there is a potential for bleeding. For example, vaporization of polycystic ovaries with the fiber permits greater destruction of the ovarian stroma than one can achieve with the $CO_2$ laser in the same amount of time, and with much less smoke. Cutting through dense adhesions can be done with less risk of bleeding and with less plume accumulation. The uterosacral ligaments can also be rapidly transected with less risk of bleeding.

Terminal neosalpingostomy, which can be done with the $CO_2$ laser, is easier to accomplish with a fiber tip. There is less risk of damage to the contralateral internal side of the fallopian tube when using the fiber because of the tendency of the $CO_2$ laser to damage underlying tissue if a backstop is not used. The risk of bleeding is also reduced with the KTP laser, which coagulates better than the $CO_2$ laser as it cuts through tissue.

There are several more advantages in using the KTP laser for laparoscopic surgery over the $CO_2$ laser or the other nonlaser techniques. The most immediate advantage is the ease of delivery of the system with the flexible fiber. The surgeon does not have to acquire special couplers or delivery devices, which are expensive, cumbersome to use, and require constant maintenance. All that is needed is a simple probe through which the fiber can be passed or, in a pinch, the fiber can be introduced through a standard operating laparoscope with no need for any other ancillary equipment. The green beam generated by the KTP is much easier to see in the pelvis than the helium:neon beam used for aiming the $CO_2$ laser. The ability to shoot through fluids allows a better use of irrigating fluids and reduces the accumulation of smoke that is a major problem with the $CO_2$ laser. Because the laser energy is passing from the tip of a fiber without a focusing lens, there is a marked falloff in the power densities as the tip moves away from the tissue. This means that a

**TABLE 11–2.**
Comparison of Results of Laparoscopic Neosalpingostomy With KTP and $CO_2$ Lasers: 1983–88 With 1 Year Minimum Follow-up

| Type Laser | Total Patients | Open Tubes at Hystero-salpingography | Attempting Pregnancy | Pregnancy Results | | |
|---|---|---|---|---|---|---|
| | | | | Intrauterine | Abort | Ectopic |
| $CO_2$ | 104 | 58/71(82%) | 88 | 22(25%) | 11(13%) | 11(13%) |
| KTP | 36 | 24/28(86%) | 32 | 10(31%) | 3( 9%) | 5(16%) |
| Totals | 140 | 82/99(83%) | 120 | 32(28%) | 14(12%) | 16(13%) |

backstop is not necessary unless you are working within 1 cm of underlying vital structures. Certainly, a steerable backstop probe can be very valuable when working close to the bowel or other vital structures, but the need for a backstop probe is minimized considerably compared to what is required for the $CO_2$ laser. The tissue effects of the KTP laser differ from those of the $CO_2$ laser in that greater tissue coagulation is produced. This means that there is less bleeding when vascular structures are vaporized or incised with the KTP laser.

The ability to put the laser in the corner of the room away from the operating field is another major advantage. We have found this particularly helpful because we usually have at least one assistant, in addition to the scrub nurse, present at the operating table.

## DISADVANTAGES OF THE KTP LASER SYSTEM FOR LAPAROSCOPY

As with all things, there are also some disadvantages to the KTP system. The major disadvantage is the need to use an eyefilter; this means another cord coming into the field and reduces the diameter of the field of vision slightly. The present eyefilter only slightly reduces visibility, but it still can reduce the accuracy of visual control. The need for running water and special electrical hookups limits the number of operating rooms that can be used with this laser compared to the mobile $CO_2$ laser, which can be plugged into an outlet in any operating room without needing access to water.

Another disadvantage of this laser is its cost of approximately $70,000, which is higher-priced than the $CO_2$ laser used for laparoscopy. The reusable fibers cost several hundred dollars, but if used carefully, they can be used for 30 to 40 procedures, thus reducing the cost per procedure tremendously. There is the risk that a piece of fiber could break off in the abdomen and be lost. This should not happen if proper precautions are taken never to introduce more than 1 cm of the fiber into the peritoneal cavity beyond the probe tip.

## SAFETY PRECAUTIONS AND TRAINING IN USE OF THE KTP LASER

Because the KTP laser is a visible-light laser, the potential for inadvertent injury to the eye is minimized. If the filter is not used or is short-circuited accidentally, the surgeon will immediately see the bright lime-green beam and close his eyes. This same phenomenon occurs for observers in the operating room, since the eye immediately detects the bright lime color. Unfortunately, retinal injury may occur during this brief interval. The Nd:YAG laser, which is infrared and therefore not visible, is potentially much more dangerous to the surgeon. The other potential danger of this laser is to the patient, in that the energy does penetrate more deeply than the $CO_2$ laser does. This can theoretically increase the risk of inadvertent damage to the bowel, ureter, or bladder if the laser is applied too long while in direct contact over these organs in the pelvis. However, the safety of this laser is greater than with the $CO_2$ laser because of the easier delivery system and the placement of the tip of the fiber near or on the tissue. With the $CO_2$ laser, unfortunately, there is a long open space in the peritoneal cavity through which the laser beam passes. The potential exists with the $CO_2$ laser for the bowel or other vital structures to enter this space and be inadvertently damaged much more easily than with the KTP laser. From November 1985 to April 1988 we performed 510 laparoscopic and 36 hysteroscopic procedures with the KTP laser without a single complication.

**TABLE 11–3.**
Percent of Operative Procedures Performed at Laparoscopy

| | Endometriosis | Hydrosalpinx | Adhesions | Ectopic |
|---|---|---|---|---|
| 1980 (before lasers) | 50 | 10 | 60 | 5 |
| 1987 (after lasers) | 80 | 90 | 90 | 95 |

Because of the short period of time that this laser has been available clinically, it is not yet widely used in residency programs. Therefore, interested gynecologists should take special courses or participate in workshops to learn safe techniques and to become familiar with its tissue effects. Just because a surgeon is experienced with the tissue effects of the $CO_2$ laser does not mean that he can immediately understand and safely begin using the KTP laser. These lasers perform at totally different wavelengths with different effects on tissue, and each must be carefully evaluated and fully appreciated before its specific application is made. At our hospital we recommend that physicians who wish to use the KTP laser clinically first be competent operative laparoscopists. They must then take an approved course that includes didactic exposure to the laser with hands-on experience involving animal use with the laser, and, finally, serve in a preceptorship role with another gynecologist trained and approved for use of the KTP laser. This three-step credentialing process is critical for maintaining a high level of safety for all, especially in this day of medical/legal high risk for hospitals and surgeons.

The manufacturers of the KTP laser have made a strong commitment to education and support courses for nurses and physicians interested in using this technology. These courses offer animal surgery experience and preceptorships with physicians trained in use of the KTP laser in laparoscopy.

## CONCLUSIONS

With the trend toward conservative surgical care and the development of new technology, this is an exciting time in endoscopic gynecologic surgery. Many patients who previously had to undergo major operations can now obtain effective treatment with outpatient or 1-day surgery. The use of lasers has tremendously changed this author's personal patterns of gynecologic surgery in the past 7 years (Table 11–3) via (1) the replacement of hysterectomy for menorrhagia with Nd:YAG laser ablation, (2) laparoscopic treatment of ectopic pregnancies, hydrosalpinges, adhesions, and endometriosis, and (3) laparoscopic removal of tubes and ovaries via operative laparoscopy. All advanced operative laparoscopic procedures tend to save patients time, money, and discomfort and are of benefit to all of us involved in health care today.

## REFERENCES

1. Daniell JF: Laparoscopic evaluation of the KTP/532 laser for treating endometriosis - Initial report. *Fertil Steril* 1986; 46:373.
2. Daniell JF, Meisels S, Miller W, et al: Laparoscopic use of the KTP/532 laser in nonendometriotic pelvic surgery. *Colpo Gynecol Laser Surg* 1986; 2:107–111.
3. Daniell JF, Osher S, Miller W: Hysteroscopic resection of uterine septi and visible light laser energy. *Colpo Gynecol Laser Surg* 1987; 3:217.

Chapter 12

# Laser Laparoscopy: Nd:YAG

Stephen L. Corson, M.D.

The neodymium:yttrium-aluminum garnet laser (Nd:YAG) has a radiation emission in the near infrared portion of the electromagnetic spectrum at1.06 μm. The laser medium is a dilute solution of $Nd^{3+}$ ions in a YAG crystal; $Nd^{3+}$ ions are substituted for $Y^{3+}$ ions within the crystal matrix. Because of its low efficiency (about 2%), high-pressure krypton or xenon arc lamps are required to pump the medium, which in turn requires an efficient heat transfer system because the lamp uses approximately 5 kW. This is accomplished by water cooling within the unit.

In a pulsed mode, the Nd:YAG can create pulse trains of $5 \times 10^{-9}$ seconds with megawatt power ranges. The wavelength of the Nd:YAG allows for transmitting the energy through optical fibers with little loss. When high wattage is used, such as 100 watts, a strong lens must be used to focus the output and the diameters of the fibers must be increased. Most fibers used for gynecology are 0.6 mm.

Because the Nd:YAG laser penetrates deeply into soft tissue when used through a bare fiber, little value was seen for the system in conjunction with laparoscopic surgery, although Lomano[1] did describe using a bare fiber to ablate endometriotic implants. The scatter is appreciable not only in forward and lateral directions but backward as well. Nevertheless, the Nd:YAG system has many properties that are more useful for laparoscopy, especially for treating endometriosis, than carbon dioxide ($CO_2$) laser systems.

The chief advantage of the Nd:YAG laser at laparoscopy is its ability to use a small flexible fiber to avoid the problems associated with the rigid arm delivery system of the $CO_2$ laser. Because blood absorbs the YAG output twice as well as avascular tissue, pigmented endometriotic lesions would be better targeted for destruction, although pigmentation is not required. Also of importance is the limited amount of smoke produced when the YAG laser is used to coagulate tissue; this is important when operating in a closed space. Since the extinction length in water is 60 mm for the YAG laser versus 0.03 mm for the $CO_2$ laser, procedures can be done in a liquid environment, such as through a hysteroscope with liquid media distension. Laparoscopically, this feature offers the capability of working within an endometrioma cavity with constant irrigation. The YAG laser has much greater inherent hemostatic properties than the $CO_2$ laser. The YAG can be delivered to tissue using either a no-touch or a touch technique, with the latter being more comfortable for most pelvic surgeons.

The drawbacks of the Nd:YAG compared with the $CO_2$ laser are that the $CO_2$ laser is better at vaporization than coagulation (when focused) and has more precise scalpel-like cutting qualities without scatter into adjacent tissue. These differences underscore the comment that there is no laser system ideal for every gynecologic application.

## INSTRUMENTATION

The introduction of sapphire probes to the YAG laser fiber by Joffe[2] completely changed the practice of YAG laser surgery. First, the envelope of energy distribution became dependent upon the configuration of the probe employed and various shapes could be used to truly tailor the tip to the indication (Fig 12–1). Second, the scatter became tremendously reduced and, with the energy now focused by the probe, smaller generators could be employed and the extent of tissue damage depth better modulated (Fig 12–2). Surgeons felt more comfortable with a true touch technique, and safety increased because energy levels 1 cm away from the sapphire probe were so low that inadvertent damage could be avoided; backstops and the precautions necessary for use of the $CO_2$ laser were not necessary. Smoke production was further decreased (Fig 12–3). Thus, the "shotgun" energy distribution of YAG laser emission, a desirable property for endometrial ablation or tumor bed destruction, could be converted to that of a fine-bore rifle for the precise destruction of endometriotic implants near sensitive structures and lesions on the bladder and bowel wall. In this author's experience and in animal studies blood loss can also be dramatically reduced when operating in a vascular bed (Fig 12–4).[2, 3] The cutting of tissue can now be performed using scalpel tips such that histologic studies show little apparent difference from $CO_2$-generated lesions (Fig 12–5) with respect to the depth and the width of necrosis seen in the adjacent tissue.

Because the sapphire probe must be cooled, handles were developed with coaxial conduits for gas or liquid cooling. Although there are a number of manufacturers of these devices, only the system from Surgical Laser Technologies (SLT) (Malvern, Pennsylvania) will be described in detail.

The generator operates on a 220 volt single-phase line (Fig 12–6). It is internally water-cooled so no plumbing connections are necessary in the operating room. The touch-sensitive keyboard is computer driven, which is especially helpful to the nursing staff who

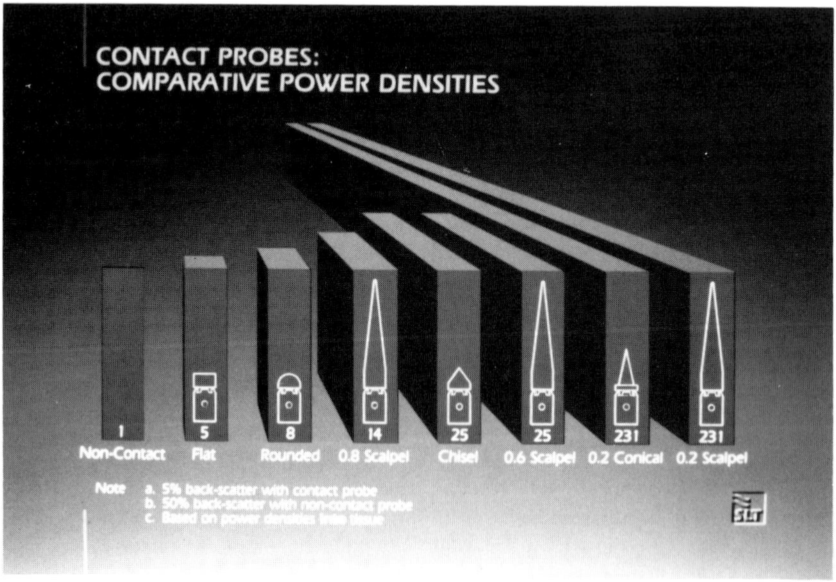


**FIG 12–1.**
YAG laser sapphire probes for laparoscopic surgery and their relative power densities.

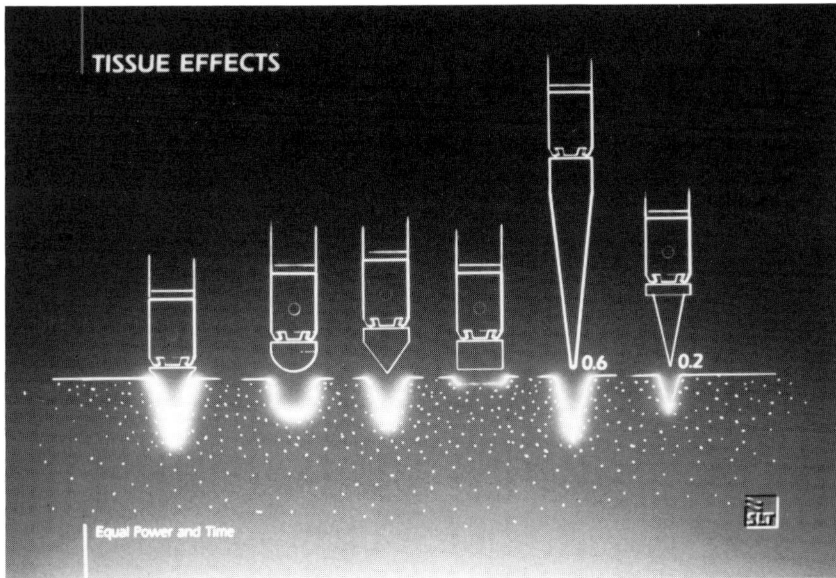


**FIG 12–2.**
Envelope of tissue effect according to probe.

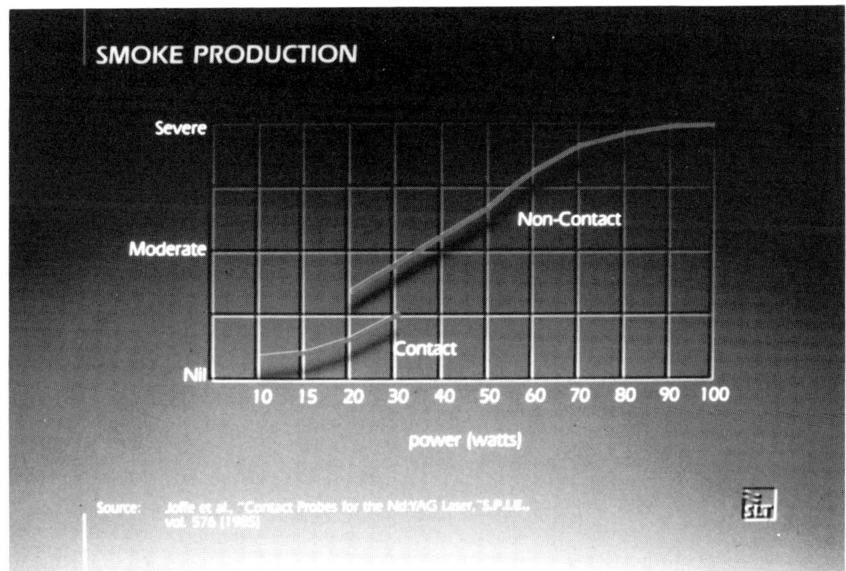


**FIG 12–3.**
Reduction of smoke. Contact versus bare fiber in the canine liver.
(Adapted from Joffe SN, Daikuzono N, Osborn J, et al: Contact probes for the Nd:YAG laser. *SPIE* 1985; 576:42.)

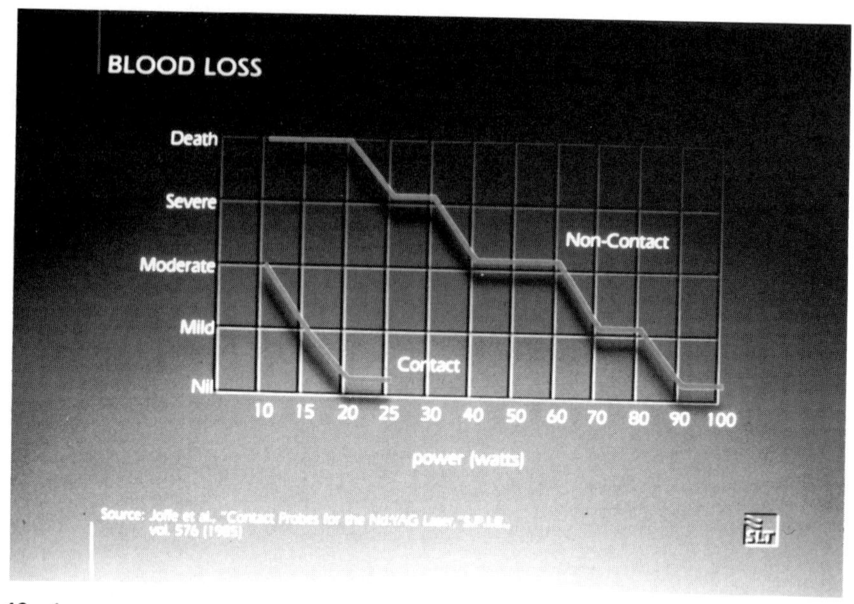


**FIG 12–4.**
Blood loss. Contact versus bare fiber in the canine liver.
(Adapted from Joffe SN, Daikuzono N, Osborn J, et al: Contact probes for the Nd:YAG laser. *SPIE* 1985; 576:42.)

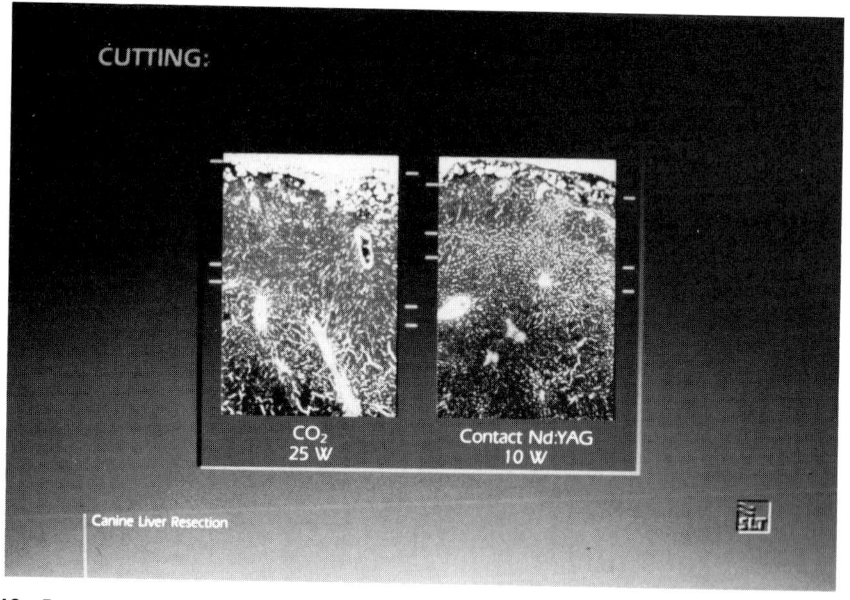


**FIG 12–5.**
Section through tissue cut with $CO_2$ laser and with YAG laser. Canine liver resection.
(Adapted from Joffe SN, Daikuzono N, Osborn J, et al: Contact probes for the Nd:YAG laser. *SPIE* 1985; 576:42.)

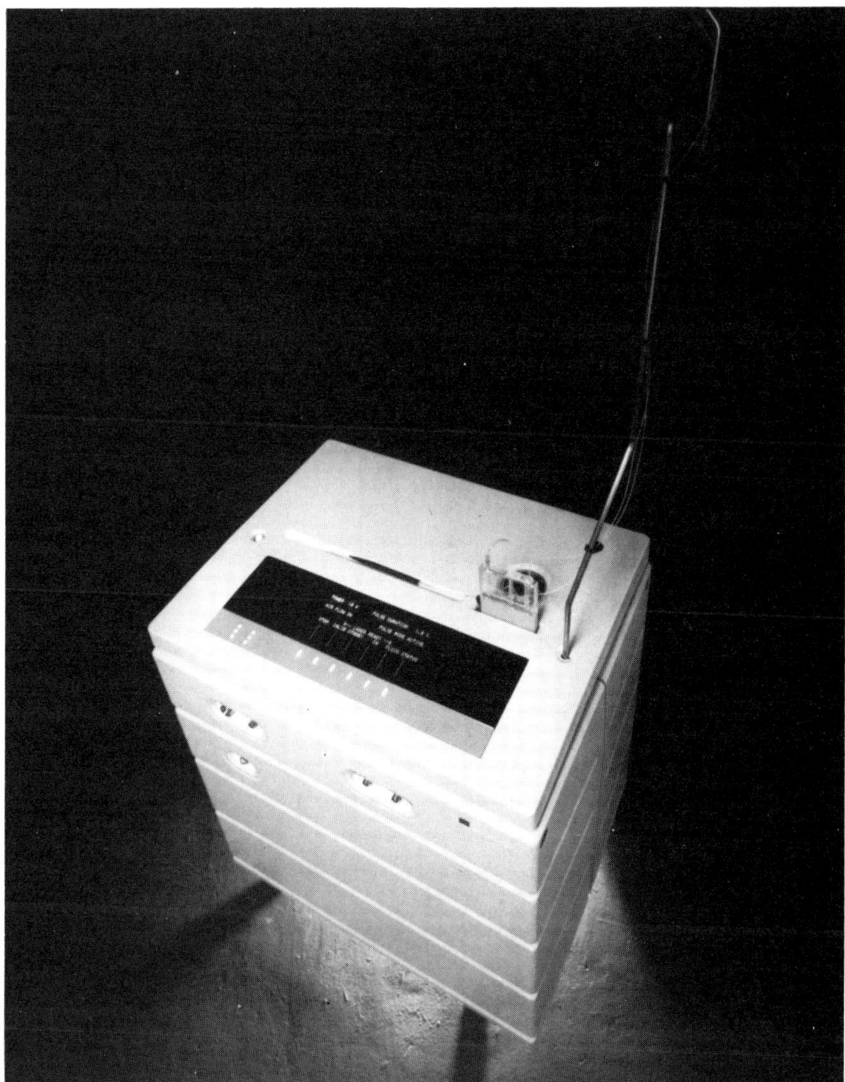

**FIG 12–6.**
YAG laser generator. Surgical Laser Technologies (SLT), (Malvern, Pennsylvania).

may be unfamiliar with the particular unit. The console essentially talks one through the process of turning on the laser, warming up the lamp, and calibrating output.

Laser handles for laparoscopy come in various sizes and lengths for introduction through an operating laparoscope or side sheath (Fig 12–7). The handles pass through a 3-mm sheath and are disposable. Each disposable unit is calibrated in the laser source so that the efficiency of fiber energy transfer can be determined. The generator then compensates internally and automatically so that the output wattage desired at the end of the fiber is obtained.

Cooling of the probe can be accomplished with carbon dioxide or a liquid cartridge (Fig 12–8). Because we use the laser hysteroscopically as well, and because the flow of carbon dioxide through the fiber is high enough to be unsafe for that procedure, we use the liquid cooling cartridge exclusively, although carbon dioxide cooling for laparoscopy is

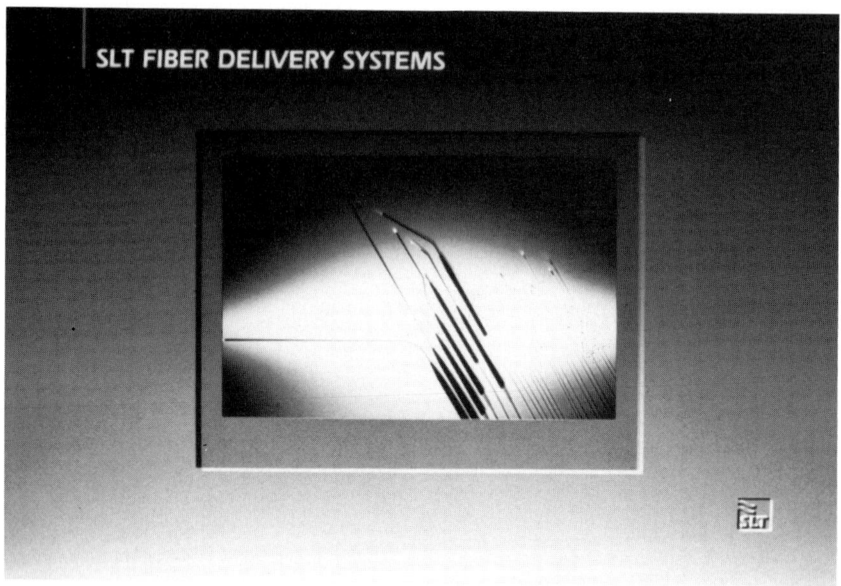


**FIG 12–7.**
Rigid handles for laparoscopic, hysteroscopic, or manual delivery system.

quite acceptable. The operator has a choice of various sterile liquids. Flow rates are adjustable.

Because of the wavelength, regular eyeglasses will not suffice to avoid retinal damage from reflected energy passing through the laparoscopic lens system. A break in the fiber unnoticed by operating personnel could also result in direct absorption. Special green–tinted glasses with an optical density of at least 5 must be worn. Energy reflected

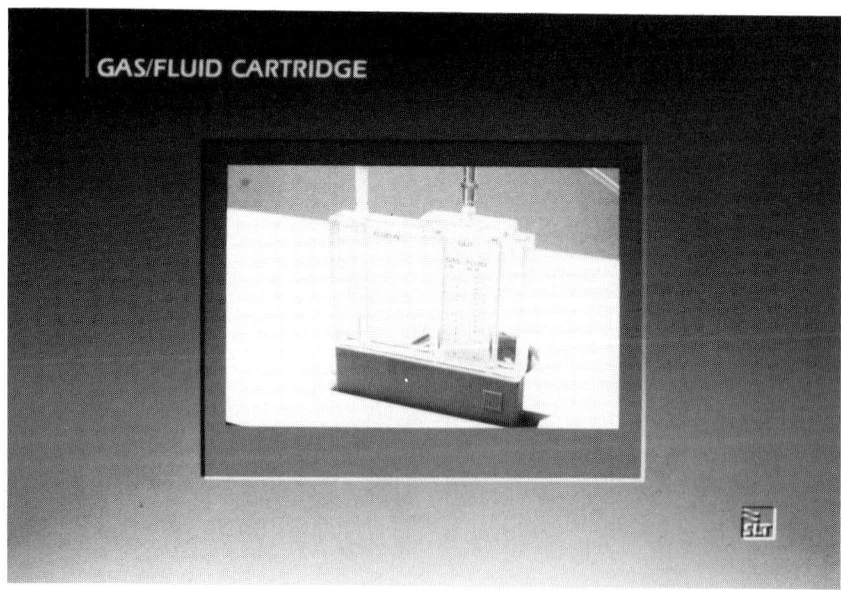


**FIG 12–8.**
SLT liquid or gas cartridge for probe cooling.

from peritoneal structures passing back through the laparoscope can be made harmless by putting a filter in the laparoscopic ocular. If a video system without a beam splitter is used on the telescope, the filter is not needed.

## ANIMAL STUDIES

In a laboratory experiment, five adult New Zealand female rabbits were used to study the immediate and delayed effects of the YAG laser on ovarian and uterine tissue.[3] The contact sapphire "chisel probe" was used at the usual clinical setting of 20 W. Using a continuous application of energy for 2 to 6 seconds, lesions were made in the uterine wall and in the ovaries. One ovary then was removed for the immediate studies, while the other was examined at 14 to 21 days. The width and depth of the lesion were measured microscopically after routine histologic preparation. Lesions made in the uterine horn with a 2-second pulse at 20 W showed a depth of 357 μm to 612 μm and a width of 612 μm to 816 μm (Plate 11). The immediate ovarian lesions made with the same probe and settings had depths between 714 μm and 1112 μm and widths between 1020 μm and 1122 μm, and were less dependent on the duration of the probe-tissue contact than on the angle of application and adequacy of contact (Plate 12).

The delayed study (Plate 13) showed that by 21 days the ovary was essentially completely healed, with the restoration of good epithelial covering.

## CLINICAL TECHNIQUES

As with any other laparoscopic laser system, certain accessories are necessary for the Nd:YAG laser. A high-resolution laparoscope with good light-conducting properties is essential. The light source must be adequate and substantial. Elaborate systems for venting the plume, as with $CO_2$ lasers, are not necessary. Usually no venting is required during an operation. Because procedures are usually multipunctured and may be prolonged (45 to 60 minutes), a gas source with high flow capabilities is helpful and an irrigation system allowing for speedy lavage and aspiration of high volumes of lactated Ringer's solution is also necessary.

The SLT probes can be used through the operating laparoscope or through an accessory sheath. This author prefers the latter. We use the SSRH9 handle with a 600-μm fiber and usually use the chisel probe MD 3.5 or the ball probe MTR 3.5. The chisel probe can be used for entering the endometrioma cavity, for destroying the cyst wall lining, and for uterosacral denervation; hence, it is essentially an all-purpose probe. The ball probe is especially helpful for peritoneal implants.

Endometriomas are steadied by an assistant with laparoscopic forceps under video-monitor guidance. The chisel probe is used at 20 to 22 W for entry into the lesion. The forceps then widen the aperture created, and the irrigating cannula tip is inserted directly into the cavity. Copious irrigation with 500 to 3,000 mL of lactated Ringer's solution follows and the cul-de-sac is aspirated.

Then the cyst wall is destroyed in situ by "painting" it, using a touch technique with the laser probe, in contradistinction to $CO_2$ laser techniques in which the cyst wall and overlying ovarian stroma and tunic are removed or the cyst wall is stripped out laparoscopically. This latter technique can be arduous, time-consuming, and associated with significant bleeding. In comparison, the technique with the Nd:YAG laser outlined above is not associated with bleeding, consumes less operating time, and needs no ovarian sutures for hemostasis or reconstruction because the edges of the cyst wall collapse on themselves, for no tissue (save a biopsy specimen) has been removed.

When extensive adhesions are encountered, a scalpel tip may be employed to lyse these. Although this is satisfactory, there is no question in my mind that the $CO_2$ laser is much superior for fine cutting. However, this advantage seems to be significantly outweighed by the disadvantages of the $CO_2$ system discussed earlier. Ideally, the surgeon should have access to both systems, but the YAG system for endometriosis uncomplicated by severe adhesions is much easier to use.

## CLINICAL RESULTS

The next question is whether one technique is better than the other in the area of results. Efficacy may be gauged by relief of pain or fecundity rates or both. First, no modality has been proven superior to another, including comparisons with electrosurgical techniques. Sulewski, et al.,[4] and Daniell and Christianson[5] reported pregnancy rates of 40% and 57%, respectively, with up to a 5-year follow-up after laparoscopic electrosurgery for endometriosis. $CO_2$ laser laparoscopists have reported rates of 48% through 61%.[6–8] Keye, et al.,[9] reported a 34% pregnancy rate with argon laser therapy of endometriosis.

Comparisons of these results are difficult, if not impossible, because of differences in staging systems, the distribution of those stages in the population studied, differing durations of follow-up, and, most important, the additional therapies given postoperatively, including ovulation stimulation, insemination, and so on. Projected cumulative pregnancy rates actually predicated on short-term follow-up assume constant fecundity over an interval of time that may not be valid.

The uterosacral ligament interruption described by Doyle[10] often has a salutary effect on the pain associated with endometriosis, irrespective of the manner in which division is accomplished. Using the chisel tip or scalpel, this can be accomplished quite easily with the Nd:YAG laser.

We recently reviewed a series of 84 patients with endometriosis who had YAG laser laparoscopy for pain or infertility or for an asymptomatic mass that proved to be an endometrioma. Patients ranged in age from 21 through 46, with a mean of 33 years. Although 22 had previously been pregnant, only four had delivered. Pain had been present for ±42.1 months or infertility for ±49.2 months, or both. The mean American Fertility Score (AFS) score[11] was 8.8 with a median score of 12. AFS stages were divided as IV = 15 patients, III = 34, II = 20, and I = 15.

Total anesthesia time was 48.4 ± 15.5 minutes, with a range of 20 to 91 minutes and a median of 47 minutes. Wattage was 20.7 and the chisel probe was the one most often used. Total energy equaled 1,856 ± 1,260 joules, usually as a continuous application rather than pulsed.

Twenty-six patients had at least one endometrioma with a mean size of 4.6 cm and a median size of 5 cm. Lesions as large as 10 cm were treated laparoscopically. No complications relative to the laser procedure were encountered.

Follow-up for infertile patients was 8.7 ± 6.2 months (median 8 months) and was 10.2 ± 6.5 (median 8.5 months) for those with pain.

Within the group of 84 patients, 65 had previous endometriotic laparoscopic procedures and 22 had prior laparotomy, 12 with salpingo-oophorectomy. Danazol (Winthrop Laboratories, New York, New York) had been used by 44 patients, progestins by 25 patients, and gonadotropin-releasing factor analog by 1 patient. In the infertile group, gamete intrafallopian transfer (GIFT) had been used in 3 patients, clomiphene citrate in 20 patients, human menopausal gonadotropins in 4 patients, and insemination in 1 patient. Obviously then, this was a hard-core infertile population (49.2 months) in which endometriosis had been treated vigorously prior to entering into this study group. Moreover, a male factor was found in 26 patients, ovulatory deficiency in 8 patients, tubal disease in 2 patients, myomas in 7 patients, the DES syndrome in 3 patients, and other factors in 4 patients.

In 16 patients, preoperative danazol was used (generally for 3 months) to reduce the size of bulky endometriomas and was used postoperatively in 9 patients because of the feeling that there was retroperitoneal disease that could not be treated laparoscopically. Concomitant surgical procedures included lysis of adhesions (59), laparoscopic tubal repair (4), submucous myomectomy via hysteroscopy (2), uterosacral division (23), and simultaneous GIFT (2).

Laser treatment was directed to the anterior cul-de-sac (17), small bowel (1), colon (3), tube (15), ovary (56), peritoneum (53), posterior cul-de-sac (58), and 23 patients had uterosacral division. Twenty-three infertile patients conceived (39.7%) during a relatively short follow-up interval, with nine having some form of additional active therapy.

Pain relief was subjectively graded by the patients. In the 48 patients who were followed for at least 6 months (exclusive of those who conceived before 6 months), the postoperative distribution was 29 patients with total relief, 15 patients with good results, 3 patients with only mild relief, and 1 patient with no change.

One patient conceived who was not in the infertile group. Second-look procedures were done in 14 patients; in 2 patients because of pain, in 11 patients as part of a GIFT protocol, and in 1 patient to rule out ectopic pregnancy. No active endometriosis was found in the 2 patients who had poor relief of pain; their initial AFS scores had been 38 and 3. In the others, 6 had no active disease; previous scores had ranged from 6 through 20. AFS scores were higher in 1, unchanged in another, and lower in 12. Thus of the 14 patients, 8 had zero AFS scores at 7 to 16 months after the initial procedure.

## ADDITIONAL YAG LASER LAPAROSCOPIC PROCEDURES

### Ovarian Wedge Resection

Huber[12] described the use of the YAG laser for a laparoscopic wedge procedure but did not specify if a contact probe was employed. Previous workers have demonstrated resumption of ovulation in patients resistant to clomiphene citrate with electrosurgery to the ovarian cortex only.[13, 14] Resumption of ovulation was accompanied by the expected endocrine changes and, in Greenblatt and Casper's series,[15] four of six patients conceived. Since this latter approach would seem to have the propensity for less adhesion formation than does a classical wedge resection, drilling 10 to 20 small openings in the subcapsular cysts of a typical polycystic ovary with a YAG contact probe seems like a good idea in these patients, especially if they do not wish to be treated with human menotropins. This can be accomplished at the time of a diagnostic laparoscopic procedure as part of the general workup.

**TABLE 12–1.**
Comparison of Laser Systems

| | $CO_2$ Laser | Nd:YAG Laser Sapphire Probe |
|---|---|---|
| Delivery system | Rigid system | Flexible fiber |
| Absorption by liquids | Great | Small |
| Need for mirror alignment | Frequent | Rare |
| Production of smoke | Great | Small |
| Delivery | Focused beam | Touch |
| Vaporization | Great | Small |
| Coagulation | Small | Great |
| Propensity for tissue damage past intended target | Great | Small |

## Destruction of Non-endometriotic Ovarian Cysts

In addition, other ovarian pathology can be treated with the YAG laser. I have destroyed a few cystic teratomas that were found incidentally at the time of laparoscopy. The lesions have been drained, lavaged, and a biopsy taken of the wall, after which the cyst was eradicated with the YAG laser contact probe. To date, none have recurred, and patients have been followed with serial ultrasonography. Whether this is a legitimate therapeutic alternative remains to be seen.

## Myomectomy

Because of the ability to both cut and effectively coagulate, a laparoscopic myomectomy can be accomplished with the YAG laser contact conical probe. The problem then becomes one of removing the lesion from the abdomen after its separation from the surface of the uterus. Stalked lesions are readily treated in this fashion. One cannot easily vaporize a large volume of tissue; therefore, removal either with a morcellator or a colpotomy incision usually follows. The morcellator incision tends to be tedious, while the colpotomy incision runs a small risk of pelvic infection. The wisdom of these "incidental" myomectomies can certainly be questioned and, at this time, prophylaxis against further growth is the usual indication.

## Ectopic Pregnancy

Ampullary tubal pregnancy is a condition very amenable to laparoscopic YAG laser therapy. Hemostasis with the YAG is excellent, and linear salpingotomies are virtually bloodless. Of course, this is not the only way in which this can be accomplished; other lasers or the unipolar electric needle are also adequate. One can also seal the vessels in the broad ligament with the laser and remove either a segment of tube as with an isthmic ectopic gestation, or indeed the entire tube itself.

# SUMMARY

In summary, the advantages of YAG laser laparoscopy versus a $CO_2$ system for endometriosis are presented in Table 12–1. The efficacy for pain relief seems to be excellent.

In a short-term follow-up, the pregnancy rate has been 39.7%, but 9 of the 24 pregnancies were in conjunction with additional treatment in a group with long-standing infertility, previous therapies, and often multiple findings. YAG laser treatment via laparoscopy of ectopic gestation, ovarian cysts, and some stalked myomas is also possible and may offer alternatives to laparotomy.

## REFERENCES

1. Lomano JM: Photocoagulation of early pelvic endometriosis with the Nd:YAG laser through the laparoscope. *J Reprod Med* 1985; 30:77.
2. Joffe SN: The Neodymium:YAG laser in general surgery. *Contemp Surg* 1985; 27:17.
3. Corson SL, Unger M, Kwa D, et al: Laparoscopic laser treatment of endometriosis with the Nd:YAG sapphire probe. *Am J Obstet Gynecol* 1989; 160:718–723.
4. Sulewski JM, Crucia FD, Brenitskey C, et al: The treatment of endometriosis at laparoscopy for infertility. *Am J Obstet Gynecol* 1980; 138:128.
5. Daniell JR, Christianson C: Combined laparoscopic surgery and danazol therapy for pelvic endometriosis. *Fertil Steril* 1981; 35:521.
6. Feste JR: Advanced gynecologic endoscopic surgery. Syllabus material, pp 162–163, Maui, Hawaii, July 1987 (manuscript in preparation).
7. Martin DC: $CO_2$ laser laparoscopy for endometriosis associated with infertility. *J Reprod Med* 1986; 31:1089.
8. Nezhat C, Crowgey SR, Garrison CP: Surgical treatment of endometriosis via laser laparoscopy. *Fertil Steril* 1986; 45:778.
9. Keye WR Jr, Hansen LW, Astin W, et al: Argon laser therapy of endometriosis: A review of 92 consecutive patients. *Fertil Steril* 1987; 47:208.
10. Doyle JB: Paracervical uterine denervation by transection of the cervical plexus for the relief of dysmenorrhea. *Am J Obstet Gynecol* 1955; 780:1.
11. American Fertility Society: Revised American Fertility Classification Categories for Endometriosis. *Fertil Steril* 1985; 43:351.
12. Huber J, Hosmann J, Spona J: Polycystic ovarian syndrome treated by laser through the laparoscope. *Lancet*, 1988, :215.
13. Gjonnaess H: Polycystic ovarian syndrome treated by ovarian electrocautery through the laparoscope. *Fertil Steril* 1984; 41:20–25.
14. Sumioki H, Utsunomyiya T, Matsuoka K, et al: The effect of laparoscopic multiple punch resection of the ovary on a hypothalamo-pituitary axis in polycystic ovary syndrome. *Fertil Steril* 1988; 50:567–572.
15. Greenblatt E, Casper RF: Endocrine changes after laparoscopic ovarian cautery in polycystic ovarian syndrome. *Am J Obstet Gynecol* 1987; 156:279–285.

Chapter 13

# The Nd:YAG Laser in Fetal/Placental Surgery

Julian E. De Lia, M.D.

Over 6 years have passed since DeVore, et al., undertook their novel experiment of inserting a fetoscope into the uterus of a pregnant ewe and demonstrated the feasibility of in utero fetal surgery with a neodymium:YAG laser.[1] In this experiment the laser was used to photocoagulate and amputate various structures on the fetus in an amniotic fluid medium. Despite the importance of this innovative experiment, no specific anomaly of the fetus comes to mind that would benefit from this therapeutic tool. It is my impression from discussions at the International Fetal Medicine and Surgical Society meeting in 1987 that obstructive hydrocephalus and uropathies, and congenital diaphragmatic hernia appear to be the only structural anomalies deserving continued attention in the realm of fetal surgery. Additionally, the trend has been to move away from using the fetoscope itself for fetal skin and blood sampling as techniques have been perfected using ultrasound needle guidance. Nevertheless, linking the neodymium:YAG laser with a fetoscope does enable investigators to perform in utero cutting and coagulating under direct visualization in the pregnancy.

Despite the rare indications for using this technology on the fetus, the placenta might be the site of pregnancy complications that seem to be ideally suited to this technology. For example, Kurt Benirschke has maintained for some time that the vascular communications present in monochorionic twin placentas may be the underlying source of most poor outcomes in twin pregnancies.[2] Indeed, blood shunted between twins with monochorionic placentas may lead to circulatory overload or anemia (twin transfusion syndrome), hydramnios, and intrauterine death or the premature delivery of otherwise normal fetuses. The more serious manifestations of this complication occur between 20 to 28 weeks' gestation and have extremely poor outcomes. To date, therapies for this condition have ranged from a nihilistic hands-off approach to radical procedures (feticide) with isolated anecdotal successes.[3] Despite the various clinical manifestations of monochorionic twin placentation, the common denominator remains the placental vascular communications (chorioangiopagus). Fetoscopic delivery of a neodymium:YAG laser for photocoagulation of the placental vessels and for separation of the fetal circulations affords an obvious theoretical advantage to various forms of feticide and other drastic therapies. For instance, with the death of one twin (whether spontaneous or via therapeutic measures), the release of thromboplastin or placental fragments and their transplacental passage through the patent communications remains a significant risk to the surviving twin who may experience significant structural loss as a consequence.[4]

This chapter reviews the work we have done thus far in pursuing the feasibility of separating the circulations of monochorionic twins. In addition, it provides some answers to the questions posed by DeVore in the first edition of this text regarding tissue damage, long-term effects on the fetus and the pregnancy, the issue of fetal eye exposure, and current instrumentation.

## ANIMAL STUDIES

### The Sheep Experiments

Our initial experiments were aimed toward establishing the dosimetry necessary to occlude placental vessels of various sizes.[5] Four ewes of approximately 100 to 125 gestational days were examined radiographically to document pregnancy and gestational age. In the first two sheep, cesarean delivery under general thiopental anesthesia was performed to expose the placental vasculature. Placental vessels were measured, and a hand-held 600 μ quartz fiber was used to determine the dose necessary to occlude vessels of various diameters. A Molectron 8000 neodymium:YAG laser was used with a spot size of 2 mm and a power setting of 80 W (2,000 W/cm$^2$). The vessels and the fiber were kept submerged in amniotic fluid with the fiber held 1 cm from the tissues. (We had assumed that the depth of focus of most fetoscopes would be approximately 2 cm and that the fiber would be held 1 cm from the tissues for adequate visualization.) The vessels were coagulated for a distance of 1 cm. Placental vessels 1 to 3 mm in diameter required 3 seconds (6,000 joules/cm$^2$) to show no evidence of bleeding when incised. Vessels 4 to 7 mm required up to 6 seconds to occlude. Umbilical vessels (1 cm diameter) remained patent despite photocoagulation for over 15 seconds.

For the next two sheep, the fiber was passed through the side port of a pediatric cystoscope (Karl Storz, Endoscopy America, Inc., Culver City, CA). The scope was inserted into the uterus via a stab wound, and attempts were made to identify and coagulate vessels under direct fetoscopic visualization. Although some difficulty was encountered because of the cotyledonary nature of the sheep placenta, several vessels were identified and coagulated, using the above dosimetry, which also showed occlusion upon incision.

Figure 13–1 shows the histologic appearance of an occluded vessel. The basic structure of the vessel was maintained, but it showed shrinkage and edema. In light of these histologic findings, we assumed that the vessels were heated to 60° to 70°C, at which temperature denaturing of proteins and loss of cell membrane integrity would occur.

Despite these encouraging findings, two immediate problems remained. The sheep placenta (cotyledonary) differs from the human placenta (discoid) enough to make this initial experiment only marginally relevant. In addition, the sheep were sacrificed immediately after the experiment so that long-term, permanent occlusion remained to be proven, along with any long-term effects on the placenta and surrounding tissues.

### The Monkey Experiments

In order to resolve these questions and to design an experiment that would parallel the human situation more closely, we sought a more satisfactory animal model. There seems to be no suitable animal model that consistently demonstrates monochorionic twin placentation. However, the rhesus monkey placenta does share similar structural and circulatory

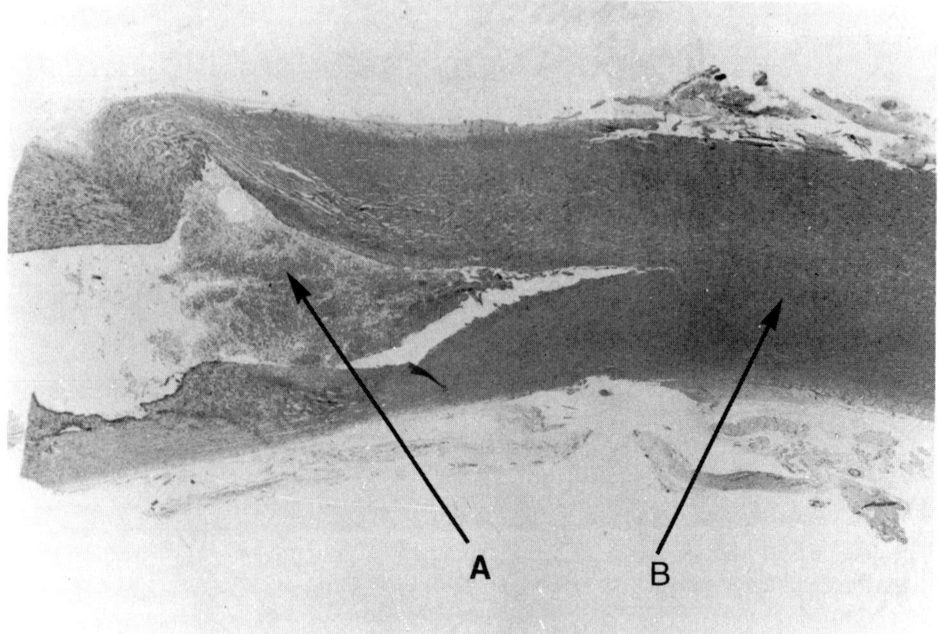


**FIG 13–1.**
Sheep placental vessel showing progression from normal (*A*) to occlusion (*B*) at region of laser impact (From De Lia, et al: *Am J Obstet Gynecol* 1985; 151:1126. Used by permission).

patterns with the human placenta. In addition, in 80% of singleton pregnancies, the placenta is bidiscoid with arterial and venous communications running between the placental disks (Fig 13–2). Because open surgical ligation of the communicating vessels has been performed in this animal without miscarriage,[6] long-term occlusion of the photocoagulated vessels could be assessed, along with untoward effects on the surrounding tissues and fetus.

The twelve experiments were performed at the California Primate Research Center over the course of 2 years (four monkeys, each during three separate breeding cycles).[7] The animals were examined ultrasonographically to determine gestational age, bilobed placentation, and the location of the primary disk (by umbilical cord insertion). We planned on photocoagulating the communicating vessels over the edge of the primary disk to mimic the placental (chorionic plate) location of the communicating vessels in the human monochorionic twin placenta. Additionally, the effects of the laser energy on the placenta itself could be assessed histologically.

At the end of the second trimester (91 to 116 days), the animals were anesthetized and, using sterile techniques, a laparotomy was performed to expose and exteriorize the uterus. Uterine transillumination was performed to determine the best entry site for the fetoscope (Olympus Selfoscope, 1.7-mm outside diameter). Initially, a second puncture was planned for a 600-μ fiber to be inserted through a 16-gauge spinal needle; but after being unable to coordinate the fiber and the scope over the placental vessels in the first experiment, the fiber was attached with suture to the side of the scope for the remaining experiments (Fig 13–3). For the first four experiments, a 600-μ quartz fiber was used, with the laser output set at 80 watts (Model 8000, Cooper LaserSonics); for the last eight experiments, a 400-μ fiber and 40 watts were used.

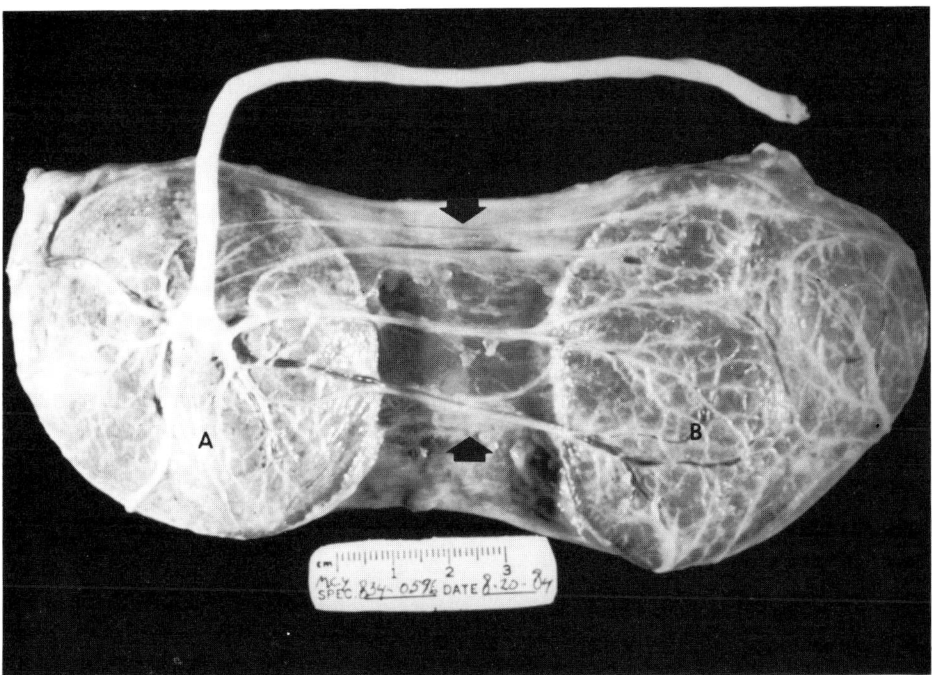


**FIG 13–2.**
Bidiscoid singleton rhesus monkey placenta showing communicating vessels (*arrows*) running from primary disk (*A*) to secondary disk (*B*).

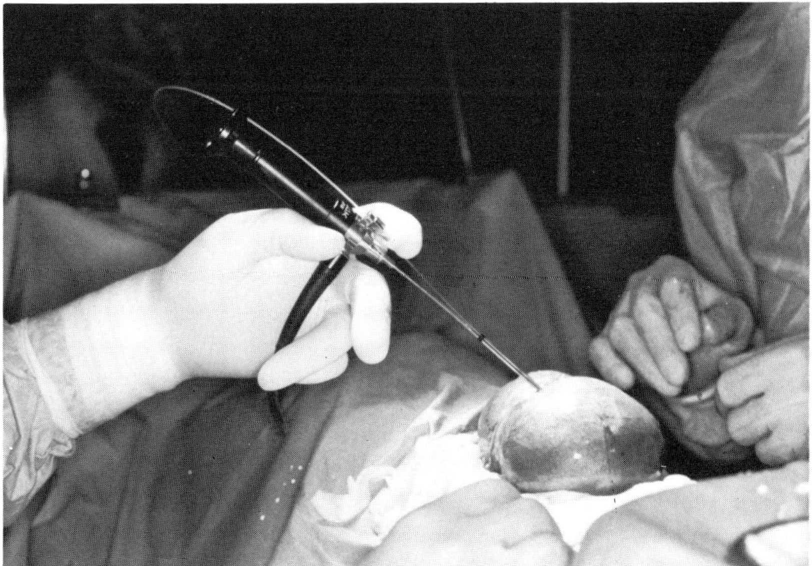

**FIG 13–3.**
Intraoperative photograph of the laser fiber and fetoscope passed through a stab wound in the uterine wall of the monkey.

After photocoagulating all apparent communications (which measured between 0.5 and 1.5 mm in diameter), the instruments were removed and the hysterotomy oversewn. Because the rhesus mother commonly consumes the placenta immediately postpartum, all animals were scheduled to undergo elective cesarean section near term (151 to 157 days) so that we could examine the fetus and placenta.

Although technical problems were encountered in four animals, the technique was successful in eight. One case ended in spontaneous labor 2 weeks postocclusion, and one spontaneous stillbirth occurred at term (148 days, placenta consumed). All treated vessels showed occlusion, both grossly and histologically (Fig 13–4). In addition, thermal degenerative changes including coagulation necrosis, stromal consolidation, and focal areas of mineralization were seen extending 2 to 4 mm below the chorionic plate. All fetuses were considered normal for gestational age on close physical examination regardless of the outcome of the surgery.

## COMMENT

These experiments allowed us to make the following observations: (1) The neodymium:YAG laser can be used in an amniotic fluid medium to photocoagulate placental vasculature under direct fetoscopic visualization; (2) the placental vessels remain sealed for the duration of the pregnancy after photocoagulation; (3) the minimal damage to the underlying placenta appears to be of no consequence; and (4) the fetus appears to be at small risk from the effects of the laser applied to the placenta.

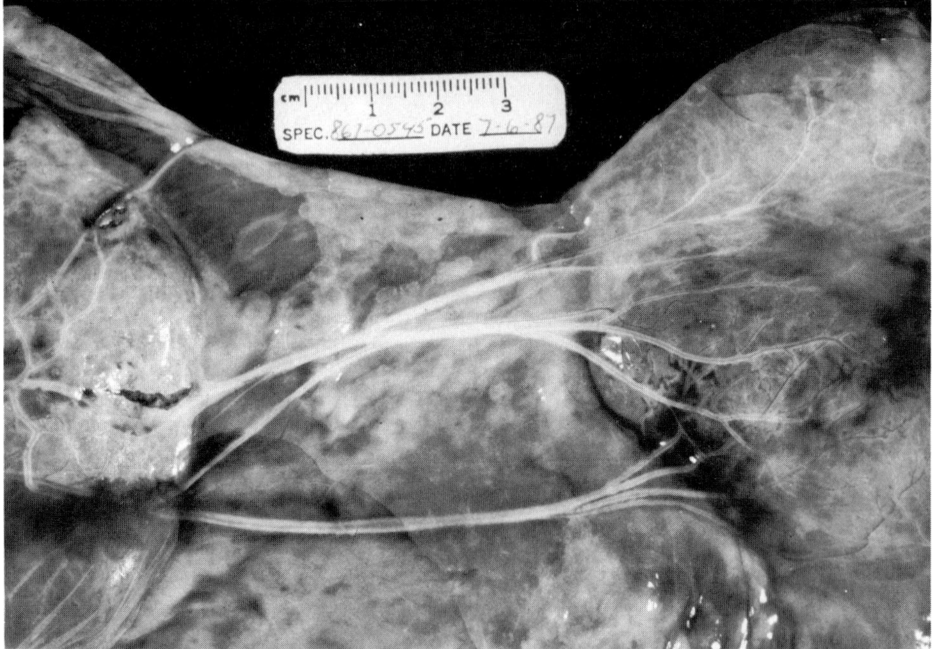


**FIG 13–4.**
Close-up view of the placenta from the ninth case. Two laser impact sites are seen on the edge of the primary disk (*left*), with a nontreated vessel group below. Segmental degeneration is seen in the secondary disk (*right*).

With the near-routine use of ultrasound in pregnancy, more cases of twin transfusion will be diagnosed during early gestation where an acceptable therapeutic intervention might decrease the near 70% reported mortality and untold morbidity of these fetuses. Extrapolating from the studies of Benirschke[2] and Rausen, et al.,[8] this author calculates the number of twin fetuses that succumb to the sequelae of chorioangiopagus to be 2,200 per year in the United States alone. To accomplish this interruption of the vascular anomaly in humans with current fetoscopic/laser technology, several problems and issues have been identified and remain as follows:

1. There is a theoretical risk of damage to the fetal eye from the reflections of the laser energy. However, if the surgery is performed between the 18th and 25th weeks, when the most severe expressions of twin transfusion become evident, the fused fetal eyelids should give considerable, if not total, protection from retinal damage. Ultimately, the biologic effect of the reflected laser beam depends on many factors including the light intensity and absorption characteristics of the tissue and the type of laser used. The absorptive and reflective properties of the amniotic fluid and the divergence angle of the laser beam at the fiber tip in our open experiments suggest that the fetus would be exposed to low power densities unless it was within 2 cm of the laser impact site.

2. There is some concern about the ability to identify the offending vessels. Studies have shown that these vessels are generally found along the "vascular equator" of the monochorionic placenta and are invariably visible to the naked eye.[9] Generally, their diameters vary inversely to the distance between the umbilical cords. Placental mapping relative to the cord insertions by ultrasound may direct the operator to the area of the equator where the vessels may be more easily located. It is the experience of this author that the

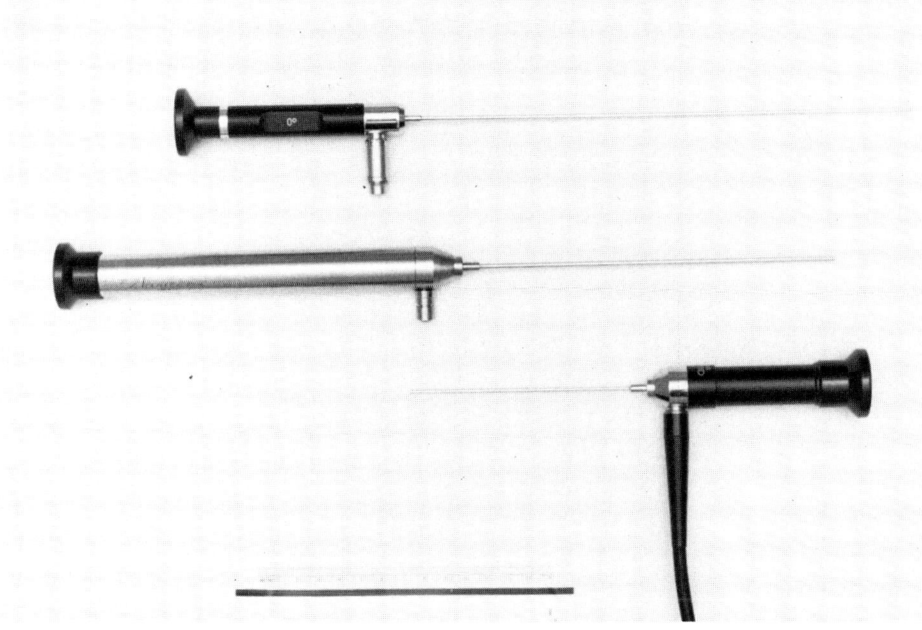

**FIG 13–5.**
Available fetoscopes include the Olympus Selfoscope (*bottom*—although their shorter arthroscope of similar diameter is shown), the Dyonics Needlescope (*middle*), and the Bryan prototype with its 25-cm telescope (*top*).

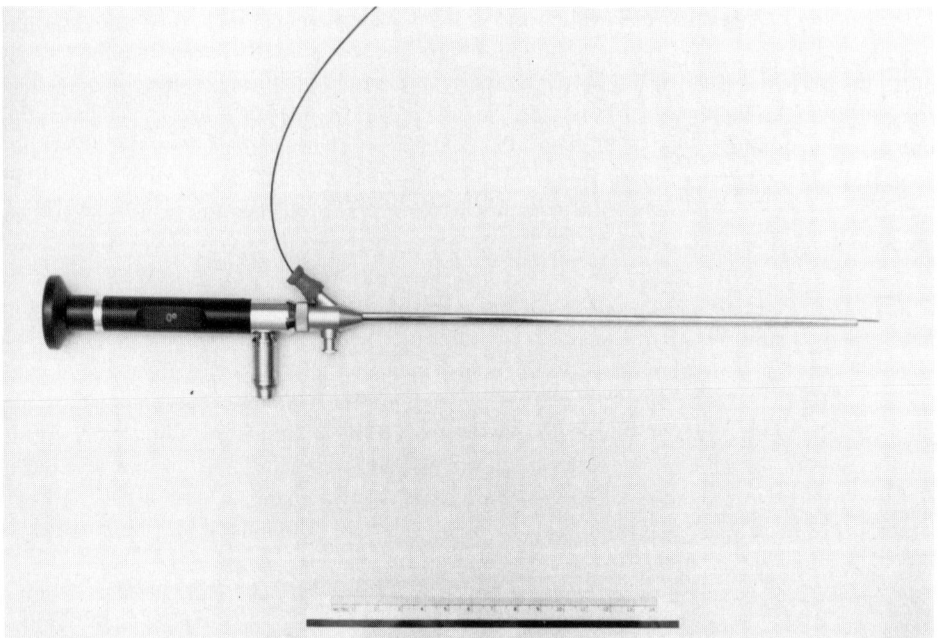

**FIG 13–6.**
The Bryan fetoscope and sheath with a 400-μ quartz rod running within the side channel. The outside diameters of the scope and sheath are 3.8 by 25 mm.

worst manifestations of this condition are associated with the fewest (single A-V) anastomoses. However, there is one type of common villous district sharing where direct communications are not seen (these are identified by observing a vessel dipping into the chorionic plate without its corresponding artery or vein). Kypros Nicolaides of King's College School of Medicine in London (personal communication) has suggested dividing the placenta in half by coagulating *all* vessels along the theoretical median, sacrificing some cotyledons if necessary. The substantial placental reserve should allow for sufficient fetal sustenance.

3. Because of the rigidity of the available fetoscopes, only those cases with posteriorly implanted placentas currently allow for visualization and photocoagulation of communicating vessels without laparotomy. Additionally, current fetoscopes may be inadequate in length to perform placental evaluation in those affected pregnancies where the amniotic sac may be overdistended with hydramnios. Figures 13–5 and 13–6 show both the currently available fetoscopes (although none are in production in 1988) and the prototype fetoscope made for placenta visualization by the Bryan Corporation (Woburn, Mass.). In order to perform an evaluation by sweeping its entire diameter, mini-laparotomy may be necessary to achieve adequate maneuverability.

## CONCLUSION

The experiments described herein support the feasibility of satisfactory treatment of placental vascular anomalies in pregnancies at risk. However, specific laser surgical procedures on the fetus itself remain elusive to this author. Given the well-quantitated poor outcomes for the pregnancy complications described above, the risks of these procedures seem greatly outweighed by the risks of these poor outcomes.

## REFERENCES


1. DeVore GR, Dixon JA, Hobbins JC: Fetoscope-directed neodymium-YAG laser: A potential tool for fetal surgery. *Am J Obstet Gynecol* 1983; 145:379–380.
2. Benirschke K, Chung KK: Multiple pregnancy (first of two parts). *N Engl J Med* 1973; 288:1276–1284.
3. Wittman BK, Farquharson DF, Thomas WE, et al: The role of feticide in the management of severe twin transfusion syndrome. *Am J Obstet Gynecol* 1986; 155:1023–1026.
4. Jung JH, Graham JM, Schultz N, et al: Congenital hydranencephaly/porencephaly due to vascular disruption in monozygotic twins. *Pediatrics* 1984; 73:467–469.
5. De Lia JE, Rogers JG, Dixon JA: Treatment of placental vasculature with a neodymium-yttrium-aluminum-garnet laser via fetoscopy. *Am J Obstet Gynecol* 1985; 151:1126–1127.
6. Panigel M, Meyers RE: Histologic and ultrastructural changes in rhesus monkey placenta following interruption of fetal placental circulation by fetectomy or interplacental umbilical vessel ligation. *Acta Anat* 1972; 81:481–506.
7. De Lia JE, Cukierski MA, Lundergan DK, et al: Neodymium-YAG laser occlusion of rhesus placental vasculature via fetoscopy. *Am J Obstet Gynecol* 1989; 160:485–489.
8. Rausen AR, Seki M, Strauss L: Twin transfusion syndrome. A review of 19 cases studied at one institution. *J Pediatr* 1965; 66:613–628.
9. Bleisch VR: Placental circulation of human twins. Constant arterial anastomoses in monochorionic placentas. *Am J Obstet Gynecol* 1965; 91:862–869.

Chapter 14

# The Future of Lasers in Gynecology: The Free-Electron Laser and Photodynamic Therapy*

Richard C. Straight, Ph.D.
John Hunter, M.D.
John Dixon, M.D.

Gynecologic laser applications have matured rapidly since the first edition of this text. Indications and contraindications have become more clearly defined, relative advantages and disadvantages have been investigated, and new procedures and instruments have been developed.

Of the many unique features of the laser, three major characteristics will form the basis for future developments: (1) the ability to cut and coagulate without touching tissue, (2) the ability to deliver many wavelengths of laser energy through flexible fiberoptic wave guides, and (3) the selective absorption and interaction of each laser wavelength and tissue type.

Advances in medical lasers during the next decade will be in the following areas: (1) the development of more powerful and, in some cases, smaller lasers, (2) the use of new wavelengths, (3) the development of new delivery systems, (4) the use of chemicals to sensitize pathologic tissues to laser energy, and (5) the exploration of non-thermal effects of lasers.

## DEVELOPMENT OF MORE POWERFUL LASERS

During the past 5 years existing clinical lasers have become more powerful. Through the development of the superpulse, $CO_2$ lasers can now deliver peak powers of over 100 watts, and the KTP/532 and argon lasers can deliver powers of more than 15 watts. How-

*Work supported in part by the Veterans Administration Medical Research Program, by the Department of Defense SD10 Medical Free Electron Laser Program, and by the Utah Laser Institute, University of Utah.

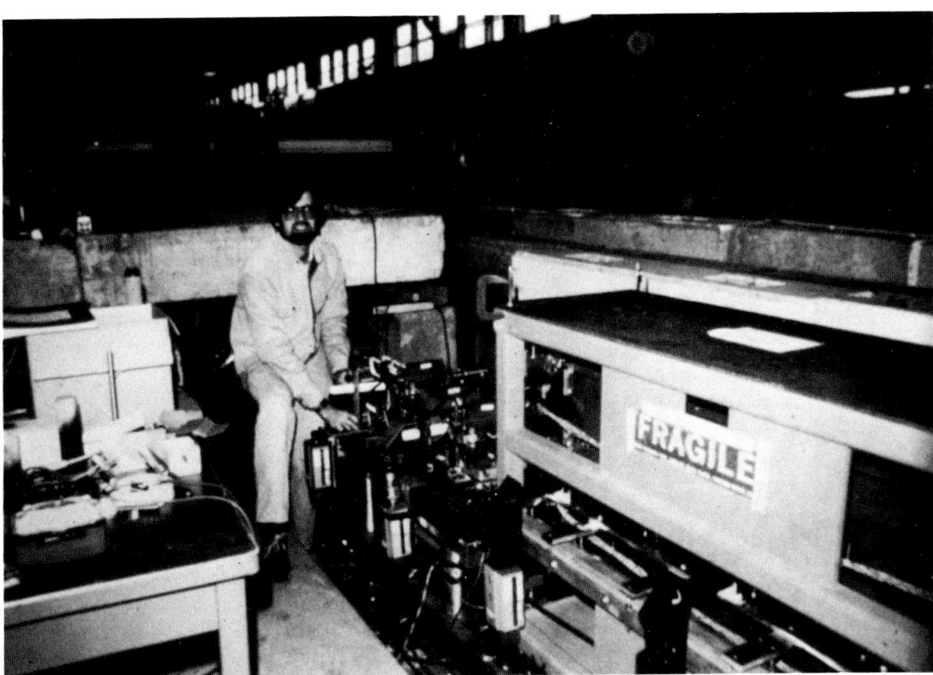


**FIG 14–1.**
Stanford Mark III Free Electron Laser. Electron beam "gun" near operator. Note surrounding walls and shielding.

ever, the free-electron laser (FEL) will provide the opportunity to investigate average powers of 300 watts or greater and peak powers in the gigawatt range during pulses as short as 500 femtoseconds. The FEL, developed by John Madey at Stanford University in the 1970s,[1] has captured the imagination of basic science and medical scientists (Fig 14–1). It is best known for its role in the Department of Defense Strategic Defense Initiative (SDI), or Star Wars Program. The FEL is driven by a synchroton accelerator, which generates a beam of electrons that are passed between powerful magnets called wigglers. As the polarity and strength of the magnets are varied, an almost infinite number of wavelengths of amplified laser energy can be produced and tuned (Fig 14–2). The FEL is unique because of its tunability over a wide range of wavelengths and its ability to deliver

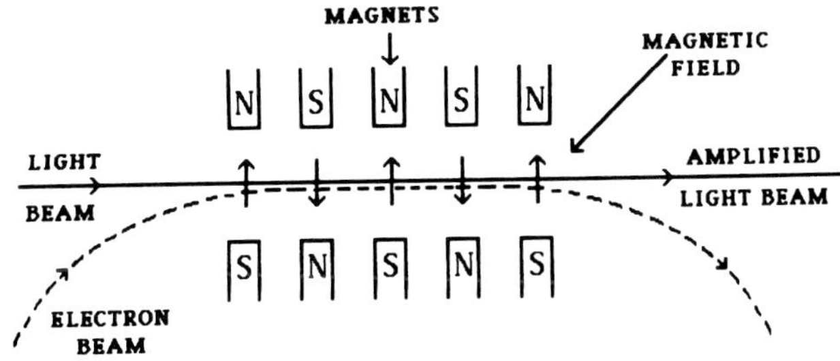


**FIG 14–2.**
Free electron laser diagram. Beam of electrons passed through "wigglers" varying wavelength of light produced.

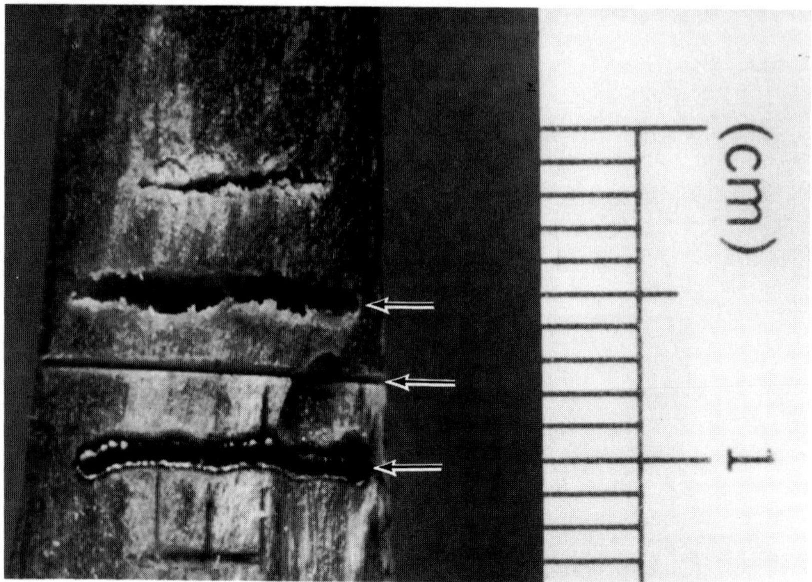


**FIG 14–3.**
Comparison of bone incisions. *Top arrow:* Standard bone saw. Note wide incision, fragmentation. *Middle arrow:* Free electron laser at 3.1 μ, 50 mJ/pulse. Note narrow incision, absence of thermal injury. *Bottom arrow:* $CO_2$ laser. Note extensive thermal damage with carbonization.

energy of high powers for very short periods of time. This will make it possible to study the non-thermal effects of laser energy. In 1984, the United States Congress recognized the potential applications of this technology in the medical sciences and allocated approximately $15 million each year for the Medical Free Electron Program. Although it is not likely to be generally available because of cost ($5 million), size, and complexity, this laser is an excellent tool for screening new wavelengths and pulses of higher power and shorter duration. For example, using low powers of a laser beam with a wavelength near 3 microns, we have been able to cut through bone without gross mechanical or thermal damage to the surrounding bone (Fig 14–3).[2] The ability to deliver laser energy in high-powered, short bursts may make it possible to dissect and ablate gynecologic tissues with greater precision and less unintended thermal injury to surrounding tissues than is currently possible.

As some lasers become more powerful, others will become much smaller, more efficient, and less costly. These trends will be made possible because of the use of superconductors and diodes. For example, diode lasers, which can produce different wavelengths of laser energy, are compact, demonstrate a high electrical-to-optical conversion efficiency, and are potentially less expensive than today's commercially available medical lasers. In addition, computers and sophisticated software will be incorporated into lasers to control the parameters of power, wavelength, spot size, and pulse characteristics to match the goals of the surgery and the characteristics of the tissue.

## DEVELOPMENT OF NEW WAVELENGTHS

While most gynecologists are familiar with the $CO_2$, Nd:YAG, argon, and frequency-doubled Nd:YAG laser, there are several other wavelengths currently being investigated for their gynecologic applications. Recent reports suggest possible roles in medicine and gynecology for mid-infrared and heavy metal vapor lasers such as the erbium:YAG laser, the gold vapor laser, the copper vapor laser, the argon pumped dye laser, and the helium holmium chromium:YAG laser. The process of exploring new wavelengths is complicated by the cost and difficulty of developing individual lasers to study each wavelength of interest. The more practical approach may involve a tunable laser, such as the FEL, which can be tuned continuously from 4 μm to 300 μm. The FEL will make it possible to explore, with a single machine, the biological effects of many wavelengths. Examples of research with new wavelengths include the photochemical destruction of viruses (perhaps in the future HIV, human papillomavirus, hepatitis virus, or herpes virus) and of malignant tissues. In addition, studies are now planned to investigate the use of new wavelengths to influence cellular (fibroblast migration and collagen deposition) and subcellular (rate of cell division or protein production) processes. One might envision that the exposure of human gametes or pre-embryos to laser energy may enhance the success rates of in vitro fertilization or cryopreservation.

## DEVELOPMENT OF NEW DELIVERY SYSTEMS

The initial enthusiam that followed the introduction of the $CO_2$ laser in gynecologic surgery was soon followed by frustration with the bulky and delicate articulating arm that limited its use at laparoscopy. As a result, the use of a flexible fiberoptic delivery system for the delivery of the argon laser at laparoscopy was tried.[3] The use of fiberoptics greatly simplified the endoscopic use of lasers for the treatment of pelvic diseases. Soon thereafter, the Nd:YAG laser was used through an optical fiber at laparoscopy (see Chapter 9), hysteroscopy (see Chapter 7), and fetoscopy (unpublished data). Unfortunately, the characteristics of the Nd:YAG laser-tissue interaction limited its use in the pelvis. These limitations led to the development of a sapphire probe which, when coupled to the end of the quartz fiber, made it possible for the surgeon to actually touch the tissue with the fiber (see Chapter 12). As a result, one could produce a limited, safe, and predictable pattern of thermal damage, which included vaporization as well as coagulation.

While initial attempts to develop a flexible fiber for the delivery of the $CO_2$ laser at laparoscopy were unsuccessful,[4] there have been two recent developments that have simplified the endoscopic delivery of the $CO_2$ laser. The first was the development of a rigid wave guide, which, when introduced through the operating channel of the single-puncture laparoscope, eliminated the unpredictable nature of focusing tubes and improved the efficiency of the laparoscopic delivery of the $CO_2$ laser (see Chapter 9).

The most recent development has been a flexible fiber for delivery of the $CO_2$ laser by Fuller Research. The fiber, which measures 1 mm outside diameter, is nontoxic and capable of delivering argon and Nd:YAG laser energy as well as the $CO_2$ laser. It can bend in a very small radius, is reusable, and is projected to be very reasonable in cost. Hopefully, the fiber will be commercially available by 1990.

Thus, there have been a number of changes in delivery systems during the past 10 years. The delivery systems in the future will be designed for specific surgical procedures (e.g., specialized fiberoptic tips specially designed to simultaneously ablate large areas of the endometrium). Others may give off circumferential (360°) beams or a 180° beam that will uniformly destroy the walls of ovarian cysts, the core of uterine myomas, or malignant pelvic nodules. Other delivery systems may facilitate tissue welding of vessels, fallopian tubes, or the surface of the uterus or ovary to decrease adhesion formation. The development of new flexible laser delivery systems will most likely parallel the increasing use of photodynamic therapy.

Another advance in the delivery of laser energy will be the development of micromanipulators capable of creating spot sizes of 5 to 10 microns or smaller. With these small spot sizes, lasers may be used to drill the zona pellucida of human oocytes to facilitate sperm penetration or to dissect a blastomere from a blastocyst for biochemical or genetic analysis.

## THE USE OF LASERS IN ACTIVATING PHOTOSENSITIVE REACTIONS

Perhaps one of the most exciting areas for the future of lasers in gynecology involves photodynamic laser therapy. Photodynamic action (PDA), refers to sensitized photooxidation in which light interacts with either endogenous biomolecules[6] (phototherapy) or exogenous administered photoactivatable chemicals (photochemotherapy).[7]

Phototherapy as a result of the light absorbed by an *endogenous* biomolecule is older than recorded history. As a science, phototherapy was developed by Niels Finsen (Nobel Prize, 1903) and others when they successfully used ultraviolet (UV) radiation from sunlight and artificial sources in the treatment of lupus vulgaris, a form of skin tuberculosis.[8] Ultraviolet phototherapy is used today to treat a variety of skin diseases and infections.[6] Phototherapy involving the photochemical destruction of bilirubin with visible blue light is routinely used to treat hyperbilirubinemia in infants.[7]

Selective phototherapy of the microvessels in port wine stains and other blood vessel abnormalities has been achieved recently with lasers (argon, dye, copper, vapor) that generate light at wavelengths absorbed by endogenous hemoglobin.[9] The heme in hemoglobin acts as an endogenous absorber and photothermal sensitizer that helps to confine the thermal damage to the blood and blood vessels or vascularized lesions.

In photodynamic therapy (PDT), light or other forms of electromagnetic radiation is absorbed by an *exogenous* photosensitizer or nontoxic drug that is retained in the target tissue (e.g., tumor). PDT is typically carried out using laser "light" in the 400-nm to 800-nm (0.4 to 0.8 micrometers) wavelength range, with most of the clinical studies done with red light above 600 nm. The photosensitizer, e.g., hematoporphyrin derivative (HPD), absorbs a photon of light energy and initiates the photophysical and photochemical changes that lead to the therapeutic effect.

Because the light energy (wavelength), intensity, and location of absorption can be controlled, the therapist has control over the extent of damage to the target tissue and the ability to limit damage to surrounding tissues. Thus, PDT has fewer side effects than most other modalities for tumor therapy.

## MECHANISMS OF PHOTODYNAMIC THERAPY

### Photochemical Mechanisms

Photodynamic action (PDA) refers to the photobiological phenomena (e.g., enzyme inactivation, cell killing, skin phototoxicity, tumor destruction) that are observed when a biological target is exposed to a photosensitizer, light, and molecular oxygen. Molecular oxygen is consumed in the process, but the photosensitizer is usually not consumed.

Photodynamic therapy depends primarily on the photochemical mechanisms shown in Figure 14–4. Light is absorbed by an exogenous sensitizing drug (a colored light-activat-

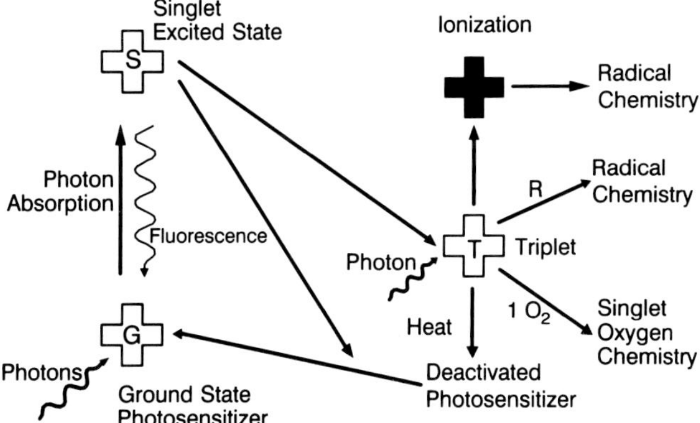


**FIG 14–4.**
The photochemical mechanism of photodynamic therapy is initiated with the absorption of light by an exogenous photosensitizer *(G)*. The electronically and vibrationally excited and unstable sensitizer *(S)* molecule rapidly ($10^{-12}$ to $10^{-9}$ sec) dissipates the energy of the absorbed photon by one of several pathways, including fluorescence; conversion to a lower energy, triplet excited state *(T)*; or thermal deactivation to a ground state *(G)*. The more stable, triplet excited state molecule *(T)* will either interact with oxygen ($^3O_2$) to form excited oxygen singlet state ($^1O_2$) or react electronically with a biomolecule in about $10^{-7}$ to $10^{-3}$ sec. Usually the sensitizer is not consumed in these reactions but returns to its stable ground state *(G)* and can absorb another photon. With sufficiently intense photon fluxes, *(G)* or *(T)* may absorb a second photon that can result in photosensitizer ionization and destructive radical chemistry.

able compound); the energy absorbed is then transferred to molecular oxygen or tissue biomolecules and the oxidation of the biomolecules in the target tissues takes place.[7] Mild thermal effects (a rise in bulk temperature of 1° to 10°C and chemical reactions of the sensitizer with biomolecules may also play a role.[7, 10, 11] Sensitized photooxidations primarily involve the formation of a reactive oxygen molecule called "singlet" oxygen ($^1\Delta gO_2$), although reactive biomolecules (free electron radicals) may also be formed. Both lead to the photodynamic destruction of tumors or other tissue containing hematoporphyrin derivative (HPD) or other colored compounds as sensitizers.

The photochemical and photobiological effects are readily produced by low energy photons of light (630 nm) at relatively low irradiances using lasers that generate continuous-wave (CW) light such as the argon-pumped dye laser. Pulsed lasers, such as the metal vapor lasers (gold, copper) with low-energy, high-repetition rate (8 kHz) pulses, are equally effective.[12]

These initial reactions are the photochemical basis of all photodynamic actions and all photodynamic therapies.[7] The various photobiological and physiological effects that are seen in PDT depend on where the photosensitizer is located in the biological target (organ, tissue, cell type, membrane, cytoplasm, mitochondria, nuclei) and on which biomolecule(s) are damaged initially. Selecting photosensitizers that are preferentially retained at certain locations in the target tissue (e.g., capillary endothelial cells of tumors) may produce selective biochemical damage, selective biological effects (vascular disruption), and the desired phototherapy.

## The Nature of Photodynamic Sensitizers

The physical, chemical, photochemical, and photobiological properties of photosensitizers are basic to their use in the PDT of tumors. Many dyes and pigments, including the porphyrins, are photodynamic sensitizers, but not all photodynamic sensitizers are useful for photodynamic therapy.

The properties of photosensitizers that are important to PDT include (1) their solubility and transport in blood; (2) the capacity to localize and be retained in tumor tissue or other lesions in vivo; (3) the ability to absorb light efficiently above 600 nm; (4) the ability to produce necrosis of tumor tissue upon exposure to light and to fluoresce in vivo; (5) toxicity in the dark; and (6) skin phototoxicity. Porphyrins were among the first naturally occurring compounds shown to photosensitize living organisms to visible light.[13–16] Porphyrins are unique photosensitizers that can be useful in tumor detection and photochemotherapy because of their retention and fluorescence in tumor tissue and their ability to produce necrosis in tumor tissue upon exposure to light.[17–21] Laboratories have been working to determine the chemical nature of HPD to separate and identify the various porphyrin components, and to find out which components are most effective.

The main component of HPD before it is treated with base is hematoporphyrin diacetate[22]; other components are HP monoacetate (two isomers), isomeric hydroxyethyl vinyl deuteroporphyrins, isomeric acetoxyethyl vinyl deuteroporphyrins, and protoporphyrin. All HPD components are photodynamic sensitizers in vitro.

Purpurins are a group of newly sensitized photosensitizers that have demonstrated significant in vivo tumoricidal activity when combined with red light.[22–25] One of the major absorption peaks of the purpurins lies in the red region of the visible spectrum, an area of excellent tissue transmission. The purpurins have strong absorption at wavelengths greater than 650 nm and can be synthesized with a high degree of purity. They would appear to be a new class of very useful photosensitizers for PDT. A third class of dyes, the sulfonated phthalocyanines, are also photodynamic sensitizers that may have clinical applications.

All the photodynamic sensitizers that have shown the most activity against tumors in vivo are large, macrocyclic, negatively charged, colored compounds that self-aggregate or bind, or both, to serum proteins in vitro and in vivo. The colloidal properties of these colored compounds may play some role in their localization and retention in tumors and other sites of abnormal vasculature. The actual mechanisms by which these different classes of negatively charged dyes and pigments localize and are retained in tumors and other lesions are not known.

There are also photodynamic sensitizers that are either neutral or positively charged that have been shown to destroy tumors photodynamically in vivo. These include the dyes rhodamine 123, merocyanine 540, and the cyanine dyes.[26–27] These sensitizers appear to be retained in tumors and to produce a phototoxic reaction by a different mechanism than the negatively charged photosensitizers.

## The Pharmacology of Photosensitizers in Tumor Tissue

The properties of tumors in vivo that result in the localization and retention of photosensitizers, especially porphyrins, remain to be determined. There is some evidence that leaky capillaries, capillary endothelial cells, and extracellular components of tumor tissue play a major role.[28–29]

**Localization and Retention.**—Apparently, an active component of HPD in vivo is an aggregate of monomers, dimers, and polymers derived from hematoporphyrin. These aggregates compete with the binding of porphyrins to plasma proteins (albumin, hemopexin, lipoprotein) and tumor tissue proteins. Their aggregation may play a key role in the uptake and retention of fluorescent and photoreactive dyes and colorants in tumor tissue.[27, 30–34] Aggregated photosensitizers including the porphyrins may circulate in blood with very weak protein binding and be deposited via altered capillary permeability in tumor tissue. The porphyrin aggregates may then localize and dissociate within tumors through strong binding with the extracellular and cellular components of the tumor tissue. Localization and retention in tumor or any other tissue would then depend on the relative efficiency of the tissue components (e.g., collagen and other extracellular and cellular proteins) and blood proteins to bind the porphyrin aggregates. Aggregated porphyrins may also accumulate in normal tissues whose structure allows ready access to colloids and proteins and in pathological but non-tumorous tissues that have an altered and increased vascular permeability. In fact, after injection of HPD (24h), we and others have observed tissue concentrations among normal tissues in rodents as follows: liver > kidney ~ spleen > tumor > skin > lung > muscle > fat.[35–36] The distribution of colloidal dyes, proteins, and dyes bound to proteins is similar in tumors[17, 37, 38] and in other tissues with altered vascular permeability, such as inflammation,[39] wound healing,[40] and embryogenesis (Plate 14)[41] It has been suggested that the localization of injected HPD in tumors is due to the relatively high influx, and the inefficient removal and trapping, of the colloidal or the protein-bound components of HPD for extended periods, thus allowing more time for equilibration with tumor cells.[42] Other evidence suggests that the capillary endothelial cell and cellular and extracellular components of microvascular septae in addition to the tumor cell are important binding sites for photosensitizers and are targets for photodynamic action (Plate 15).[28, 29]

It has long been known that many of the aggregated or colloidal dyes (e.g., trypan blue) that localize and are retained in tumor tissue are found primarily in the stroma associated with the capillary system of tumors and in the phagocytic cells (macrophages) associated with tumors.[17, 43–46] In general, the tumor cells of both carcinomas and sarcomas are only faintly stained by colloidal dyes, including HPD, in contrast to the heavily stained stroma and phagocytic cells associated with the tumor mass (see Fig 14–1, A and B).[27, 47]

By mechanisms that are still unknown, tumor tissue generally remains fluorescent in in vivo porphyrins longer than in normal tissue. Tumor cells in vitro have been reported to retain HPD longer than do normal cells.[42] The mechanism, in vivo, has not been tested with pure compounds and there are other observations that suggest the retention in tumor tissue involves sites other than tumor cells. A fundamental issue is whether the tumor cell itself retains the photosensitizer and is therefore directly destroyed by the photooxidation reactions, or whether it is within the tumor tissue that the photosensitizer is localized and bound to the extracellular components or to the capillary endothelial cells, mast cells, macrophages, fibroblasts, or to them all.

**Photodynamic Action.**—The tumor is destroyed by ischemia as a result of the photooxidation reactions occurring within these tumor components (especially within the vascular compartment) (Plate 16). Under the conditions of clinical PDT with HPD or DHE injected intravenously, the vascular endothelial cells and the vascular system may be the most important targets for photodynamic action and the tumor cell may be only a secondary target. In the case of topical application of the photosensitizer, all cells within the tumor mass are likely to take up the photosensitizer and to be photosensitive.

Other factors may also play a role in the selective binding and retention of porphyrins in tumor tissue, such as metal chelation, covalent binding, pH, phagocytosis, and lipoprotein receptor binding.[47, 48] The relative importance of these factors is unknown.

Host responses may also play a key role in porphyrin localization, retention, and photodynamic therapy. Inflammatory wound repair responses and neovascularization are two processes in tumor-host interactions that may be important in porphyrin localization and retention, tumor detection, and photonecrosis. The connective tissue stroma of the host in contact with the dividing and invading tumor cells undergoes major changes and plays a role in the inflammatory response and neovascularization associated with tumors.[49, 50] The host extracellular matrix contains several types of macromolecules, including collagen, elastin, fibronectin, glycosaminoglycans, and proteoglycans, that are modified in tumor growth and could be involved in porphyrin retention.[18, 27, 30–34] Tumor-localizing porphyrins have been shown to bind to collagen, elastin, and fibrin, especially the polar substituted porphyrin (TPPS). Porphyrins are localized around blood vessels and stroma in tumor tissue.[50, 51] The binding of the fluorescent porphyrins to the noncellular stroma of tumor tissue may play a more significant role in the detection of tumors than in tumor photodynamic therapy, and the binding to the vascular component of tumor tissue may play a more significant role in the site and mechanism of photodynamic therapy.

## Photobiological Reactions to Photodynamic Therapy

Porphyrins may localize in either the cell membrane or in subcellular compartments. Studies show that cell membranes are the major targets of photodynamic action when cells in culture are exposed to the hydrophobic, 2-carboxyporphyrins associated with HPD and are irradiated.[52] The photooxidation reactions manifest themselves at the cell surface as membrane blebbing, lysis, enzyme inactivation, and protein cross-linking. They may also occur at the mitochondrial, microsomal, and lysosomal membranes, and perhaps at the nuclear membrane. Damage to the DNA appears to be minimal. In contrast to the lipophilic, subcellular localization of the 2-carboxyporphyrins, the more polar, hydrophilic uroporphyrin and TPPS appear to concentrate in cell lysosomes.[53] Lysosomal enzymes are released and photoinactivated to some extent when the lysosomes are irradiated.

The role of the capillary endothelial cells, mast cells, and other nonmalignant cells may be especially important as primary sites of the photooxidation reactions with the retained porphyrins in tumors in vivo.

In vivo, the initial photooxidative damage in PDA often occurs at the site of the capillary.[54–63] Acute skin phototoxicity in mice rendered protoporphyric by feeding with griseofulvin was found to be caused by the selective destruction of vascular endothelial cells, whereas the other dermal components were not damaged directly.[61] The pattern of vascular photodamage was very similar to that observed in tumor tissue.[60]

Several investigators have suggested that damage to the vascular supply of a tumor may be of major importance in tumor destruction and in the control of tumor growth.[64–66] Studies with injected radioactive microspheres have found a specific disruption of blood flow to HPD-light–treated rat tumors.[56]

Tumor capillaries differ from normal ones in several ways. They usually have larger diameters (>10 μm) and their endothelial linings and basement membranes are often irregular, discontinuous, and leaky. In some cases, tumor cells appear to serve as vessel or sinusoidal walls. At any rate, the vascular network of solid tumor tissue produced by tumor-host interaction represents a favorable site for controlling tumor growth, even at the state of preneoplastic lesions.[66]

The vascular effect appears to be a true photobiochemical phenomenon, although hyperthermia may play an additional and synergistic role.[64] The simultaneous application of photodynamic action and hyperthermia by laser irradiation selectively to solid tumors retaining porphyrins is a practical, two-pronged method of (1) *directly* destroying tumor cells by thermolysis and photooxidation and (2) *indirectly* destroying tumor cells by thermolysis and photooxidations at the endothelial cell level by producing ischemia. The latter may be a more general phenomenon than previously thought.

## CLINICAL APPLICATIONS OF LASER TUMOR PHOTODYNAMIC THERAPY

### Factors Influencing Clinical Efficacy

Photodynamic therapy (PDT) is now being used worldwide with hematoporphyrin, hematoporphyrin derivative, or the high molecular weight fraction (DHE) of HPD and other negatively charged photosensitizers for the clinical treatment of tumors.[65–71] The response to PDT depends on several factors: (1) the concentration (microconcentration) and optical absorption properties of the photosensitizer in the tumor tissue; (2) the concentration and availability of molecular oxygen; (3) the intensity, frequency, and pulse parameters of the activating laser light; and (4) the immunological and biological status of the patient. Although most of these factors are not yet adequately defined, several thousand human and veterinary patients have been treated.[65–71, 73–76]

In order to be effective, light at a wavelength that falls within the absorption band of the photosensitizer used must reach it with sufficient intensity to initiate enough photooxidation reactions to produce the photobiological response. We know that there is a window of light between 600 nm and 1,200 nm that is most effective for PDT.[77]

The light absorption by endogenous tissue chromophores (heme, bilirubin, melanin, flavins) must be minimal so that the activating light will be able to penetrate and reach the sensitized tissue. Above 600 nm, the molar absorption coefficients of the endogenous chromophores are at their lowest values[77]; thus, this wavelength range permits the maximum depth of tissue penetration by the activating light while restricting unwanted tissue absorption. However, some superficial tumors may be treated at still lower wavelengths (410 to 580 nm). The depth of penetration of different wavelengths of light for different tissues has been determined.[79] For example, at 400 nm, 0.4 mm of white skin will reduce the light to 1% of the incident intensity, but at 600 nm, 2.54 mm of white skin is required to reduce the light to 1%, and at 1,000 nm, 7.36 mm of white skin is required.

The radius of effective action in porphyrin-sensitized, nonpigmented tumor tissue at 630 nm (50 mW) with HPD (10 to 20 mg/kg of body weight) is about 4 mm.[80] The radius would be expected to increase significantly at higher light intensities and HPD drug doses. The photosensitizer currently approved for clinical use is a preparation of HPD or the high molecular weight fraction DHE. The absorption spectra of these porphyrins, when localized in tumor tissue, typically show four absorption bands in the visible spectrum in addition to the strong Soret band at about 400 nm. The only band available above 600 nm peaks at about 632 nm. Unfortunately, this band has the lowest absorption coefficient and is therefore the least efficient for exciting the porphyrin to the triplet state. The Soret band at 400 nm would be at least ten times more efficient for photooxidation. Other photosensitizers, such as the chlorins and the phthalocyanines, with absorption bands between 600 nm to 750 nm, have absorption coefficients on the order of the Soret band.[81] It has yet to be shown that these photosensitizers are more effective for tumor PDT.

The efficiency of PDT may be enhanced by manipulating the absorption spectrum of the photosensitizer to maximize the absorptivity, and by tuning the wavelength and intensity of the laser to match the peak wavelength of the sensitizer. The control of the pulse parameters (pulse duration, pulse frequency) may also be useful in PDT, but this has only recently been studied.[82–86]

The concentration of oxygen may be a factor limiting the reaction to photoactivated PDT although, generally speaking, the photosensitized oxidation reactions are efficient in vitro even at low oxygen concentrations ($10^{-6}$ to $10^{-8}$ M).[87–88] However, this has not been studied in animal models.

Temperature is not expected to have any significant effect on the photochemical process but may affect the rates of dark reactions and may be an important parameter for combined PDT and hyperthermia.[80, 82, 89]

Manipulating and controlling these factors of laser PDT are basic for establishing treatment protocols for clinical use. The results of early trials indicate that several types of cancer may be controlled or eradicated by PDT. Issues that require further research include finding a photosensitizer that will eliminate the prolonged skin phototoxicity that occurs with HPD. Other photosensitizers with less skin phototoxicity may be found[22, 81, 84, 90] or the phototoxic reaction may be inhibited by other agents (e.g., beta-carotene).[91] New sensitizers also need to be found that are more effective in vivo, both for the direct destruction of tumor cells and for the destruction of the tumor vascular system. In addition, PDT has the potential for being used with one or more other cancer treatment modalities, including chemotherapy, surgical therapy, phototherapy, and heat therapy, and protocols should be developed to determine the most effective combinations. Phase I and Phase II clinical trials are needed. The transient immune suppression that has been reported in mouse model experiments with HPD may not be clinically significant but should be studied in more detail.[92, 93] Finally, the synergistic effect of pulsed laser irradiation compared to CW irradiation in the PDT of tumors should be investigated further.[86] Continued developments in optical fibers, procedures for irradiation, and protocols for multiple light exposures are needed.

## Gynecologic Applications of Photodynamic Diagnosis and Therapy

Since an early report in 1957 by Mack, et al., who treated 24 patients with cancer of the cervix with a combination of hematoporphyrin and radiation therapy, we have known that porphyrins would accumulate in these lesions and serve as a fluorescent diagnostic marker.[94] The hematoporphyrin-treated group received doses of hematoporphyrin ranging from 20 to 1,000 mg. One of the consistent observations made was that the tumors invariably became fluorescent and, although the fluorescence seemed to be related to the dose of the drug, the type of tumor also played a major role in the amount of porphyrin necessary to produce the fluorescence in the tumor. Although these authors did not use light and photodynamic therapy to treat the tumors, they did observe the side reaction of skin photosensitivity in all the patients. Again, the skin photosensitization was variable from patient to patient and was not necessarily directly related to the dose of porphyrin.

Lipson, et al., had previously shown that hematoporphyrin derivative accumulates in malignant tissue[95, 96] and that its fluorescence could be a valuable adjunct to the endoscopic detection of malignant neoplasms.[97–99] They also evaluated the use of the fluorescent technique in studies of neoplastic lesions of the cervix.[98] Recently, Fioretti, et al. noted a greater uptake and retention of hematoporphyrin derivative in cervical cancer than in normal surrounding tissues.[100]

In 1985, McCaughan, et al. injected five patients with various gynecologic neoplasms with hematoporphyrin derivative, then treated them using photodynamic therapy and 630 nm light from an argon dye laser.[101] In this series, one patient with multifocal squamous cell cancer of the vagina had no evidence of the disease 15 months after her first PDT. At autopsy 9 months after the first treatment of another patient with multifocal invasive cancer of the vagina and perimetrium, there was no evidence of tumor on the surface of the vagina. In another, there was no evidence of Bowen's disease of the vulva and thigh 8 months after treatment of an area 8 × 12 cm. Vaginal bleeding from breast cancer metastatic to the endometrium was controlled by one treatment until that patient died 5 months later from her disease. Adenocarcinoma metastatic to the vaginal cuff showed partial response when vaginectomy was performed 5 weeks after photodynamic therapy.

In McCaughan's study, interstitial irradiation from the argon dye laser was used through cylindrical-type fibers about 2.5 cm long, and the irradiances used were on the order of 600 to 700 mW/cm per fiber. Light doses varied from less than 30 to 200 J/cm$^2$. These authors pointed out that in each case the treatment had to be individualized for each patient to determine the best way to deliver the light. The total dose required was difficult to establish in a consistent way.

There are a few other scattered reports in the literature of the treatment of gynecological cancers with PDT. These include a study by Ward, et al.,[102] who reported treating five gynecologic cancers with PDT, using the technique of multiple insertions of quartz fibers directly into the tumor, with 300 to 500 mW delivered from the tip of the fiber. Multiple applications were performed in this series on multiple days; some of the tumors were also treated with external radiation by holding the fiber tip approximately 1 cm from the tumor. They reported no evidence of recurrence of one tumor at 12 months, another patient free of tumor at 10 months, and varying degrees of response from the other three patients.

Kennedy, in 1983, also reported experience with vaginal cancer using a tunable dye laser and a slide-projector light source with a solid lucite cone to deliver the light. He reported substantial palliation in the treatment of vaginal cancer by this method.[103]

Soma and Nutahara reported the results of treating five patients with cancer of the vagina and the vulva, five patients with carcinoma in situ of the uterine cervix, and three patients with cancer metastatic to the vagina.[104] They used a tunable dye laser system through a colposcope, maintaining the tip at a distance of 5 cm from the lesion to produce a spot of 2.8 to 5.5 cm in diameter. Treatments usually lasted 20 to 40 minutes with a power output of 10 to 400 mW, delivering an estimated dose of 80 to 346 J/cm$^2$. However, because of the excellent cure rates of cervical intraepithelial carcinoma with the $CO_2$ laser with few complications, there would appear to be little use for photodynamic therapy for this disease.

## FUTURE DEVELOPMENTS FOR LASER PHOTOCHEMOTHERAPY

The parallel development of (1) new laser systems for generating light at many wavelengths with a wide range of pulse characteristics, (2) photosensitizing drugs and drug delivery systems that can be used to selectively target tissue components, and (3) optical fibers and devices to irradiate and treat a biological target almost anywhere in the body is providing exciting new therapeutic and diagnostic tools for surgery and medicine.

For example, viral lesions and infections may be treated by laser photodynamic therapy. It is well known that positively charged dyes such as proflavine, neutral red, and acridine orange photodynamically inhibit viral replication.[105] Photochemotherapy with such sensitizers has been used to treat herpesvirus lesions clinically.[106] However, the procedure has been criticized by some as being ineffective and potentially mutagenic and carcinogenic.[107] Despite the reduction in infectious virions after proflavine photodynamic treatment of herpesvirus-infected cells, neither viral nor cell DNA synthesis was inhibited.[108]

In contrast to proflavine and the other positively charged photosensitizers, the negatively charged photosensitizers, such as the carboxyporphyrins in HPD, sensitize the inactivation of herpesvirus by a different mechanism.[109] HPD-photoinactivated virions are no longer able to infect cells or to penetrate the nuclei of susceptible cells.[110] Although the photodynamic action of HPD can result in single-strand breaks in viral DNA, this does not seem to occur during HPD photoinactivation of herpesvirus in suspension when irradiated with either blue light (400 nm) or red light (630 nm).[108, 109] It is also unlikely to occur in vivo. Instead, it appears that the target is either the lipid, the protein, or both, on the viral envelope surface, which when damaged photochemically prevents the virus from binding and infecting cells. Preliminary studies suggest that the herpesvirus is more sensitive than human cells to HPD phototherapy and that in vivo clinical laser phototherapy of viral lesions should be evaluated in animal studies to determine efficacy and potential benefits and hazards.[110] The treatment of herpes lesions by laser HPD (topically or systemically applied) photochemotherapy may become a useful clinical procedure.

Other viral lesions of clinical importance that may be treated by HPD-sensitized laser PDT are human papillomavirus (HPV) lesions, including laryngeal and genital papillomas, that are rapidly growing benign epithelial neoplasms that persistently recur after surgical or medical therapy. Abramson, et al., were recently able to completely destroy cottontail rabbit papillomavirus in Dutch Belt rabbits.[111] If further animal studies are equally successful, PDT treatment of viral papillomas in humans may be possible. Five patients with laryngeal papilloma lesions have been treated in Australia using HPD and PDT with very encouraging results. A larger series (70 patients) with genital lesions treated with HPD-PTD should be reported in the near future.

Microbial infections may also be treated by photochemotherapy. Clinically important bacterial, yeast and fungal infections have been treated with laser photochemotherapy. However, more widespread use of PDT to treat microbial infections or to prevent infections after surgery will depend on the development of successful protocols. For example, *Staphylococcus aureus* is activated in vitro and in vivo in animal models by HPD-sensitized PDT.[112] Mycoplasma cells are also killed by HPD-sensitized photodynamic action.[113] The cell membrane is the site of damage in both *Mycoplasma hominis* and *Acholeplasma laidlawii*. Eukaryotic microorganisms, including yeast cells *(Saccharomyces cervisiae)*, are killed on exposure to light in the presence of HPD.[114] No genetic changes are found in yeast as a result of HPD-sensitized PDT.[115] The HPD-sensitized photooxidation damages the cell membrane but not the DNA of yeast cells. The human pathogenic fungi *Candida albicans* and *Cryptococcus neoformans* are killed by exposure to HPD that is followed by irradiation with visible light for 30 minutes.[116] It is likely that clinical yeast infections could be treated by PDT; however, further animal and clinical studies are needed.

The visible and occult lesions of endometriosis also have been shown recently to take up HPD in both a rabbit and a rhesus monkey model. The lesions were treated with argon laser light and PDT was demonstrated. These preliminary unpublished studies were carried out at the University of Adelaide and by the Utah Laser Institute in collaboration with the Oregon Primate Research Center. Further studies are underway to determine whether successful treatment of occult endometrial lesions is possible.

Finally, Schneider and his colleagues at the University of Cincinnati and the Jewish Hospital Laser Laboratory have demonstrated the rapid uptake of dihematoporphyrin derivative by the endometrium of estrogen-treated ovariectomized rats. When exposed to the gold vapor laser (628 nm) at 50J with a power of 200 mW for 12 minutes at a distance of

12 cm and a spot size of 2 cm, selective necrosis of the endometrium and inner portion of the myometrium occurred in 9 of 10 animals when mated pregnancy failed to occur in these animals. These preliminary animal studies suggest that photodynamic therapy may be of use in the ablation of the endometrium in women with menorrhagia. The technique using a quartz rod passed into the uterine cavity through the cervix would be simpler than the current technique using the Nd:YAG laser and could possibly be performed in the office without anesthesia.

### Non-thermal Effects of Lasers

In addition to photochemical tissue ablation, future applications of lasers may involve other photochemical actions of lasers. For example, the selection of an appropriate wavelength may make it possible to influence the rate of wound healing by altering the rate of fibroblast migration and collagen deposition. Or perhaps by selecting an appropriate wavelength, we may be able to influence the rate of cell division and differentiation, the function of individual cells or gametes, the rate of protein synthesis within cells, the activation or inactivation of genetic material, or other intracellular or intercellular functions.

## SUMMARY

### Changing Role of Lasers in Gynecology

Along with the development of new lasers and laser accessories, the role of lasers in gynecology will also change. To date, the major role for the intra-abdominal use of lasers has been in the treatment of infertility. The laser and its accessory equipment have been adapted to lyse adhesions, to treat polycystic ovaries, to open up obstructed fallopian tubes, and to destroy endometriosis. However, as the success of the assisted reproductive technologies (in vitro fertilization, gamete intrafallopian transfer, zygote intrafallopian transfer, and cryopreservation) improve, the role of the laser in infertility surgery will decrease. Instead of performing a neosalpingostomy to achieve a 5% to 20% pregnancy rate, women may choose in vitro fertilization with a pregnancy rate of 25% to 40%. Additionally, extensive adhesiolysis will be performed for the relief of pain, not for the treatment of infertility.

As the laser assumes its place among the traditional and standard surgical instruments and devices that we have used for decades, the mystique of the laser will disappear and it will become an adjunct to more traditional devices. Freestanding laser units will cease to exist as they are incorporated into standard hospital or outpatient surgical administrative units. Training in lasers will become a standard part of residency training, and the demand for postgraduate education and the need for certification will level off. As lasers find their proper place in gynecologic surgery, the American Board of Laser Surgeons will die a peaceful and to some a welcome death. Hopefully, the extraordinary claims, the blatant examples of self-promotion, and the occasional unjustified fees that have accompanied the introduction of lasers in gynecology will also cease.

Finally, non-laser technologies, such as electrocautery and ultrasonography, will be modified to accomplish many of the tissue effects now achieved with lasers at a fraction of the cost of lasers. For example, electrosurgical probes will be introduced to coagulate and incise tissue with the same degree of precision and greater safety than with the laser. As a result, the use of lasers in gynecology to merely coagulate and vaporize may decline as the use of photodynamic therapy increases.

While the use of lasers in gynecology has grown rapidly during the past decade, the developments of the next decade will be even more dramatic and rapid. It behooves gynecologists to become familiar with the current generation of lasers and laser procedures so that they will be well positioned to take advantage of the next generation of lasers and their applications.

## REFERENCES

1. Madey MJ: Free electron laser technology. *J Appl Physiol* 1971; 42:1906–1909.
2. Dixon JA, Straight RC: Free electron laser fragmentation of calcified tissue. *Lasers Surg Med* 1987; 7:87–88.
3. Keye WR, Dixon JA: Photocoagulation of endometriosis by the argon laser through the laparoscope. *Obstet Gynecol* 1983; 383–386.
4. Fuller TA: Mid-infrared fiberoptics. *Lasers Surg Med* 1986; 6:399–403.
6. Morison WL: *Phototherapy and Photochemotherapy of Skin Diseases*. New York, Praeger Publishers, 1983.
7. Straight RC, Spikes JD: Photosensitized oxidation of biological molecules, in Frimer A (ed): *Singlet $C_2$, IV*. Boca Raton, CRC Press, 1985, pp 91–143.
8. Spikes JD: The historical development of ideas on applications of photosensitized reaction in the health sciences, in Bensasson RV, Jori, G, Land EJ, Truscott TJ (eds): *Primary Photoprocesses in Biology and Medicine*. New York, Plenum Press, 1985, pp 209–227.
9. Parrish JA, Anderson RR, Harrist T, et al: Selective thermal effects with pulsed irradiation from lasers: From organ to organelle. *J Invest Dermatol* 1983; 80:755–805.
10. Parrish JA, Stern RS, Pathak MA, et al: Photochemotherapy of skin diseases, in Regan JD, Parrish JA (eds): *The Science of Photomedicine*. New York, Plenum Press, 1982, pp 595–623.
11. Henderson BW, Dougherty TJ, Malone PB: Studies on the mechanism of tumor destruction by photoradiation therapy, in Doiron DR, Gomer CJ (eds): *Porphyrin Localization and Treatment of Tumors*. New York, Alan R Liss, Inc, 1984, pp 601–612.
12. LaPlant M, Parker J, Stewart B, et al: Comparison of the optical transmission properties of pulsed and continuous wave light in biological tissue. *Lasers Surg Med* 1987; 7:336–338.
13. Hausmann W: Ober die sensibilisierende Wirking tierischer Farbstoffe und ihre physiolois-che bedeatung. *Biochem Z* 1908; 14:275–278.
14. Hausmann W: The sensitizing action of hematoporphyrin. *Biochem Z* 1911; 30:176–189.
15. Meyer-Betz F: Untersuchungen uber die biologische (photodynamische) Wirkung des Hematoporphyrins und ander derivate des Blut 3und Gallenfarbstoffe. *Dtsch Arch Clin Med* 1913; 112:476–503.
16. Jori G, Spikes JD: The photochemistry of porphyrins, in Smith KD (ed): *Topics in Photomedicine*. New York, Plenum Publishing Corp, 1984, pp 183–318.
17. Duran-Reynals F: Studies on the localization of dyes and foreign proteins in normal and malignant tissues. *Am J Cancer* 1939; 35:98–106.
18. Figge FHJ, Weiland GS, Manganiello LJ: Cancer detection and therapy. Affinity of neoplastic, embryonic and traumatized regenerating tissue for prophyrins and metalloporphyrins. *Proc Soc Exp Biol Med* 1948; 68:640–641.
19. Rasmussen-Taxday DS, Ward GE, Figge FHJ: Fluorescence of human lymphatic and cancer tissues following high doses of hematoporphyrin. *Cancer* 1955; 8:78–82.
20. Altman KF, Salomon K: Localization of a halogenated porphyrin in mouse tumors. *Nature* 1960; 187:1124–1127.
21. Zanelli GD, Kaelin AC: Synthetic porphyrins as tumor-localizing agents. *Br J Radiol* 1981; 54:403–407.

22. Morgan AR, Tertel NC: Observations on the synthesis and spectroscopic characteristics of purpurins. *J Org Chem* 1986; 51:1347–1350.
23. Selman SH, Morgan AR, Kreimer-Birnbaum M, et al: Photodynamic therapy of transplantable FANFT-induced urothelial tumors using the purpurin NT-2 and light. *Surg Forum* 1986; 37:659–665.
24. Morgan AR, Garbo GM, Kreimer-Birnbaum M, et al: Morpholotic study of the combined effect of purpurin derivatives and light on transplantable bladder tumors. *Cancer Res* 1987; 47:496–498.
25. Selman SH, Garbo GM, Keck RW, et al: A dose response analysis of purpurin derivatives used as photosensitizers for the photodynamic treatment of transplantable FANFT-induced urothelial tumors. *J Urol* 1987; 137:1255–1257.
26. Kalyanaraman B, Sieber F: On the mechanism of merocyanine 540 mediated photosensitization. *Photochem Photobiol* 1986; 43:28S.
27. Musser DA, Datta-Gupta N: Inability to elicit rapid cytocidal effects on L1210 cells derived from porphyrin-injected mice following *in vitro* irradiation. *J Natl Cancer Inst* 1984; 72:427–433.
28. Spikes JD, Straight RC: Photodynamic behavior of porphyrins in model cell, tissue and tumor systems, in Jori G, Perria C (eds): *Photodynamic Therapy of Tumors and Other Diseases*. Padova, Edisioni Liberia Progetto, 1985, pp 45–53.
29. Straight RC, Spikes JD: Preliminary studies with implanted polyvinyl alcohol sponges as a model for studying the role of neointerstitial and neovascular compartment of tumors in the localization, retention, and photodynamic effects of photosensitizers, in Kessel D (ed): *Methods in Porphyrin Photosensitization*. New York, Plenum Press, 1985, pp 77–89.
30. Straight RC, Dixon JA, Spikes JD: Laser photodynamic therapy of tumors: Tumor, brain and skin phototoxicity of tumor localizing chromophores. *Lasers Surg Med* 1985; 5:139.
31. Musser DA, Wagner JM, Datta-Gapta N: The interaction of tumor localizing porphyrins with collagen and elastin. *Res Commun Chem Pathol Pharmacol* 1982; 36:251–259.
32. Musser DA, Wagner JM, Weber FJ, et al: The binding of tumor localizing porphyrins to a fibrin matrix and their effects following photoirradiation. *Res Commun Chem Pathol Pharmacol* 1980; 28:505–525.
33. El-Far MA, Pimston NR: Tumor localization of uroporphyrin isomers I and III and their correlation to albumin and serum protein binding. *Cell Biochem Funct* 1983; 1:156–160.
34. Straight RC, Dixon JA, Spikes JD: Isolation of protein bound porphyrins from tranplanted tumors, fibrin clots and implanted polyvinyl alcohol sponges in porphyrin injected mice. *Photochem Photobiol* 1984; 39:675.
35. Gomer CJ, Dougherty TJ: Determination of $^3$H - and $^{14}$C hematoporphyrin derivative distribution in malignant and normal tissue. *Cancer Res* 1979; 39:146–151.
36. Straight RC, Spikes JD: Tumor and tissue levels of fluorescent porphyrins and the effect of liposomes on porphyrin distribution *in vivo*, in Bensasson RV, Land EJ, Jori G, Truscott TG (eds): *Primary Photoprocesses in Biology and Medicine*. New York, Plenum Press, 1985, pp 361–365.
37. Goldacre RJ, Sylven B: On the access of blood-borne dyes to various tumor regions. *Br J Cancer* 1962; 16:306–322.
38. Peterson HI, Appelgren KL: Experimental studies on the uptake and retention of labeled proteins in a rat tumor. *Eur J Cancer* 1973; 9:543–546.
39. Majno G, Palade GE: Studies on inflammation. The effect of histamine and serotonin on vascular permeability: An electron microscopic study. *J Biophys Biochem Cytol* 1961; 11:571–577.
40. Schoefl G: Studies on inflammation III. Growing capillaries: Their structure and permeability. *Virchows Arch Pathol Anat Physiol Klin Med* 1963; 337:97–141.
41. Haar JL, Ackerman GA: A phase and electron microscope study of vasculogenesis and erythropoiesis in the yolk sac of the mouse. *Anat Rec* 1971; 170:199–206.

42. Cozzani I, Jori G, Reddi E, et al: Distribution of endogenous and injected porphyrins at the subcellular level in rat hepatocytes and in ascites hepatoma. *Chem Biol Interact* 1981; 37:67–70.
43. Weil R: Chemotherapeutic experiments on rat tumors. *J Cancer Res* 1916; 1:95–106.
44. Ludford RJ: The vital staining of normal and malignant cells - II. The staining of malignant tumors with trypan blue. *Proc R Soc Lond Biol* 1929; 104:493–511.
45. Simpson BT, Marsh MC: Chemotherapeutic experiments with coal-tar dyes on spontaneous mouse tumors. *J Cancer Res* 1926; 10:50–60.
46. Lewis MR, Goland PP, Sloviter HA: Selective action of certain dye stuffs on sarcomata and carcinomata. *Anat Rec* 1946; 96:201–220.
47. Bugelski PJ, Porter CW, Dougherty TJ: Autoradiographic distribution of hematoporphyrin derivative in normal and tumor tissue of the mouse. *Cancer Res* 1981; 41:4606–4612.
48. Kessel D: Review of photosensitization with derivatives of haematoporphyrin. *Int J Radiat Biol* 1986; 49:908–1003.
49. Van den Hoof A: Connective tissue changes in cancer, in *International Review of Connective Tissue Research*, vol 10. New York, Academic Press, 1983, pp 395–432.
50. Pauli BU, Schwartz DE, Thonar EJ-M, et al: Tumor invasion and host extracellular matrix. *Cancer Metastasis Rev* 1983; 2:129–133.
51. Kelley JF, Snell ME: Hematoporphyrin derivative: A possible aid in the diagnosis and therapy of carcinoma of the bladder. *J Urol* 1976; 115:15–154.
52. Kessel D: Hematoporphyrin and HPD: Photophysics, photochemistry and phototherapy. *Photochem Photobiol* 1984; 39:851–859.
53. Sandberg D, Romslo G, Hovding G, et al: Porphyrin-induced photodamage as related to the subcellular localization of the porphyrins. *Acta Derm Venereol [Suppl]* 1982; 199:75–80.
54. Castellani A, Pace GP, Concioli M: Photodynamic effect of haematoporphyrin on blood microcirculation. *J Path Bacteriol* 1963; 86:99–102.
55. Star WM, Marijnissen JPA, Van Den Berg-Blok AE, et al: Destructive effect of photoradiation on the microcirculation of a rat mammary tumor growing in "sandwich" observation chambers, in Doiron DR, Gomer CJ (eds): *Porphyrin Localization and Treatment of Tumors*. New York, Alan R Liss, Inc, 1984, pp 637–645.
56. Selman SH, Kreimer-Birnbaum M, Klaunig JR, et al: Blood flow in transplantable bladder tumors treated with hematoporphyrin derivative and light. *Cancer Res* 1984; 44:1924–1927.
57. Zhou C, Yang W, Ding Z, et al: The biological effects of HPD-PDT treatment on the brain in normal mice: A light and electron microscopic study, in Jori G, Perria C (eds): *Photodynamic Therapy of Tumors and Other Diseases*. Padova, Liberia Progetto Editore, 1985, pp 167–176.
58. Star WM, Marijnissen JPA, Van Den Berg-Blok AE, et al: *In vivo* observations on the effects of HPD-photosensitization on the microcirculation of rat mammary tumor and normal tissues growing in transparent chambers, in Jori G, Perria C (eds): *Photodynamic Therapy of Tumors and Other Diseases*. Padova, Liberia Progetto Editore, 1985, pp 239–242.
59. Henderson BW, Dougherty TJ, Malone PB: Studies on the mechanism of tumor destruction by photoradiation therapy, in Doiron DR, Gomer CJ (eds): *Porphyrin Localization and Treatment of Tumors*. New York, Alan R Liss, Inc, 1984, pp 601–612.
60. Waner M, Straight RC, Gluckman JL, et al: The mechanism of photodynamic therapy in relation to the tumor microvascular compartment. *Lasers Surg Med* 1986; 6:162.
61. Konrad K, Honigsman H, Gschnait F: Mouse model for protoporphyria. II. Cellular and subcellular events in the photosensitivity flare of the skin. *J Invest Dermatol* 1975; 65:300–310.
62. Wise BL, Toxdal DR: Studies of the blood brain barrier utilizing haematoporphyrin. *Brain Res* 1967; 10:387–392.
63. Bonnett R, Berenbaum MC, Kaur H: Chemical and biological studies on haematoporphyrin derivative; an unexpected photosensitization in brain, in Andreoni A, Cubeddu R (eds): *Porphyrins in Tumor Phototherapy*. New York, Plenum Press, 1984, pp 361–368.
64. Denekamp J: Vasculature as a target for tumor therapy. *Prog Appl Microcirc* 1984; 4:28–38.

65. Folkman J: Anti-angiogenesis: New concept for therapy of solid tumors. *Ann Surg* 1972; 175:409–416.
66. Andreoni A, Cubeddu R (eds): *Porphyrins in Tumor Phototherapy*. New York, Plenum Press, 1984.
67. Doiron DR, Gomer CJ (eds): *Porphyrin Localization and Treatment of Tumors*. New York, Alan R Liss, Inc, 1984.
68. Berns MW: *Hematoporphyrin Derivative Photoradiation Therapy of Cancer*. New York, Alan R Liss, Inc. 1984.
69. Bensasson RV, Land EJ, Jori G, et al (eds): *Primary Photoprocesses in Biology and Medicine*. New York, Plenum Press, 1985.
70. Jori G, Perria C (eds): *Photodynamic Therapy of Tumors and Other Diseases*. Padova, Edisioni Liberia Progetto, 1985.
71. Kessel D (ed): *Methods in Porphyrin Photosensitization*. New York, Plenum Press, 1985.
72. Lim HW, Gigli I: Role of complement in porphyrin-induced photosensitivity. *J Invest Dermatol* 1981; 76:4–9.
73. Dougherty TJ: Photodynamic therapy, in Kessel D (ed): *Methods in Porphyrin Photosensitization*. New York, Plenum Press, 1984, pp 313–328.
74. Dougherty TJ, Weishaupt KR, Boyle DG: Photoradiation therapy of malignant tumors, in Devita VT, Hellman S, Rosenberg SA (eds): *Cancer: Principles and Practice of Oncology*. Philadelphia, JB Lippincott Co, 1982, pp 1836–1844.
75. Hayata Y: *Laser Photoradiation for Tumor Detection and Treatment*. Tokyo, Igaku-Shoin, Ltd, 1984.
76. Kessel D: Porphyrin localization: A new modality for detection and therapy of tumors. *Biochem Pharmacol* 1984; 33:134–138.
77. Parrish JA: Photobiologic considerations in photoradiation therapy, in Kessel D, Dougherty TJ (eds): *Porphyrin Photosensitization*. New York, Plenum Press, 1983, pp 91–108.
79. Doiron DR, Svaasand LO, Profio AE: Light dosimetry in tissue: Application to photoradiation therapy, in Kessel D, Dougherty TJ (eds): *Porphyrin Photosensitization*. New York, Plenum Press, 1983, pp 63–76.
80. Kinsey JH, Cortese DA, Neel HB: Thermal considerations in murine tumor killing using hematoporphyrin derivative phototherapy. *Cancer Res* 1983; 43:1562–1566.
81. Spikes JD: Phthalocyanines as photosensitizers in biological systems and for the photodynamic therapy of tumors. *Photochem Photobiol* 1986; 43:691–699.
82. Cowled PA, Graco JR, Forbes IJ: Comparison of the efficacy of pulsed and continuous-wave red laser light in induction of photocytotoxicity by hematoporphyrin derivative. *Photochem Photobiol* 1984; 39:115–117.
83. Parrish JA, Anderson RF, Harvist T, et al: Selective thermal effects with pulsed irradiation from lasers: From organ to organelle. *J Invest Dermatol* 1983; 80:75S.
84. Bellnier DA, Lin CW, Parrish JA, et al: Hematoporphyrin derivative and pulse laser photoradiation, in Doiron DR, Gomer CJ (eds): *Porphyrin Localization and Treatment of Tumors*. New York, Alan R Liss, Inc, 1984, pp 533–540.
85. Berns MW, Hammer-Wilson M, Walter RJ, et al: Uptake and localization of HPD and "active fraction" in tissue culture and in serially biopsied human tumors, in Doiron DR, Gomer CJ (eds): *Porphyrin Localization and Treatment of Tumors*. New York, Alan R Liss, Inc, 1984, pp 501–520.
86. Waner M, Straight RC, Gluckman JL: Studies on the effect of pulsed light on neoplastic tissue. *Lasers Surg Med* 1986; 6:168.
87. See KL, Forbes IJ, Betts WH: Oxygen dependency of photocytotoxicity with haematoporphyrin derivative. *Photochem Photobiol* 1984; 39:631–634.
88. Freitas I: Tumor hypoxia and associated drawbacks to photodynamic therapy, in Jori G, Perria C (eds): *Photodynamic Therapy of Tumors and Other Diseases*. Padova, Edizioni Liberia Progetto, 1985, pp 413–420.

89. Svaasand LO, Doiron DR: Thermal distribution during photoradiation therapy, in Kessel D, Dougherty TJ (eds): *Porphyrin Photosensitization*. New York, Plenum Press, 1983, pp 77–90.
90. Barltrop J, Martin BB, Martin DF: Ptychodiscus brevis as a model system for photodynamic action. *Microbiog* 1983; 37:95–103.
91. Mathews-Roth MM: Carotenoid pigments and protection against photosensitization: How studies in bacteria suggested a treatment for a human disease. *Perspect Biol Med* 1984; 28:127–129.
92. Elmets CA, Bowen KD: Immunological suppression in mice treated with hematoporphyrin derivative photoradiation. *Cancer Res* 1986; 46:1608–1611.
93. Lynch DH, Straight RC, Jolles CJ, et al: The cellular mechanisms by which severe systemic immunosuppression induced by photodynamic therapy is mediated. *Photochem Photobiol* 1988; 47:385.
94. Mack HP, Diehl WK, Tek GC, et al: Evaluation of the combined effects of hematoporphyrin in radiation. I. Treatment of carcinoma of the cervix. *Cancer* 1957; 10:529–539.
95. Lipson RL, Baldes EJ: The photodynamic properties of a particular hematoporphyrin derivative. *Arch Dermatol* 1960; 82:508–511.
96. Lipson RL, Baldes EJ: Photosensitivity and heat. *Arch Dermatol* 1960; 82:517–520.
97. Lipson RL, Baldes EJ, Olson AN: The use of a derivative of hematoporphyrin in tumor detection. *J Natl Cancer Inst* 1961; 26:1–5.
98. Lipson RL, Pratt JH, Baldes EJ, et al: Hematoporphyrin derivative for the detection of cervical cancer. *Ob Gyn* 1964; 24:78–84.
99. Lipson RL, Baldes EJ, Olson AN: Hematoporphyrin derivative: A new aid for endoscopic detection of malignant disease. *J Thorac Surg* 1961; 42:623–626.
100. Fioretti P, Facchini V, Gadducci A: Monitoring of hematoporphyrin injected in humans and clinical prospects of its use in gynecologic oncology; *Med Biol Environ* 1984; 12:355–361.
101. McCaughan JR, Schellhashf JS, Lomano J: Photodynamic therapy of gynecologic neoplasms after presensitization with hematoporphyrin derivative. *Lasers Surg Med* 1985; 5:491–498.
102. Ward VG, Forbes KG, Cowled TA: The treatment of vaginal recurrences of gynecologic malignancy with phototherapy following hematoporphyrin derivative pre-treatment. *Am J Obstet Gynecol* 1982; 142:356–361.
103. Kennedy J: HPD photoirradiation therapy for cancer at Kingston and Hamilton, in Kessel D, Doherty TJ (eds): *Porphyrin and Photosensitization*. New York, Plenham Publishing Corp, 1983, p 53.
104. Soma H, Nutahara S: Cancer of the female genitalia, in Hyata Y, Doherty TJ (eds): *Lasers and Hematoporphyrin Derivative in Cancer*. Tokyo, Igaku-Shoin Ltd, 1983, pp 97–109.
105. Wallis C, Melnick JL: Photodynamic inactivation of animal viruses: A review. *Photochem Photobiol* 1965; 4:159–170.
106. Melnick JL, Wallis C: Photodynamic inactivation of herpes simplex virus: A status report. *Ann NY Acad Sci* 1977; 284:171–181.
107. Bockstahler LE, Coohill TP, Hellman KB, et al: Critical review and risk evaluation of photodynamic therapy for herpes simplex, in Shugar D (ed): *International Encyclopedia of Pharmacologic Therapy and Viral Chemotherapy*, vol 1. Oxford, Pergamon Press, 1984, pp 479–509.
108. Khan NC, Melnick JL, Biswal N: Photodynamic treatment of herpes simplex virus during its replicative cycle. *J Virol* 1977; 21:16–23.
109. Schnipper LE, Lewin AA, Swartz M, et al: Mechanisms of photodynamic inactivation of herpes simplex viruses. *J Clin Invest* 1980; 65:432–438.
110. Straight RC, Stroop WG, Spikes JD, et al: Photodynamic inactivation of herpes simplex virus and laser photodynamic therapy of virus lesions with porphyrin photosensitizers, in Jori G, Perria C (eds): *Photodynamic Therapy of Tumors and Other Diseases*. Padova, Edizioni Liberia Progetto, 1985, pp 353–358.
111. Abramson AL, Shikowitz M, Steinberg B: The effects of hematoporphyrin derivative-photodynamic therapy on experimental viral papilloma. The First International Conference on

the Clinical Applications of Photosensitization for Diagnosis and Treatment. Tokyo, 1986, p 59.

112. Martinett P, Gariglio M, Pancani I, et al: Hematoporphyrin photodynamic effects "in vitro" and "in vivo" microbiological experiments after laser and daylight exposure, in Jori G, Perria C (eds): *Photodynamic Therapy of Tumors and Other Diseases*. Padova, Edizioni Liberia Progetto, 1985, pp 367–370.
113. Bertoloni G, Viel A, Grossato A, et al: The photosensitizing activity of haematoporphyrin on mollicates. *J Gen Microbiol* 1985; 131:2217–2223.
114. Kvello-Stenstrom AG, Moan J, Brunborg G, et al: Photodynamic inactivation of yeast cells sensitized by hematoporphyrin. *Photochem Photobiol* 1980; 32:349–352.
115. Ito T: Photodynamic action of hematoporphyrin on yeast cells - a kinetic approach. *Photochem Photobiol* 1981; 34:521–524.
116. Judy MM, Department of Pathology, Baylor University Medical Center, Dallas, Texas, personal communication.

# Index


**A**

Absorption
  as function of wavelength for hemoglobin, melanin and water, 29
  of laser energy within tissue, 29
  of radiation, 17
Acanthosis: with papillomatosis, 58
Adhesiolysis
  argon laser in, 217–218
  $CO_2$ laser laparoscopy in, 203–204
    with titanium rod, 203
  laser for, 176–178
Aerodigestive mucosae: affected by papillomavirus, 49–50
Anogenital mucosae: affected by papillomavirus, 49–50
ANSI Z136.3, 11
Anus
  condyloma acuminatum, $CO_2$ laser for, 32
  condylomata covering, 118
  exophytic growth, 115
  perianal (*see* Perianal)
Argon laser
  advantages, 218–220
  beam, flexible optical fiber to deliver, 211
  characteristics, 20
  for conization of cervical intraepithelial neoplasia, 144–148
  disadvantages, 218–220
  in ectopic pregnancy, 218
  endometriotic implant appearance after, 216
  fiber
    distance to tissue, 211
    power density and, 212
    spot size and, 211
    tip position near peritoneal surface, 215
  future applications, 220
  for laparoscopy (*see* Laparoscopy, laser, argon)
  Model 20, 210
  in neosalpingostomy, 218
  operating room set-up for use of, 213

**B**

Beam (*see* Laser, beam)
Biopsy: $CO_2$ laser excisional cone, for cervical intraepithelial neoplasia, 140–142
Biotechnicians: for laser unit, 8
Blood loss: and Nd:YAG laser, 234
Bone incisions: comparison of, 252
Bowenoid carcinoma: of temporal area, 51
Bryan telescope, 247–248

**C**

Cancer, genital, papillomavirus in
  as casual or causal, 60–61
  other co-carcinogens in, 60–61
  evidence implicating, 60
Cannulating: vestibular gland with sialogram, 87
Carbon dioxide (*see* $CO_2$)
Carcinoma
  temporal area, ulcerated bowenoid, 51
  vulva, in situ, 106
    extending down hair follicle shaft, 109
    extensive, 110–112
    involving labia minora tip, 108
Cell-virus interaction
  different types, 59
  in papillomavirus, different patterns, 76
Certificate of need: for laser unit, 6
Cervix, 130–150
  condyloma (*see* Condyloma, cervix)
  destroyed by laser "ablative conization," 89

Cervix *(cont.)*
disease, preinvasive
high grade and low grade, laser in, 79–81
and papillomavirus, 64–73
laser for, 130–150
historical perspective, 130–131
laser surgery, depth control, 90–91
neoplasia, intraepithelial, 131–148
biology of, 132–133
$CO_2$ laser excision plus laser ablation for, 142–143
$CO_2$ laser excisional cone biopsy in, 140–142
$CO_2$ laser for, follow-up, 144
$CO_2$ laser vaporization, 134–140
$CO_2$ laser vaporization procedure, 136–138
$CO_2$ laser vaporization, volume and configuration of tissue destroyed by, 135
"cold" coagulation of, 134
combination procedure for, 142–143
cryotherapy, 133–134
ectocervical, combination procedure for, 142–143
electrocoagulation diathermy of, 134
endocervical, combination procedure for, 142–143
epidemiology, 131–132
laser therapy, 134–148
laser treatment, argon for conization, 144–148
laser treatment, $CO_2$ (*see* $CO_2$ laser *above*)
laser treatment, KTP-532 for conization, 144–148
laser treatment, ND:YAG, for conization, 144–148
natural history, 132–133
three characteristic configurations, tissue defects appropriate for, 135
papillomavirus infection of, 53
minimally expressed, 57
subclinical, 69
transformation zone, subclinical papillomavirus involving, 126
$CO_2$ laser
in cervical intraepithelial neoplasia (see Cervix, neoplasia, intraepithelial, $CO_2$ laser)
characteristics, 20
for condyloma acuminatum
anal, 32
of vulva, 119
end beam delivery instruments for, 24
handpiece
with defocused beam, 170
with focused beam, 169
for laparoscopy (*see* Laparoscopy, laser, $CO_2$)
in neosalpingostomy, 228
for papillomavirus (*see* Papillomavirus, $CO_2$ laser for)
for vaginal intraepithelial neoplasia, results, 124
vaporization of cervical intraepithelial neoplasia, 134–140
Coagulation
"cold," of cervical intraepithelial neoplasia, 134
with Easly-Keplinger forcep with $CO_2$ laser, 189
in menorrhagia (*see* Menorrhagia, Nd:YAG laser for endometrial photovaporization and coagulation)
necrosis, 92
Co-carcinogens: and papillomavirus in genital cancer, 60–61
Coital friction: and papilloma, 62
"Cold" coagulation: of cervical intraepithelial neoplasia, 134
Colpophotograph: of labia major neoplasia, 101
Colposcopic index: combined, 71
Colposcopy
of condyloma, 66
vulva, 104–107
Committees: for laser unit, 5
Conception: time from surgery to, after laser laparoscopy for endometriosis, 197
Condyloma acuminatum
anus, $CO_2$ laser for, 32
anus covered by condylomata, 118
hybridization and, in situ, 78
mons pubis covered by condylomata, 118
papillomavirus and, 61–62
vagina, 124–128
laser surgery technique, 125–126
postoperative care, 128
results, 128
vulva, 113–121
contiguous mass covering, 118
laser surgery principles, 115
laser technique, 116–120
laser vaporized, 117
mature-appearing, 114
postoperative management, 120
results, anticipated, 120–121
Condyloma: benign, papillomatosis in, 58
Condyloma, cervix
acuminatum, 126–128
flat, 127
florid, 127
clinically important, minor-grade lesions, 66–72

clinically important, minor grade lesions, vascular patterns of, 71
clinically inapparent, high-grade dysplasias, 72–73
exophytic, 64–66, 70
filiform vascular, 65
with keratotic plaque, 67
papillary, 65
type-specific disease association, 67
Condyloma: colposcopic magnification of, 66
Condyloma: vagina, benign, 81–82
Condyloma, vulva, 52
benign, 81–82
Cone
biopsy, in cervical intraepithelial neoplasia, 140–142
excision of cervical intraepithelial neoplasia, 135
Conization: of cervical intraepithelial neoplasia, 144–148
Coordinator: for laser unit, 3–4
Costs (*see* Laser unit, costs)
Credentialing of physicians: for laser unit, 6–8
Cryotherapy: of cervical intraepithelial neoplasia, 133–134
Cyst
ovarian, non-endometriotic, Nd:YAG laser for, 240
paratubal, destruction of, 178

**D**

Delivery systems: new, development of, 253–254
Dental mirrors: rhodium-surfaced angled, 175
Design: for laser unit, 5–6
Development
future, for laser photochemotherapy, 261–263
of more powerful lasers, 250–252
of new delivery systems, 253–254
of new wavelengths, 252–253
Diathermy: electrocoagulation, of cervical intraepithelial neoplasia, 134
Director: for laser unit, 3
DNA: organization of papillomavirus, 48
Dye laser: characteristics, 20
Dyonics Needlescope, 247
Dysmenorrhea: uterosacral ligament ablation for, 199–200
Dysplasia
epidermo-, verruciformis, temporal area carcinoma and, 51
high-grade, in condyloma of cervix, 72–73
perianal, refractory, 94
pilosebaceous duct, 93

**E**

Ectasia: vascular, of central vulval dermis, 86
Ectopic (*see* Pregnancy, ectopic)
Education: and laser unit, 6–11
Educational coordinator: for laser unit, 4
Electrocoagulation diathermy: of cervical intraepithelial neoplasia, 134
Electromagnetic mode patterns: transverse, 22
Electromagnetic spectrum, 15
Electron beam: TEM patterns, 22
Emission: of radiation, 17
Endometrioma: ovarian, destruction with argon laser, 215–217
Endometriosis, pelvic, $CO_2$ laser laparoscopy in, 194–199
life-table analysis of patients, 199
pregnancy outcome after, 197
pregnancy rates after, 197
results, early, 194–199
technique, 194–199
time from surgery to conception, 197
vaporization, 196
Endometriotic implant: after argon laser, 216
Endometrium
ablation with Nd:YAG laser, 31
coagulation (*see* Menorrhagia, Nd:YAG laser endometrial photovaporization and coagulation)
photovaporization (*see* Menorrhagia, Nd:YAG laser for endometrial photovaporization)
Energy (*see* Laser, energy)
Engineer: for laser unit, 4
Epidermo-dysplasia verruciformis: and temporal area carcinoma, 51
Erythema: vestibular, painful, 85

**F**

Fallopian tube laser, 166–186
accessories, 171–173
advantages, 182–183
animal studies, 173–176
complications, 183
cysts, paratubal, destruction of, 178
historical review, 166–167
instrumentation, 168–171
laser physics and tubal surgery, 167–173
micromanipulator, 170
Pyrex rods for, 172, 177
reanastomosis of tube, 179–180
reimplantation of tube, 181
results, clinical, 181–182
training for, 183–184
uses, clinical, 176–181

Fetal surgery: Nd:YAG laser in, 242–249
Fetoscope(s), 245, 247
  Bryan, 247–248
  Dyonics Needlescope, 247
  Olympus Selfoscope, 247
Filter: in-line, 175
Fimbrioplasty, 178
Finances: for laser unit, 9–11
Food and Drug Administration: and laser unit, 11
Forcep: Easly-Keplinger, with $CO_2$ laser, 189
Free-electron laser, 250–269
  diagram of, 251
  Stanford Mark III, 251
Future
  developments for laser photochemotherapy, 261–263
  of lasers in gynecology, 250–269

G

Gated pulsing techniques: for $CO_2$ laser within papillomavirus, 90
Gaussian laser beam: effective diameter of, 26
Genetic function (*see* Papillomavirus, genetic function)
Genital cancer (*see* Cancer, genital)
Graves laser speculum, 145
Gynecology
  lasers in
    changing role, 263–264
    future of, 250–269
  photodynamic diagnosis and therapy applications in, 260–261

H

Hair follicle
  relationship to sebaceous gland and sweat gland
    apocrine, 103
    eccrine, 104
  shaft, vulvar carcinoma in situ extending down, 109
Hand warts, 51
Handles: rigid, for laparoscopic, hysteroscopic, or manual delivery system, 236
Handpiece (*see* $CO_2$ laser, handpiece)
Healing: of vulvar intraepithelial neoplasia, 110–112
Hemoglobin: absorption as function of wavelength for, 29
HeNe laser: characteristics, 20
Hospital laser committee, 5
HPV (*see* Papillomavirus)
Hybridization of papillomavirus, 75–78
  dot blot, 76, 77
  filter in situ, 76
  in situ, 76–78
    of condyloma acuminatum, 78
  Southern blot, 75–76, 77
    in 16 and 18 papillomavirus, 56
Hysteroscopic delivery system: rigid handles for, 236

I

Immunosuppressed population: vulvar warts in, exophytic acuminata, 114
Immunosuppression: and cutaneous HPVs, 50
Inoculation: in papillomavirus, 50–51
Institutional Review Board: and laser unit, 12
Intrauterine laser, 151–165
  future of, 163–164

K

Keratotic plaque: in cervical condyloma, 67
KIP laser: characteristics, 20
Koilocytotic atypia: in cervical papillomavirus infection, 57
KTP laser
  advantages, 228–229
  disadvantages, 229
  discussion of, 222–223
  532
    for conization of cervical intraepithelial neoplasia, 144–148
    control panel of, 224
    design, schematic representation, 225
  for laparoscopy (*see* Laparoscopy, laser, KTP)
  in neosalpingostomy, 228
  results with, 228
  safety precautions, 229–230
  training in, 229–230

L

Labia: minora tip involvement in vulvar carcinoma in situ, 108
Laparoscopist: Monoshutter to protect eye of, 212
Laparoscopy
  coagulation, pregnancies after, 198
  excision, pregnancies after, 198
Laparoscopy, laser
  argon, 208–221
    in adhesiolysis, 217–218
    advantages, 218–220
    destruction of ovarian endometrioma, 215–217
    destruction of superficial implants, 214–215

disadvantages, 218–220
future applications, 220
instrumentation for, 209–213
optical fiber tip position near peritoneal surface, 215
results of clinical trials, 213–214
surgical techniques, 214–218
$CO_2$, 187–207
clinical applications, 194–205
double-puncture, 192
for endometriosis (*see* Endometriosis, pelvic, $CO_2$ laser laparoscopy in)
fibers, 194
forcep for, Easly-Keplinger, 189
indications in 611 patients, 188
lenses for, 193
in neosalpingostomy, 202
probes for, 193
prototypes for, development of, 188–190
single-puncture, 190–192
systems for, present, 190–194
three-puncture, 192
wave guides, 194, 195
delivery system, rigid handles for, 236
KTP, 222–230
advantages, 228–229
clinical techniques, 225–228
clinical trials, 224–225
disadvantages, 229
initial studies, 224
results, 228
Nd:YAG, 231–241
animal studies, 237
results, clinical, 238–239
techniques, clinical, 237–238
off-set 45°, 191
parallel operative, 190
in polycystic ovarian disease, 200–201
Laser(s)
argon (*see* Argon laser)
beam
amplification occurring within resonant cavity, 19
diameter, effective, 24
emission occurring within resonant cavity, 19
focusing, configuration for, 24
Gaussian, effective diameter of, 26
green/yellow, hypothetical, spectral purity of, 16
intensity reduction, effect of, 27
spot size, 23–25
spot size, reduced focal, effect of, 27
TEM, effect on crater shape in tissue, 23
for cervix (*see under* Cervix)
characteristics, 20
$CO_2$ (*see* $CO_2$ laser)
dye, characteristics, 20
energy
absorption, 29
generating, 14–18
reflection, 29
scattering, 29
transmission, 29
for fallopian tube (*see* Fallopian tube laser)
free-electron (*see* Free-electron laser)
future, in gynecology, 250–269
Graves laser speculum, 145
in gynecology (*see* Gynecology, lasers in)
HeNe, characteristics, 20
history of, 14
KIP, characteristics, 20
KTP (*See* KTP laser)
laparoscopy (*see* Laparoscopy, laser)
metroplasty, 161–163
modes of, 21–22
more powerful, development of, 250–252
Nd:YAG (*see* Nd:YAG laser)
neurectomy, 199–200
output, 15
for papillomavirus (*see* Papillomavirus, $CO_2$ laser)
photochemotherapy, future developments for, 261–263
photodynamic therapy (*see* Photodynamic therapy)
in photosensitive reaction activation, 254
physics, 14–44
power density, 25–26
values, 27
practice standards for, 8
superpulse, understanding, 26–28
surgical
delivery systems, 22–23
types of, 19–21
system, 18–28
components, 18
surgical delivery, 22–23
-tissue interaction, 28–33
summary of basic qualitative laser effects in tissue, 28
training, for Fallopian tube laser, 183–184
types of, discussion of, 19–21
unit *(see below)*
unskilled, destroying cervix, 89
for uterus, 151–165
future of, 163–164
for vagina (*see under* Vagina)
vaporization
with scalpel excision (*see* Scalpel excision with laser vaporization)
for vulvar intraepithelial neoplasia, 109
for vulva (*see under* Vulva)

Laser unit, 1–13
administration, 1–13
ANSI Z136.3, 11–12
biotechnicians for, 8
certificate of need, 6
charging structure, 9–10
committees for, 5
coordinator, laser, 3–4
costs
incidental expenses, 10
indirect expenses, 10
purchase, total, 9
start-up, 9
credentialing of physicians for, 6–8
data collection in, 1
design for, 5–6
director, medical laser, 3
education and, 6–11
educational coordinator, 4
engineer for, 4
evaluation, 12
finances, 9–11
Food and Drug Administration and, 11
goals for, establishing and evaluating, 2
guidelines, 11–12
Institutional Review Board, 12
monitoring, 12
occupational safety in, 12
organization, 1–13
organizational structure, 3–5
profit, 10
program design, 3
program development, 1–2
quality assurance coordinator for, 5
regulations, 11–12
reimbursement, 10–11
research, 11
resources for, evaluating, 2
responsibilities for, distribution of, 3–5
safety officer for, 4, 9
space for, 5–6
support staff, 8
training in, 6–11
uses per year, 10
years of use, 10
Light: coherent vs. incoherent, 16

**M**

Macular lesions: and papillomavirus, 63
Melanin: absorption as function of wavelength for, 29
Menorrhagia: Nd:YAG laser for endometrial photovaporization and coagulation, 151–163
clinical studies, 154–161
complications, 156–160
histologic follow-up, 160–161
patient selection for, 154–155
preliminary studies, 153–154
results, 156–160
surgical technique, 155–156
Metroplasty: laser, 161–163
Micromanipulator: for fallopian tube laser, 170
Mirrors: dental, rhodium-surfaced angled, 175
Monitoring: laser unit, 12
Monoshutter: to protect eye of laparoscopist, 212
Mons pubis: condylomata covering, 118
Mucosa: anogenital and aerodigestive, affected by papillomavirus, 49–50
Myomectomy: Nd:YAG laser in, 240

**N**

Nd:YAG laser
blood loss in, 234
characteristics, 20
for conization of cervical intraepithelial neoplasia, 144–148
in ectopic pregnancy, 240–241
end beam delivery instruments for, 24
endometrial ablation with, 31
in fetal surgery, 242–249
instrumentation for, 232–237
for laparoscopy (*see* Laparoscopy, laser, Nd:YAG)
in menorrhagia (*see* Menorrhagia, Nd:YAG laser)
in myomectomy, 240
for ovarian cyst destruction, non-endometriotic, 240
for ovarian wedge resection, 239
in placental surgery, 242–249
probes for
cooling of, 236
sapphire, 232
smoke reduction in, 233
surgical laser technologies, 235
tissue effects of, 30
Necrosis: coagulation, 92
Neoplasia
cervix (*see* Cervix, neoplasia)
labia major, 101
photodynamic therapy
clinical applications, 259–261
efficacy of, 259–260
photosensitizer pharmacology in tumor tissue, 256–258
vagina (*see* Vagina, neoplasia)
vulva (*see* Vulva, neoplasia)
Neosalpingostomy, 178–179
argon laser in, 218
with $CO_2$ laser laparoscopy, 202
comparison of KTP and $CO_2$ lasers in, 228
Neurectomy: laser, 199–200

## O

Occupational safety: in laser unit, 12
Olympus Selfoscope, 247
Operating room: set-up for argon laser use, 213
Ovaries
  cortex, vaporizing defects in, 201
  cysts, non-endometriotic, Nd:YAG laser in, 240
  endometrioma, destruction with argon laser, 215–217
  polycystic, laser laparoscopy in, 200–201
  wedge resection, Nd:YAG laser for, 239

## P

Pain: of vestibular erythema, 85
Papilloma: and coital friction, 62
Papillomavirus, 46–99
  active expression phase, 51–52
  cervical disease and, preinvasive, 64–73
  clinical groups of, 49–50
  $CO_2$ laser for
    advantages of, 88–95
    choice of comfortable power density, 89–90
    choosing an appropriate beam geometry, 90
    depth control during cervical surgery, 90–91
    depth control during vaginal surgery, 90
    depth control during vulvar surgery, 91–95
    gated pulsing techniques, 90
    high power outputs, 89
    maintaining average power density above carbonization levels, 89
    strategies to aid surgical control, 89–95
    strategies to limit lateral heat conduction, 88–89
    superpulse and, rapid, 88–89
  condyloma acuminatum and, 61–62
  in condyloma, benign, 58
  cutaneous
    immunocompetent population and, 49
    in immunosuppressed individuals, 50
  DNA organization, 48
  early region, 48
  18, Southern blot hybridization, 56
  expression, varying levels of disease expression, 55
  genetic function, 48–49
  in genital cancer (*see* Cancer, genital, papillomavirus in)
  host containment phase, 52–54
  hybridization of (*see* Hybridization)
  incubation phase, 51
  infection
    abortive potentially transforming, 59–60
    cervix, 53
    chronic, latent, 55–56
    individual differences in disease expression, 54–60
    laboratory diagnosis, 73–78
    minimally expressed, 56–57
    natural history stages, 50–54
    subclinical, 63
    subclinical, of cervix, 69
    subclinical, of cervix, transformation zone, 126
    in temporal area carcinoma with epidermo-dysplasia verruciformis, 51
    of vestibule, 64
    well-developed, 57–60
  inoculation, 50–51
  late phase, 54
  late region, 49
  macular lesions and, 63
  mucosae affected by, anogenital and aerodigestive, 49–50
  papular lesions and, 63
  polymerase chain reaction, 78
  replication, productive, 57
  16, Southern blot hybridization, 56
  taxonomy of, 47
  therapeutic principles, 78–88
  upstream regulatory region, 48
  vaccination, prospects, 61
  vaginal disease and, preinvasive, 61–64
  virion structure, 47
  virology of, 47–49
  vulval disease and, preinvasive, 61–64
Papular lesions: and papillomavirus, 63
Parakeratosis: with papillomatosis, 58
Paratubal cysts: destruction of, 178
Pelvis (*see* Endometriosis, pelvic)
Perianal
  dysplasia, refractory, 94
  wart, papular pedunculated, 54
Phosphate (*see* KTP laser)
Photobiological reactions: to photodynamic therapy, 258–259
Photochemical mechanisms, 254–255
  of photodynamic therapy, 255
Photochemotherapy: laser, future developments for, 261–263
Photodynamic
  action, 257–258
  diagnosis, gynecologic applications, 260–261
  sensitizers, nature of, 255–256

Photodynamic *(cont.)*
therapy
gynecologic applications, 260–261
mechanisms of, 254–261
photobiological reactions to, 258–259
photochemical mechanism of, 255
of tumors, clinical applications, 259–261
of tumors, efficacy, 259–260
Photosensitive reaction: activation with lasers, 254
Photosensitizers
localization with, 256–257
pharmacology in tumor tissue, 256–258
retention, 256–257
Photovaporization (*see* Menorrhagia: Nd:YAG laser for endometrial photovaporization)
Physicians: credentialing of, for laser unit, 6–8
Physics, laser, 14–44
tubal surgery and, 167–173
Pilosebaceous duct dysplasia, 93
Placental surgery: Nd:YAG laser in, 242–249
Polycystic ovarian disease: laser laparoscopy in, 200–201
Polymerase chain reaction: and papillomavirus, 78
Potassium (*see* KTP laser)
Practice standards: for lasers, 8
Pregnancy
ectopic
argon laser in, 218
Nd:YAG laser in, 240–241
salpingostomy in, 204–205
salpingostomy for, linear, 180–181
after laparoscopic coagulation and excision, 198
outcome after laparoscopic laser for endometriosis, 197
rates after laparoscopic laser for endometriosis, 197
Probes (*see* Nd:YAG laser, probes)
Pyrex rod, 177
for fallopian tube laser, 172

## Q

Quality assurance coordinator: for laser unit, 5

## R

Radiation
absorption of, 17
emission of, spontaneous and stimulated, 17
Reanastomosis: tubal, with laser, 179–180
Reflection: of laser energy within tissue, 29
Reimbursement: and laser unit, 10–11
Replication: productive, of papillomavirus, 57–58
Research: in laser unit, 11
Rhodium-surfaced angled dental mirrors, 175

## S

Safety
occupational, in laser unit, 12
officer, for laser unit, 4, 9
precautions for KTP laser, 229–230
Salpingostomy
in ectopic pregnancy, 204–205
linear, for ectopic pregnancy, 180–181
terminal, 201–203
Sapphire probes: for Nd:YAG laser, 232
Scalpel excision with laser vaporization of vulvar intraepithelial neoplasia, 110
results, 113
Scattering: of laser energy within tissue, 29
Sebaceous gland, relationship to hair follicle and sweat gland
apocrine, 103
eccrine, 104
Sensitizers
photodynamic, nature of, 255–256
photosensitizers (*see* Photosensitizers)
Sialography: for cannulating vestibular gland, 87
Skin
papillomavirus and (*see* Papillomavirus, cutaneous)
structure in vulvar intraepithelial neoplasia, 104
Smoke: reduction for Nd:YAG laser, 233
Southern blot hybridization: of papillomavirus, 75–76, 77
Space: for laser unit, 5–6
Spot size (*see* Laser, beam, spot size)
Stanford Mark III free electron laser, 251
Suction cannisters, 174
Superpulse
rapid, and $CO_2$ laser, 88–89
understanding, 26–28
Support staff: for laser unit, 8
Sweat gland, relationship to sebaceous gland and hair follicle
apocrine gland, 103
eccrine gland, 104

## T

Taxonomy: of papillomavirus, 47
Telescope: Bryan, 247–248
TEM
effect on crater shape in tissue, 23
patterns, 22

Temporal area: carcinoma, ulcerated bowenoid, 51
Tissue (*see* Laser-tissue interaction)
Titanium rod: for adhesiolysis, 203
Titanyl (*see* KTP laser)
Training
for fallopian tube laser, 183–184
in KTP laser, 229–230
in laser unit, 6–11
Transformation zone: true anatomy of, 80
Transverse electromagnetic mode patterns, 22
Tubal (*see* Fallopian tube)
Tumors (*see* Neoplasia)

U

Ulcer: of temporal area carcinoma, 51
Unit (*see* Laser unit)
Uterosacral ligament: ablation for dysmenorrhea, 199–200
Uterus, laser for, 151–165
future of, 163–164

V

Vaccination: for papillomavirus, prospects, 61
Vagina
anatomy, 121–122
condyloma
acuminatum (*see* Condyloma acuminatum, vagina)
benign, 81–82
disease, preinvasive, and papillomavirus, 61–64
histology, clinical, 121–122
normal, 122
laser surgery, depth control, 90–91
neoplasia, intraepithelial, 83–84, 121–124
laser procedure, 124
laser surgery, 123
postoperative care, 124
Vestibule
erythema, painful, 85
gland cannulation with sialogram, 87
papillomavirus infection of, 64
Virus(es)
-cell interaction (*see* Cell-virus interaction)
papillomavirus (*see* Papillomavirus)
Vulva
carcinoma (*see* Carcinoma, vulva)
colposcopy, 104–107
condyloma, 52
acuminatum (*see* Condyloma acuminatum, vulva)
benign, 81–82
dermis, vascular ectasia of, 86
disease, preinvasive, and papillomavirus, 61–64
exophytic growth, 115
laser surgery, depth control during, 91–95
neoplasia, intraepithelial, 82–83, 100–121
diagnostic procedures, 105
healing, 110–112
laser surgery, carbon dioxide, results, 124
laser surgery principles, 107–109
laser vaporization guidelines for, 109
laser vaporization with scalpel excision, 110
lesion locations, 100–104
management of hairy areas, 109–110
multifocal, 102
postoperative care, 110–112
skin structure, 104
III, distribution, anatomical, 102
III, distribution in hairy and non-hairy areas, 103
III involving hairy portions of vulva, 105
III, laser vaporization with scalpel excision, results, 113
III lesions at fourchette-perineal area, 101
III, perianal, 108
warts (*see* Warts, vulva)
Vulvectomy: simple, VIN 3 recurrence at, 82
Vulvodynia: idiopathic, 84–88

W

Warts
hands, 51
perianal, papular pedunculated, 54
vulva
exophytic acuminate, in immunosuppressed population, 114
multiple accuminate, 113
Water: absorption as function of wavelength for, 29
Wavelengths
absorption as function of, for hemoglobin, melanin and water, 29
new, development of, 252–253